Manual of
Exercise Testing

Manual of
Exercise Testing

Victor F. Froelicher, M.D.

Professor of Medicine
Director, ECG and Exercise Laboratory and Cardiac Rehabilitation
Division of Cardiovascular Medicine
Stanford University School of Medicine
Palo Alto Veterans Affairs Medical Center
Palo Alto, California

SECOND EDITION

with 83 illustrations

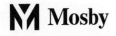 Mosby

St. Louis Baltimore Boston Chicago London Madrid Philadelphia Sydney Toronto

Mosby

Dedicated to Publishing Excellence

Publisher: George Stamathis
Editor: Stephanie Manning
Developmental Editor: Carolyn Malik
Project Manager: Carol Sullivan Wiseman
Senior Production Editor: Pat Joiner
Cover Design: GW Graphics & Publishing
Designer: Betty Schulz
Manufacturing Supervisor: John Babrick

Printed in the United States of America
Composition by The Clarinda Company
Printing/binding by Maple-Vail Book Manufacturing Group

Mosby–Year Book, Inc.
11830 Westline Industrial Drive
St. Louis, Missouri 63146

Library of Congress Cataloging in Publication Data
Froelicher, Victor F.
   Manual of exercise testing / Victor F. Froelicher.
      p.   cm.
   Includes bibliographical references and index.
   ISBN 0-8151-3346-4
   1. Treadmill exercise tests—Handbooks, manuals, etc.   I. Title.
   [DNLM: 1. Exercise Test—handbooks. 2. Electrocardiography—
handbooks.   WG 39 F926m 1994]
   RC683.5.E94F77   1994
   616.1'207547—dc20
   DNLM/DLC
   for Library of Congress

94 95 96 97 98 / 9 8 7 6 5 4 3 2 1

To Susie Q

My favorite energy previously was measured in amps and volts

but then *along came Susie* and now every day

I know how man felt with the discovery of electricity!

Preface

This second edition of this manual follows the same formula as last time; it basically is the exercise ECG testing portion of my larger book, *Exercise and the Heart,* which just came out in its third edition. The references and writing are skimmed down to a minimum for readability. Only key tables and figures are carried over, but a big addition is the 42 case presentations in Chapter 9. They are all new and are accompanied by the complete 12-lead averaged ECGs played back from the Mortara X-Scribe Exercise ECG system. These tracings are examples of rare and common exercise ECGs that should accelerate the learning process for all new trainees and provide a test for more experienced students. As always, the management of the patients presented could be debated. They certainly do not all represent my conservative approach, since the clinical decisions were often made by our health care team. Also, they were specifically chosen to have correlative test results, so they may appear "overtested."

Gilberto has died since he and I co-authored the first edition of the *Manual of Exercise Testing.* This happened back in his home in Brazil after a long illness. He is missed by many colleagues and friends as well as by the medical and academic community in South America and Portugal. The first edition came about while he was on a sabbatical with me because he suggested it and was willing to mount the exercise ECG figures. He would have been pleased to see the new computer ECG averages that Dave Mortara has made possible in this edition.

The purpose of this book is to meet the needs for trainees of all levels to learn how exercise testing should be performed and interpreted. Over 50% of internists and probably a similar number of family practitioners are now performing exercise tests. Fortunately, excellent teachers like Jerry Hizon and Corey Evans are helping educate these groups. If your purpose in reading this manual is to become active in exercise testing, you should review the accreditation guidelines published by the ACC and ACP.

There is no reason to go into the reasons why cardiologists are doing fewer routine exercise tests or even why they are transitioning from referring patients for nuclear exercise tests to doing exercise echocardiograms themselves. This appears to be a national trend. This trend actually may be very good because it could facilitate the implementation of national health care goals to appropriately direct resources by having the nonspecialist use exercise test results to serve as a gatekeeper to the cardiologist.

The most optimistic statement I have heard regarding the current financial restrictions being put on health care is that there is enough money to accomplish reasonable national goals, but to accomplish them, the amount currently available must be redirected. The financial restrictions are due in part to the AIDS epidemic, the national deficit, and the switch from a cold-war to a peace economy. I hope enlightened leadership in government will get us through these times, with appropriate attention paid to the issues that further separate the rich from the poor in our society. These issues particularily concern education, the drug abuse problem, poverty, and unemployment. Bold initiatives will be needed, perhaps even a public-works program such as the one that was so effective in getting our country out of the Great Depression. Although the debate rages over how to modify our health care system, most experts agree that a single-payer approach such as that used in Canada and a limit on the number of specialists could be good solutions.

So why write about a technologic approach when national objectives call for more general practice and less specialization? The exercise test could be used with scores based on clinical data to decide which patients need to be referred to the cardiologist. My personal perspective is not simply concern with saving money (although we should be cost conscious) but from the point of seeing that patients have only necessary procedures. Little has been written on the effects of tests and encounters on patients, but all I know is that my back never hurts as much as after I'd seen an orthopedic surgeon, and my whole approach to ordering tests changed after I had my second spinal tap.

Newer approaches that are highlighted in this manual are the exercise capacity nomograms, ramp testing, scores for predicting cardiovascular mortality, and the use of computer exercise ECG ischemia scores. Regarding the latter, we have not been able to find any that outperform standard visual interpretation. Other newer subjects, which are left out here but are covered in *Exercise and the Heart,* include expired gas analysis, nonexercise stress testing, and exercise echocardiography. All are worthy of study in other books; this manual concentrates on basic exercise ECG testing. It is my hope that primary care physicians and physicians in training find this book helpful.

Victor F. Froelicher

Contents

CHAPTER 1

Methods

INTRODUCTION

Despite technological advances in the diagnosis and treatment of cardiovascular disease, the exercise test remains an important modality. Its many applications, widespread availability, and high yield of clinically useful information make it an important gatekeeper for more expensive and invasive procedures. The numerous approaches to the exercise test, however, have been a drawback to its proper application. Excellent guidelines, which are based on research studies over the last 20 years, have been updated by organizations such as the American Heart Association (AHA), American Association of Cardiovascular and Pulmonary Rehabilitation (AACVPR), and American College of Sports Medicine (ACSM) and have led to greater uniformity in methods. Nevertheless, in many laboratories, methodology remains based on tradition, convenience, equipment, or personnel.

Key Point: Exercise is only one of many stresses to which an organism can be exposed; therefore it is more appropriate to call an *exercise test* exactly that and not a *stress test.*

Recent technology, although adding convenience, has raised new questions about methodology. For example, all commercially available systems today use computers. Do computer-averaged exercise electrocardiograms (ECGs) improve test performance, and of what should the practitioner be cautious in their use? What about the many computer-generated exercise scores? When should expired gases be measured during testing?

SAFETY PRECAUTIONS AND RISKS

The safety precautions outlined by the AHA are explicit about the requirements for exercise testing. Everything necessary for cardiopulmonary resuscitation must be available, and regular drills should be performed to ascertain that personnel

1

and equipment are ready for a cardiac emergency. The classic survey of clinical exercise facilities by Rochmis and Blackburn[1] demonstrated that exercise testing is a safe procedure, with approximately one death and five nonfatal complications per 10,000 tests. Perhaps because of an expanded knowledge concerning indications, contraindications, and endpoints, maximal exercise testing appears safer today than 20 years ago. Gibbons et al[2] have reported the safety of exercise testing in 71,914 tests conducted over 16 years. The complication rate was 0.8 per 10,000 tests. The authors suggested that the low complication rate might be a result of a cool-down walk, but a low complication rate has also been observed despite laying patients supine immediately after maximal exercise and despite exercising higher-risk patients.[3]

There are, however, reports of acute infarctions and deaths associated with exercise testing. Although the test is remarkably safe, the population referred for this procedure usually is at high risk for coronary events. Irving and Bruce[4] have reported an association between exercise-induced hypotension and ventricular fibrillation. Shepard[5] has hypothesized the following risk levels for exercise testing: (1) 3 or 4 times normal mortality rates in a cross-country footrace, (2) 6 to 12 times normal in a coronary-prone population performing unaccustomed exercise, and (3) as high as 60 times normal when exercise is performed by patients with coronary disease in a stressful environment, such as a physician's office. Cobb and Weaver[6] estimated the risk to be over 100 times in the last situation and pointed out the dangers of the recovery period. The risk of exercise testing in patients with coronary artery disease cannot be disregarded even with its excellent safety record.

CONTRAINDICATIONS

The box lists the absolute and relative contraindications to performing an exercise test. Good clinical judgement should be foremost in deciding the indications and contraindications for exercise testing. In selected cases with relative contraindications, testing can provide valuable information even if the test is performed submaximally.

HISTORY AND PHYSICAL EXAMINATION

Exercise testing should be an extension of the history and physical examination. A physician obtains the most information by being present to talk with, observe, and examine the patient with the test. A brief physical examination should always be performed to rule out significant obstructive aortic valvular disease. In this way, patient safety is ensured, and the physician obtains optimal information about the patient's condition. In some instances, such as when asymptomatic, apparently healthy subjects are being screened or a repeat treadmill test is being done on a patient whose condition is stable, a physician need not be present but should be in close proximity and prepared to respond promptly. The physician's reaction to

---

ABSOLUTE AND RELATIVE CONTRAINDICATIONS TO EXERCISE TESTING

Absolute Contraindications
Acute myocardial infarction or any recent change in the resting ECG
Unstable angina
Serious cardiac dysrhythmias
Acute pericarditis or myocarditis
Endocarditis
Severe aortic stenosis
Severe left ventricular dysfunction
Acute pulmonary embolus or pulmonary infarction
Any acute or serious noncardiac disorder
Severe physical handicap

Relative Contraindications*
Any less serious noncardiac disorder
Ventricular conduction defects
Significant arterial or pulmonary hypertension
Tachydysrhythmias or bradydysrhythmias that are not serious
Moderate valvular or myocardial heart diseases
Drug effect or electrolyte abnormalities
Fixed-rate artificial pacemaker
Left main obstruction or its equivalent
Psychiatric disease or inability to cooperate

---

*Under certain circumstances, relative contraindications can be superseded.

signs or symptoms should be moderated by the information the patient gives regarding usual activity. If abnormal findings occur at levels of exercise that the patient usually performs, it may not be necessary to stop the test. Also, the patient's activity history should help determine appropriate work rates for testing.

PATIENT PREPARATION

Preparations for exercise testing include the following:

1. The patient should be instructed not to eat or smoke at least 2 to 3 hours before the test and to come dressed to exercise.
2. A brief history and physical examination should be accomplished to rule out any contraindications to testing (see box).
3. Specific questioning should determine which drugs are being taken, and potential electrolyte level abnormalities should be considered. The physician should ask to see the labeled medication bottles so that they can be identified and recorded. Because of the life-threatening rebound phenomenon associated with beta-blockers, they should not automatically be stopped

before testing. However, if testing is performed for diagnostic purposes, they can be gradually stopped if a physician or nurse carefully supervises the tapering process.

4. If the reason for the exercise test is not apparent, the referring physician should be contacted.

5. A 12-lead ECG should be obtained in the supine and standing positions and the supine ECG compared with previous supine ECGs. The latter is an important rule, particularly in patients with known heart disease, since an abnormality may prohibit testing. Occasionally, a patient referred for an exercise test will instead be admitted to the coronary care unit. The standing ECG is important to detect individuals who develop ST-segment depression on standing and whose test results are likely to be false positive.

There should be careful explanations of reasons for the test; the testing procedure, including its risks and possible complications; and ways to perform the test, including a demonstration of getting on and off and walking on the treadmill. The patient should be told to hold on initially but should later use only the rails for balance.

TREADMILL

The treadmill should have front and side rails so that patients can steady themselves, and some patients may benefit from the help of the person administering the test. The treadmill should be calibrated at least monthly. Some models can be greatly affected by the weight of the patient and will not deliver the appropriate workload to heavy patients. An emergency stop button should be readily available to the staff only. A small platform or stepping area at the level of the belt is advisable so that the patient can start the test by pedaling the belt with one foot before stepping on. Patients should not grasp the front or side rails because this decreases the work performed and the oxygen uptake and, in turn, increases exercise time, resulting in an overestimation of exercise capacity. Gripping the handrails also increases ECG muscle artifact. When patients have difficulty maintaining balance while walking, it helps to have them take their hands off the rails, close their fists, and extend one finger to touch the rails after they are accustomed to the treadmill. Some patients may require a few moments to feel comfortable enough to let go of the handrails, but grasping the handrails after the first minute of exercise should be strongly discouraged.

CONSENT FORM

In any procedure with a risk of complications, it is advisable to make certain that the patient understands the situation and acknowledges the risks. However, some physicians feel that informing patients of the risks involved will occasionally make them overanxious or discourage them from performing the test. Because of this possibility and the fact that a signed consent form does not necessarily protect a physician from legal action, there has been less insistence on consent forms. If those performing the exercise test carefully explain the possible risks and complications in detail to each patient, a consent form should be superfluous.

LEGAL IMPLICATIONS

The legal implications of exercise testing require two major considerations. Establishment of physician-patient communication before and after performance of the exercise test should be the first consideration. A test should not be performed without first obtaining the patient's informed consent, verbally or in writing. In the process of the tester obtaining informed consent, the patient should be made aware of the potential risks and benefits of the procedure. In the absence of informed consent, a physician may be held responsible in the event of a major untoward event, even if the test is carefully performed. The argument can be made that the patient would not have undergone the procedure had he or she been made aware of the risks associated with the test. After the test, responsibility rests with the physician for prompt interpretation and consideration of the implications of the test. Communication of these results to the patient is necessary—with advice concerning adjustments in lifestyle—without delay.

The second consideration should be adherence to proper standards of care during performance of the test. Exercise testing should be carried out only by persons thoroughly trained in its administration and in the prompt recognition of possible problems. A physician trained in exercise testing and resuscitation should be readily available during the test to make judgments concerning test termination. Resuscitative equipment including a defibrillator should always be available. In 1990, a joint position statement from the American College of Physicians (ACP), American College of Cardiology (ACC), and AHA was published outlining physician competence for performing exercise testing.[7]

Key Point: Explaining the exercise testing procedure, risks, and results to the patient and significant others is essential.

BLOOD PRESSURE MEASUREMENT

Although numerous clever devices have been developed to automate blood pressure measurement during exercise, none can be recommended. The time-proven method of the physician holding the patient's arm with a stethoscope placed over the brachial artery remains most reliable. The patient's arm should be free of the handrails so that noise is not transmitted up the arm. It sometimes helps to mark the brachial artery. An anesthesiologist's auscultatory piece or an electronic microphone can be fastened to the arm. A device that inflates and deflates the cuff on the push of a button can also help. If systolic blood pressure appears to be slowly increasing or decreasing, it should be taken again immediately. If a drop in systolic blood pressure of 20 mm Hg or more occurs or if it drops below the value obtained in the standing position before testing, the test should be stopped in patients with congestive heart failure or a prior myocardial infarction and patients who are exhibiting signs or symptoms of ischemia. Systolic blood pressure must drop below the standing resting value to be associated with a poor prognosis. An increase in systolic blood pressure to 260 mm Hg and an increase in diastolic blood pressure to 115 mm Hg are also indications to stop the test.

ECG RECORDING INSTRUMENTS

Many technological advances in ECG recorders have taken place. The medical instrumentation industry has promptly complied with specifications set forth by various professional groups. Machines with a high-input impedance ensure that the voltage recorded graphically is equivalent to that on the surface of the body despite the high natural impedance of the skin. Optically isolated buffer amplifiers have ensured patient safety, and machines with a frequency response up to 100 Hz are commercially available. The lower end is possible because direct-current coupling is technically feasible.

WAVEFORM PROCESSING

Analog and digital averaging techniques have made it possible to average ECG signals to remove noise. There is a need for consumer awareness in these areas because most manufacturers do not specify how the use of such procedures modifies the ECG. Signal averaging can, in fact, distort the ECG signal. Averaging techniques are nevertheless attractive because they can produce a clean tracing despite poor skin preparation. However, the clean-looking ECG signal produced may not be a true representation of the waveform and in fact may be dangerously misleading. Also, the instruments that make computer ST-segment measurements are not entirely reliable because they are based on imperfect algorithms.

Computerization

The advantages of digital versus analog data processing include more precise and more accurate measurements, less distortion in recording, and direct accessibility to digital computer analysis and storage techniques. Other advantages include rapid mathematical manipulation (averaging), avoidance of the drift inherent in analog components, digital algorithm control permitting changes in analysis schema with ease (software rather than hardware changes), and no degradation with repetitive playback. The advantages of digital processing when outputting data include higher plotting resolution and easy repetitive manipulation.

Computerization also helps meet the the two critical needs of exercise ECG testing: the reduction of the amount of ECG data collected during the testing and the elimination of electrical noise and movement artifact associated with exercise. Because an exercise test can exceed 30 minutes and many physicians want to analyze all 12 leads during and after testing, the resulting quantity of ECG data and measurements can quickly become excessive. The three-lead vectorcardiographic (or three-dimensional, [i.e., aV_F, V_2, V_5]) approach would reduce the amount of data; however, clinicians favor the 12-lead ECG. The exercise ECG often includes random and periodic noise of high and low frequency that can be caused by respiration, muscle artifact, electrical interference, wire continuity, and electrode–skin contact problems. In addition to reducing noise and facilitating data collection, computer processing techniques may also make precise and accurate measurements, separate and capture dysrhythmic beats, perform spatial analysis, and apply optimal diagnostic criteria for ischemia.

Although cardiologists agree that computerized analysis simplifies the evaluation of exercise ECG, there has been disagreement about whether accuracy is enhanced.[8] A comparison of computerized resting ECG analysis programs with each other and with the analyses of expert readers led to the conclusion that physician review of any reading is necessary.[9] Although computers can record very clean representative ECG complexes and neatly print a wide variety of measurements, the algorithms they use are far from perfect and can result in serious differences from the raw signal. The physician who uses commercially available computer-aided systems to analyze the results of exercise tests should be aware of the problems and always review the raw analog recordings to see whether they are consistent with the processed output.

Even if computerization of the original raw analog ECG data could be accomplished without distortion, the problem of interpretation still remains. Numerous algorithms have been recommended for obtaining the optimal diagnostic value from the exercise ECG. These algorithms give improved sensitivity and specificity compared with standard visual interpretation. Often, this improvement has been documented and substantiated only by the investigator who proposed the new measurement. Thus none of these can be recommended for widespread use. It is hoped that the ability to store the entire exercise ECG in digital format will enable extraction of information to improve diagnosis. Perhaps neural networks and other discriminant function techniques will uncover new criteria.

CAUSES OF NOISE

Many of the causes of noise in the exercise ECG signal cannot be corrected, even by meticulous skin preparation. *Noise* is defined here as any electrical signal that is foreign to or distorts the true ECG waveform. Based on this definition, the types of noise that may be present can be caused by any combination of line-frequency (60 Hz), muscle, motion, respiration, contact, or continuity artifact. Line-frequency noise is generated by the interference of the 60-Hz electrical energy with the ECG. This noise can be reduced by using shielded patient cables. If in spite of these precautions this noise is still present, the simplest way to remove it is to design a 60-Hz notch filter and apply it in series with the ECG amplifier. A notch filter removes only the line frequency; that is, it attenuates all frequencies in a narrow band around 60 Hz. This noise can also be removed by attenuating all frequencies above 59 Hz; however, this method of removing line-frequency noise is not recommended because it causes waveform distortion and results in a system that does not meet AHA specifications. The most obvious manifestation of distortion caused by such filters is a decrease in R-wave amplitude; therefore a true notch filter is advisable.

Muscle noise is generated by the activation of muscle groups and is usually of high frequency. This noise, with other types of high-frequency noise, can be reduced by signal averaging. Motion noise, another form of high-frequency noise, is caused by the movement of skin and the electrodes, which causes a change in the contact resistance. Respiration causes an undulation of the waveform amplitude, so the baseline varies with the respiratory cycle. Baseline wander can be reduced by low-frequency filtering; however, this results in distortion of the ST segment and can cause artifactual ST-segment depression and slope changes. Other baseline removal approaches have been used, including linear interpolation between isoelectric regions, high-order polynomial estimates, and cubic-spline techniques, which can each smooth the baseline to various degrees.

Contact noise appears as low-frequency noise or sometimes as step discontinuity baseline drift. It can be caused by poor skin preparation resulting in high skin impedance or by air bubble entrapment in the electrode gel. It is reduced by meticulous skin preparation and by rejecting beats that show large baseline drift. Also, by using the median rather than the mean for signal averaging, this type of drift can be reduced. Continuity noise caused by intermittent breaks in the cables is rarely a problem because of technological advances in cable construction, except, of course, when cables are abused or overused.

Most of the sources of noise can be effectively reduced by beat averaging. However, two types of artifact can actually be caused in the signal-averaging process by the introduction of beats that are morphologically different from others in the average and the misalignment of beats during averaging. As the number of beats included in the average increases, the level of noise reduction is greater. The averaging time and the number of beats to be included in the average have to be compromised, though, because the morphology of ECG waveforms changes over time.

Key Point: Consider the raw ECG data first, and then use the averages and filtered data to aid interpretation if no distortion is obvious.

ECG PAPER RECORDING

For some patients, it is advantageous to have a recorder with a slow paper speed option of 5 mm/sec. This speed makes it possible to record an entire exercise test and reduces the likelihood of missing any dysrhythmias when specifically evaluating patients with these problems. A faster paper speed of 50 mm/sec can be helpful for making accurate ST-segment slope measurements.

Thermal head printers have nearly replaced all other types of printers. These recorders are remarkable in that they can use blank thermal paper and write out the grid and ECG, vector loops, and alpha-numerics. They can record graphs, figures, tables, and typed reports. They are digitally driven and can produce very high-resolution records. The paper price is comparable with that of other paper, and these devices have a reasonable cost and are very durable, particularly because a stylus is not needed.

Z-fold paper has the advantage over roll paper in that it is easily folded, and the study can be read in a manner similar to paging through a book. Exercise ECGs can be microfilmed on rolls, cartridges, or fiche cards for storage. They can also be stored in digital or analog format on magnetic media or optical disks. The latest technology involves magnetic optical disks that are erasable and have fast access and transfer times. These devices can be easily interfaced with microcomputers and can store megabytes of digital information.

EXERCISE TEST MODALITIES

Three types of exercise can be used to stress the cardiovascular system: isometric, dynamic, and a combination of the two. Isometric exercise, or constant muscular contraction without movement (such as a handgrip), imposes a disproportionate pressure load on the left ventricle relative to the body's ability to supply oxygen. Dynamic exercise, or rhythmic muscular activity resulting in movement, initiates a more appropriate increase in cardiac output and oxygen exchange. Because a delivered workload can be accurately calibrated and the physiological response easily measured, dynamic exercise is preferred for clinical testing. Using progressive workloads of dynamic exercise, patients with coronary artery disease can be protected from rapidly increasing myocardial oxygen demand. Although bicycling is a dynamic exercise, most individuals perform more work on a treadmill because a greater muscle mass is involved and most subjects are more familiar with walking than cycling.

Key Point: Dynamic exercise is preferred to isometric exercise for testing because it can be graduated and controlled and puts a volume stress on the heart rather than a pressure stress. However, most activities usually combine both types of exercise in varying degrees.

Numerous modalities have been used to provide dynamic exercise for exercise testing, including steps, escalators, and ladder mills. Today, however, the bicycle ergometer and the treadmill are the most commonly used dynamic exercise devices. The bicycle ergometer is usually cheaper, takes up less space, and makes less noise. Upper body motion is usually reduced, but care must be taken so that isometric exercise is not performed by the arms. The workload administered by the simple bicycle ergometer is not well calibrated and depends on pedaling speed. It is too easy for a patient to slow pedaling speed during exercise testing and decrease the administered workload. More expensive electronically braked bicycle ergometers keep the workload at a specified level over a wide range of pedaling speeds. These are particularly needed for supine exercise testing.

ARM ERGOMETRY

Alternative methods of exercise testing are needed for patients with vascular, orthopedic, or neurological conditions who cannot perform leg exercise. Arm ergometry can be used in such patients.[10,11] However, nonexercise stress techniques are currently more popular.

SUPINE VERSUS UPRIGHT EXERCISE TESTING

A great deal of the information available about intracardiac pressure responses to exercise has come from supine exercise, mostly because cardiac catheterization is required to obtain much of this information. However, there are marked differences between the body's response to acute exercise in the supine versus upright positions. During supine bicycle exercise, stroke volume and end-diastolic volume do not change much from values obtained at rest, whereas in the upright position, these values increase during mild work and then plateau. Naturally, exercise capacity is markedly lower in the supine position than in the upright cycling position. In patients with heart disease, left ventricular filling pressure is more likely to increase during exercise in the supine position than in the upright position. When patients with angina perform identical submaximal bicycle workloads in supine and upright positions, the heart rate is higher, maximal workload is lower, and angina develops at a lower double product while supine. ST-segment depression is often greater in the supine position because of the greater left ventricular volume.

BICYCLE ERGOMETER VERSUS TREADMILL

In most studies comparing upright cycle ergometer with treadmill exercise, maximum heart rate values have been roughly similar, whereas maximum oxygen uptake has been 6% to 25% greater during treadmill exercise.[12-16] Wickes et al[17] reported similar ECG changes with treadmill testing as compared with bicycle testing in patients with coronary disease. However, the treadmill is the most commonly used dynamic testing modality in the United States because patients are more familiar with walking than they are with bicycling. Patients are more likely to give the muscular effort necessary to adequately increase myocardial oxygen demand by walking than by bicycling.

EXERCISE PROTOCOLS

The many different exercise protocols in use has led to some confusion regarding how physicians compare tests between patients and serial tests in the same patient. The most common protocols, their stages, and the predicted oxygen cost of each stage are illustrated in Fig 1-1. When treadmill and cycle ergometer testing were first introduced into clinical practice, practitioners adopted protocols used by major researchers: Balke and Ware,[18] Astrand and Rodahl,[19] Bruce,[20] and Ellestad et al.[21] In 1980, Stuart and Ellestad[22] surveyed 1375 exercise laboratories in North America and reported that of those performing treadmill testing, 65% used the Bruce protocol for routine clinical testing. This protocol uses relatively large and unequal 2 to 3 metabolic equivalent (MET) increments in work every 3 minutes. Large and uneven work increments such as these have been shown to result in a tendency to overestimate exercise capacity.[23] Investigators have since recommended protocols with smaller and more equal increments.[24-26] Smokler et al[27] reported that among 40 pairs of treadmill tests conducted within a 6-month period, tests that were less than 10 minutes in duration showed a much greater percentage of variation than those that were greater than 10 minutes in duration. Buchfuhrer et al[14] performed repeated maximal exercise testing in five normal subjects while varying the work rate increment. Maximum oxygen uptake varied with the increment in work; the highest values were observed when intermediate increments were used. These investigators suggested that an exercise test with work increments individualized to yield a duration of approximately 10 minutes was optimal for assessing cardiopulmonary function. Lipkin et al,[28] on the other hand, observed that, among patients with chronic heart failure, small work increments yielding a long test duration (31 $\pm$ 15 minutes) resulted in reduced values for maximum oxygen uptake, minute ventilation, and arterial lactate levels compared with tests using more standard increments. These observations suggest that an exercise test should be individualized so that test duration is approximately 8 to 12 minutes.

RAMP TESTING

An approach to exercise testing that has gained interest in recent years is the ramp protocol, in which work increases constantly and continuously (Fig 1-2). The recent call for optimizing exercise testing would appear to be facilitated by the ramp approach. Because work increments are small and because it allows for increases in work to be individualized, a given test duration can be targeted. To investigate this approach, our laboratory recently compared ramp treadmill and bicycle tests to protocols more commonly used clinically; 10 patients with chronic heart failure, 10 with coronary artery disease who were limited by angina during exercise, 10 with coronary artery disease who were asymptomatic during exercise, and 10 age-matched normal subjects performed three bicycle tests (25 watts/2-minute stage, 50 watts/2-minute stage, and ramp) and three treadmill tests

Table of treadmill protocols (oxygen cost per stage). Each treadmill protocol cell lists MPH / %GR unless noted.

Functional Class	Clinical Status	O₂ Cost ml/kg/min	METS	Bicycle Ergometer (1 WATT ≈ 6 KPDS; for 70 kg body weight), KPDS	Bruce (3-min stages)	Kattus	Balke-Ware (% grade at 3.3 MPH, 1-min stages)	Ellestad (3/2/3-min stages)	USAFSAM (2 or 3 min stages)	"Slow" USAFSAM	McHenry	Stanford % grade at 3 MPH	Stanford % grade at 2 MPH	METS
NORMAL AND I (Healthy, dependent on age, activity; Sedentary healthy)		56.0	16		5.5 / 20									16
		52.5	15											15
		49.0	14	1500	5.0 / 18	4 / 22	26, 25	6 / 15	3.3 / 25					14
		45.5	13	1350			24, 23				3.3 / 21			13
		42.0	12	1200	4.2 / 16	4 / 18	22, 21	5 / 15	3.3 / 20		3.3 / 18	22.5		12
		38.5	11	1050	— / 14		20, 19					20.0		11
		35.0	10	900	3.4 / 14	4 / 14	18, 17	5 / 10	3.3 / 15	2 / 25	3.3 / 15	17.5		10
		31.5	9	750		4 / 10	16, 15			2 / 20		15.0		9
		28.0	8	600	2.5 / 12		14, 13	4 / 10	3.3 / 10	2 / 15	3.3 / 12	12.5		8
II (Limited)		24.5	7			3 / 10	12, 11	3 / 10			3.3 / 9	10.0	17.5	7
		21.0	6	450	1.7 / 10	2 / 10	10, 9		3.3 / 5	2 / 10	3.3 / 6	7.5	14	6
		17.5	5				8, 7	1.7 / 10				5.0	10.5	5
III (Symptomatic)		14.0	4	300	1.7 / 5		6, 5		3.3 / 0	2 / 5		2.5	7	4
		10.5	3	150	1.7 / 0		4, 3		2.0 / 0		2.0 / 3	0.0	3.5	3
IV		7.0	2				2, 1			2 / 0				2
		3.5	1											1

FIG 1-1.
The oxygen cost per stage for most of the commonly used treadmill protocols.

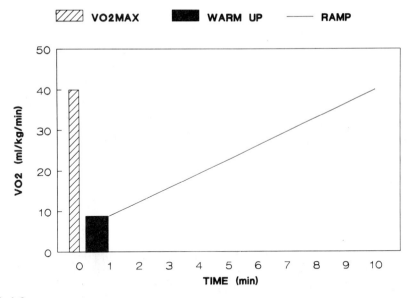

FIG 1-2.

The ramp treadmill test. After a 1-minute warm-up at 2.0 mph at 0% grade, the rate of change in speed and grade is individualized to yield a work rate (**X** axis) corresponding to an estimated exercise capacity (**Y** axis) in approximately 10 minutes.

(Bruce, Balke, and ramp) in randomized order on different days. For the ramp tests, ramp rates on the bicycle and treadmill were individualized to yield a test duration of approximately 10 minutes for each subject. Collectively, maximum oxygen uptake was significantly higher (18%) on the treadmill protocols than on the bicycle protocols, confirming previous observations. However, only minor differences in maximum oxygen uptake were observed between the treadmill protocols themselves or between the cycle ergometer protocols themselves.

The relationships between oxygen uptake and work rate (predicted oxygen uptake) suggest that oxygen uptake is overestimated from tests containing large work increments and the variability in estimating oxygen uptake from work rate is markedly greater for these tests than for a ramp test. Because the ramp approach appears to offer several advantages, we presently perform all our clinical and research testing using the ramp. If available equipment does not permit ramping, we recommend a modified Balke-Ware protocol such as the United States Air Force School of Aerospace Medicine (USAFSAM).

Key Point: The exercise protocol should be targeted for the patient rather than the reverse. Treadmill speed should be targeted to the individual's capabilities. Work increments should be even, and total time should be 8 to 10 minutes. METs, not minutes, should be reported. A ramp permits more accurate estimation of aerobic exercise capacity.

Questionnaires

The key to appropriately targeting a ramp is accurately predicting the individual's maximal work capacity. If a previous test is not available, an accurate questionnaire is critical to this process. Functional classifications are too limited and poorly reproducible. One problem is that "usual activities" can decrease, so an individual can become greatly limited without having a change in functional class. A better approach is to use the specific activity scale of Goldman et al[29] (see box), the Duke activity scale (Table 1-1), or the Veterans Administration (VA) questionnaire (refer to the box) or to question a patient regarding usual activities that have a known MET cost.[30]

BORG SCALE

Rather than using heart rate to clinically determine the intensity of exercise, it is preferable to use the 6-to-20 Borg scale or his later, nonlinear 1-to-10 scale of perceived exertion (Table 1-2).[31,32] The 6-to-20 scale was developed by noting that young men could approximate their exercise heart rate if a scale ranging from 60 to 200 was aligned with labels of very, very light for 60 to very, very hard for 200. One zero was then dropped, and the scale was used for all ages. Because sensory perception of pain or exertion is nonlinear, Borg proposed the 1-to-10 scale (Table 1-3).[3]

TABLE 1-1.

The Duke Activity Scale Index (DASI)

Activity	Weight
Can you?	
1. Take care of yourself (i.e., eating, dressing, bathing, or using the toilet)?	2.75
2. Walk indoors, such as around your house?	1.75
3. Walk a block or two on level ground?	2.75
4. Climb a flight of stairs or walk up a hill?	5.50
5. Run a short distance?	8.00
6. Do light work around the house like dusting or washing dishes?	2.70
7. Do moderate work around the house like vacuuming, sweeping floors, or carrying in groceries?	3.50
8. Do heavy work around the house like scrubbing floors or lifting or moving heavy furniture?	8.00
9. Do yard work like raking leaves, weeding, or pushing a power mower?	4.50
10. Have sexual relations?	5.25
11. Participate in moderate recreational activities such as golf, bowling, dancing, or doubles tennis or throw a basketball or football?	6.00
12. Participate in strenuous sports such as swimming, singles tennis, football, basketball, or skiing?	7.50

The index equals the sum of weights for "yes" replies.
Vo_2 (oxygen uptake) $= 0.43 \times \text{DASI} + 9.6$

SPECIFIC ACTIVITY SCALE OF GOLDMAN

Class I (≥7 METs)
A patient can perform any of the following activities:
Carrying 24 pounds up eight steps
Carrying an 80-pound object
Shoveling snow
Skiing
Playing basketball, touch football, squash, or handball
Jogging or walking 5 mph

Class II (≥5 METs)
A patient does not meet class I criteria but can perform any of the following
  activities to completion without stopping:
Carrying anything up eight steps
Having sexual intercourse
Gardening, raking, weeding
Walking 4 mph

Class II (≥2 METs)
A patient does not meet class I or class II criteria but can perform any of the
  following activities to completion without stopping:
Walking down eight steps
Taking a shower
Changing bed sheets
Mopping floors, cleaning windows
Walking 2.5 mph
Pushing a power lawn mower
Bowling
Dressing without stopping

Class IV (≤2 METs)
None of the above

TABLE 1-2.

Borg 20-Point Scale of Perceived Exertion

Points	Reaction	Points	Reaction
6		13	Somewhat hard
7	Very, very light	14	
8		15	Hard
9	Very light	16	
10		17	Very hard
11	Fairly light	18	
12		19	Very, very hard
		20	

VA ACTIVITY QUESTIONNAIRE

Draw one line <u>below</u> the activities you are able to do routinely with minimal or no symptoms such as shortness of breath, chest discomfort, fatigue.

1 MET:
Eating, getting dressed, working at a desk

2 METs:
Taking a shower
Walking down eight steps

3 METs:
Waling slowly on a flat surface for 1 or 2 blocks
Doing a *moderate* amount of work around the house such as vacuuming, sweeping the floors, or carrying groceries

4 METs:
Doing light yard work (i.e., raking leaves, weeding, or pushing a power mower)
Painting or doing light carpentry

5 METs:
Walking briskly (i.e., 4 mi/hour)
Dancing, washing the car

6 METs:
Playing nine holes of golf carrying your own clubs
Doing heavy carpentry or mowing lawn with a push mower

7 METs:
Performing heavy outdoor work (i.e., digging, spading soil)
Playing tennis (singles), carrying 60 pounds

8 METs:
Moving heavy furniture
Jogging slowly, climbing stairs quickly, carrying 20 pounds upstairs

9 METs:
Bicycling at a moderate pace, sawing wood, jumping rope (slowly)

10 METs:
Swimming briskly, bicycling up a hill, walking briskly uphill, jogging 6 mi/hr

11 METs:
Skiing cross-country
Playing basketball (full court)

12 METs:
Running briskly and continuously (level ground, 8 min/mi)

13 METs:
Doing any competitive activity, including those that involve intermittent sprinting
Running competitively, rowing, backpacking

TABLE 1-3.

Borg Nonlinear 10-Point Scale of Perceived Exertion

Points	Reaction	
0	Nothing at all	
0.5	Extremely light	(Just noticeable)
1	Very light	
2	Light	(Weak)
3	Moderate	
4	Somewhat heavy	
5	Heavy	(Strong)
6		
7	Very heavy	
8		
9		
10	Extremely heavy	(Almost maximal)
●	Maximal	

Key Point: The Borg Scale is a simple, valuable way of assessing the relative effort a patient exerts during exercise. In determining whether an effort is maximal, the Borg Scale response should be considered with patient appearance and age predictions of maximum heart rate and METs.

MEASURED EXPIRED GASES

Because of the inaccuracies associated with estimating METs (ventilatory oxygen consumption) from workload (*i.e.,* treadmill speed and grade), many investigators measure the expired gases. Although this requires additional equipment and a mouth piece in the patient's mouth during exercise, it can be done safely if the patient is taught how to use hand signs for symptoms. Although not necessary for all clinical testing, expired gas analysis also permits measurement of other perameters, including respiratory quotient, efficiency of ventilation, physiological dead space, plateauing, and ventilatory anaerobic threshold. Anaerobic threshold can also be determined by measuring blood lactate levels during exercise. This measurement is helpful because it determines the comfortable submaximal exercise limit and can be used for setting optimal exercise prescriptions. Computerization of the equipment has led to the widespread use of expired gas analysis in sports medicine to determine whether the lungs or the heart is the limiting factor in patients with combined diseases and to evaluate therapies in serial testing. Although serial testing is associated with increases in exercise workload (thus estimated METs) related to habituation or learning, measured METs are stable.

Key Point: Gas exchange measurements can supplement the exercise test by increasing precision and providing additional information concerning cardiopulmonary function during exercise. It is particularly needed to evaluate therapies using serial tests, since workload changes and estimated METs can be misleading.

SKIN PREPARATION

Proper skin preparation is essential for the performance of an exercise test. During exercise, because noise increases with the square of resistance, it is extremely important to lower the resistance at the skin-electrode interface and thereby improve the signal-to-noise ratio. Nevertheless, it is often difficult to consistently prepare the skin properly because doing so may cause the patient discomfort and minor skin irritation. However, the performance of an exercise test with an ECG signal that cannot be continuously monitored and accurately interpreted because of artifact is worthless and can even be dangerous.

The general areas for electrode placement are shaved if they have hair and are cleansed with an alcohol-saturated gauze pad; then the exact areas for electrode application are marked with a felt-tip pen. The mark serves as a guide for removal of enough of the superficial layer of skin. The placements are determined using anatomical landmarks found with the patient supine because some individuals with loose skin can have a considerable shift of electrode positions when they assume an upright position. After the placements are marked, the next step is to remove the superficial layer of skin by light abrasion with a handheld drill or fine-grain emery paper. Skin resistance should be reduced to 5000 ohms or less, which can be verified before the exercise test with an inexpensive alternating-current impedance meter driven at 10 Hz. Do not use a direct-current meter because they can polarize the electrodes. Each electrode is tested against a common electrode with an ohm meter, and when 5000 ohms or less is not achieved, the electrode must be removed and skin preparation repeated. This maneuver saves time by obviating the need to interrupt a test due to noisy tracings.

ELECTRODES AND CABLES

Many disposable electrodes perform excellently. The disposable electrodes have the advantages of quick application and no need for cleansing for reuse. A disposable electrode that has an abrasive center spun by an applicator after the electrode is attached to the skin (Quickprep) is available from Quinton Instrument Co. This approach does not require skin preparation. A clever feature of the applicator is a built-in impedance meter that stops it from spinning when the skin impedance has been appropriately lowered. Buffer amplifiers or digitizers carried by the patient are no longer advantageous. Cables develop continuity problems with use and require replacement rather than repair. We often find that replacement is necessary after 500 tests. Some systems have used analog-to-digital converters in the electrode junction box carried by the patient. Because digital signals are relatively impervious to noise, the patient cable can be unshielded and is therefore very light.

Key Point: Careful skin preparation and attention to the electrode-cable interface are necessary no matter how elaborate or expensive the ECG recording device used.

LEAD SYSTEMS

Bipolar lead systems have been used because of the relatively short time required for placement, the relative freedom from motion artifact, and the ease with which noise problems can be located. Fig 1-3 illustrates the electrode placements for most of the bipolar lead systems. The usual positive reference is an electrode placed the same as the positive reference for V_5. The negative reference for V_5 is Wilson's central terminal, which consists of connecting the limb electrodes as follows: right arm, left arm, and left leg.[33]

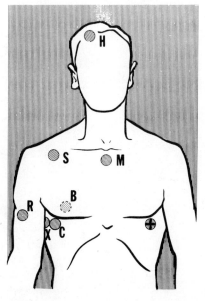

FIG 1-3.
The common bipolar ECG leads used during exercise testing.

Mason-Likar Electrode Placement

Because a 12-lead ECG cannot be obtained accurately during exercise with electrodes placed on the wrists and ankles, the electrodes are placed at the base of the limbs for exercise testing. In addition to providing a noise-free exercise tracing, their modified placement apparently shows no differences in ECG configuration when compared with the standard limb lead placement. However, this finding has been disputed by others who have found that the Mason-Likar placement causes amplitude changes and axis shifts when compared with standard placement. Because these could lead to diagnostic changes, it has been recommended that the modified exercise electrode placement not be used for recording a resting ECG. The preexercise test ECG has been further complicated by the recommendation that it should be obtained standing, since that is the same position maintained during exercise. This situation is worsened by the common practice of moving the limb electrodes onto the chest to minimize motion artifact.[34]

Fig 1-4 illustrates the Mason-Likar torso-mounted limb lead system. The conventional ankle and wrist electrodes are replaced by electrodes mounted on the torso at the base of the limbs. In this way, the artifact introduced by movement of the limbs is avoided. The standard precordial leads use Wilson's central terminal as their negative reference, which is formed by connecting the right arm, left arm, and left leg. This triangular configuration around the heart results in a zero voltage reference through the cardiac cycle. The use of Wilson's central terminal for the precordial leads (V leads) requires the negative reference to be a combination of three additional electrodes rather than the single electrode used as the negative reference for bipolar leads.[35,36]

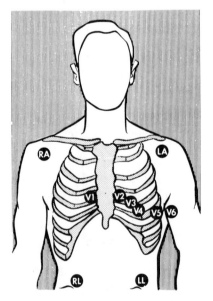

FIG 1-4.
The Mason-Likar simulated standard 12-lead ECG electrode placement for exercise testing.

The preexercise ECG is further complicated by positional differences when it is recorded.[37-40] Another complicating factor is the effect of respiration on inferior Q waves.[41,42] The results of a lead study at the University of California at San Diego clarify much of the confusion regarding the preexercise test ECG. Misplacement of the Mason-Likar arm leads is common and has even been published as the correct exercise modification. By placing the leads medially, near the midclavicular line, we have shown that the frontal plane axis shifts rightward on the average of 26 degrees (Fig 1-5). This shift caused decreased amplitudes in the Q waves in III and the R waves in I and aV_L and increased amplitudes in the Q waves in aV_L and the R waves in II, III, and aV_F. Of clinical importance is what these shifts did to the visual interpretation of the ECG. In five patients the ECG diagnosis of old inferior infarct was lost. In addition, seven patients lost significant Q waves in III alone. There were instances of Q waves gained. Eight patients had no Q waves in aV_L, one had a new Q wave in III and a new Q wave in II, one had a new Q wave in V_6, and another gained an inferior infarct diagnosis. Though these serial changes are merely artifact produced by electrode misplacement, they could be very misleading. Standing can cause many changes in the visual interpretation of the ECG, including those that would be most alarming, (i.e., the appearance of new Q waves [particularly inferiorly]). The misplacement of the arm electrodes in the midclavicular area also causes many clinical changes including the appearance of Q waves in aV_L as well as large axis shifts and amplitude changes. The correct Mason-Likar modification can also cause amplitude and duration changes, but they are less clinically important. The modified exercise electrode placement should not be used for routine ECGs. However, the changes caused by the exercise electrode placement can be kept to a minimum by keeping the arm electrodes off the chest and putting them on the

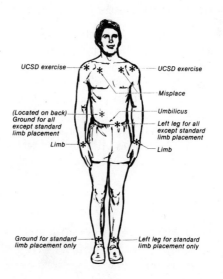

FIG 1-5.

Electrode placement of a study at the University of California at San Diego on the effects of limb lead placement and standing on the routine ECG.

shoulders and by having the patient supine. In this situation, the modified exercise limb lead placement of Mason-Likar can serve well as the resting ECG reference before an exercise test.

Inferior Lead ST-Segment Depression

Miranda et al[43] recently studied 178 men who had undergone exercise testing and coronary angiography to evaluate the diagnostic value of ST-segment depression occurring in the inferior leads. Lead V_5 had a better sensitivity (65%) and specificity (84%) than that of lead II (sensitivity and specificity 71% and 44%, respectively) at a single cutpoint. Receiver-operating characteristic curve analysis demonstrated that lead V_5 (area = 0.76) was markedly superior to lead II (area = 0.58) over multiple cutpoints. Moreover, the area under the curve in lead II was not significantly greater than 0.50, suggesting that for the identification of coronary artery disease, isolated ST-segment depression in lead II is unreliable.

The specificity of leads other than V_5 has not been demonstrated, but inferior leads may have more false-positive results and may require different criteria. This apparent lack of specificity may result from the effect of atrial repolarization in inferior leads, which causes depression of the ST segment. With adequate experience, atrial repolarization may be recognized as causing ST-segment depression. The end of the PR segment is depressed in a curved fashion to the same level that the ST segment begins. Such findings also support the concept of intercoronary artery steal during exercise; that is, ischemic areas obtain blood flow through collaterals. This phenomenon makes it impossible for ST-segment depression with multilead exercise testing to predict the location of coronary artery occlusions.

Number of Leads to Record

In patients with normal resting ECGs, a V_5 or similar bipolar lead along the long axis of the heart usually is adequate. In patients with ECG evidence of myocardial infarction or with a history suggesting coronary spasm, additional leads are needed. As a minimal approach, it is advisable to record three leads: a V_5 type of lead, an anterior V_2 type of lead, and an inferior lead such as aV_F. Alternatively, frank X, Y, and Z leads may be used. Either of these approaches is also helpful for the detection and identification of dysrhythmias. It is also advisable to record a second three-lead grouping consisting of V_4, V_5, and V_6. Occasionally, abnormalities may be seen as borderline in V_5, whereas they will be clearly abnormal in V_4 or V_6.

Key Point: Because most meaningful ST-segment depression occurs in the lateral leads (V_4, V_5, and V_6) when the resting ECG is normal, other leads are only necessary in patients who have had myocardial infarctions, those with a history consistent with coronary spasm or variant angina, or those who have exercise-induced dysrythmias of an uncertain type.

POSTEXERCISE PERIOD

If maximal sensitivity is to be achieved with an exercise test, patients should be supine during the postexercise period. It is advisable to record about 10 seconds of ECG data while patients stand motionless but still experiencing near maximal heart rates; then they lie down. Some patients must be allowed to lie down immediately to avoid hypotension. Having the patient perform a cool-down walk after the test can delay or eliminate the appearance of ST-segment depression.[44] According to the law of LaPlace, the increase in venous return and thus ventricular volume in the supine position increases myocardial oxygen demand. Data from our laboratory[45] suggests that having patients lie down may enhance ST-segment abnormalities in recovery. However, a cool-down walk has been suggested to minimize the postexercise chances of dysrhythmic events in this high-risk time when catecholamine levels are high. The supine position after exercise is not as important when the test is not being performed for diagnostic purposes. When testing is not performed for diagnostic purposes, it may be preferable to walk slowly (1.0 to 1.5 mph) or continue cycling against zero or minimal resistance (up to 25 watts when testing with a cycle ergometer) for several minutes after the test.

Monitoring should continue for at least 6 to 8 minutes after exercise or until changes stabilize. In the supine position 4 to 5 minutes into recovery, approximately 85% of patients with abnormal responses in a large series were abnormal at this time only or in addition to other times. An abnormal response occurring only in the recovery period is not unusual. All such responses are not false positives, as has been suggested. Experiments confirm mechanical dysfunction and electrophysiological abnormalities in the ischemic ventricle after exercise. A cool-down walk can be helpful when testing patients with an established diagnosis undergoing testing for other than diagnostic reasons, when testing athletes, or when testing patients with dangerous dysrhythmias.

Key Point: The recovery period is extemely important for observing ST shifts and should not be interrupted by a cool-down walk or failure to monitor for at least 5 minutes. Changes isolated in the recovery period are not more likely to be false positives.

INDICATIONS FOR TREADMILL TEST TERMINATION

The absolute and relative indications for termination of an exercise test listed in the box have been derived from clinical experience. Absolute indications are clearcut, whereas relative indications can sometimes be disregarded if good clinical judgement is used. Absolute indications include a drop in systolic blood pressure despite an increase in workload, anginal chest pain becoming worse than

---

ABSOLUTE AND RELATIVE INDICATIONS FOR TERMINATION OF AN EXERCISE TEST

Absolute Indications
1. Acute myocardial infarction or suspicion of a myocardial infarction
2. Onset of severe angina (worse than usual)
3. Drop in systolic blood pressure with increasing workload accompanied by signs or symptoms or drops below standing resting pressure or drops of 20 mm Hg
4. Serious dysrhythmias (second- or third-degree atrioventricular block, sustained ventricular tachycardia, or increasing premature ventricular contractions)
5. Signs of poor perfusion, including pallor, cyanosis, and cold and clammy skin
6. Central nervous system (CNS) symptoms, including ataxia, vertigo, visual or gait problems, and confusion
7. Technical problems with monitoring any parameters (such as with the ECG)
8. Patient's request

Relative Indications
1. Pronounced ECG changes from baseline, including more than 0.2 mV of horizontal or downsloping ST-segment depression, or 0.2 mV of ST-segment elevation (except in lead aV_R)
2. Any chest pain that is increasing
3. Pronounced fatigue and shortness of breath
4. Wheezing
5. Leg cramps or intermittent claudication
6. Hypertensive response (systolic blood pressure greater than 260 mm Hg; diastolic blood pressure greater than 115 mm Hg)
7. Less serious dysrhythmias such as supraventricular tachycardia
8. Exercise-induced bundle branch block that cannot be distinguished from ventricular tachycardia

---

usual, CNS symptoms, signs of poor perfusion (such as pallor, cyanosis, and cold skin), serious dysrhythmias, technical problems with monitoring the patient, a patient's request to stop, and marked ECG changes (e.g., 0.2 mV of ST-segment elevation and more than 0.3 mV of horizontal or downsloping ST-segment depression). Relative indications for termination include other worrisome ST or QRS changes such as excessive junctional depression; increasing chest pain; fatigue, shortness of breath, wheezing, leg cramps, or intermittent claudication; worrisome appearance; hypertensive response (systolic pressure greater than 260 mm Hg and diastolic pressure greater than 115 mm Hg); and less serious dysrhythmias, including supraventricular tachycardias. In some patients estimated to be at high risk by their clinical history, it may be appropriate to stop at a submaximal level, since the most severe ST-segment depression or dysrhythmias may occur only after exercise. If more information is required the test can be repeated later.

Most problems can be avoided by having an experienced physician, nurse, or exercise physiologist standing next to the patient, measuring blood pressure, and assessing patient appearance during the test. The exercise technician should operate the recorder and treadmill, take the appropriate tracings, enter data on a form, and alert the physician to any abnormalities that may appear on the monitor scope.

SUMMARY

Use of proper methodology is critical for patient safety and accurate results. Preparing the patient physically and emotionally for testing is necessary. Good skin preparation will cause some discomfort but is necessary for providing good conductance and for avoiding artifact. The use of specific criteria for exclusion and termination, physician interaction with the patient, and appropriate emergency equipment are essential. A brief physical examination is always necessary to rule out significant aortic valve disease. Pretest standard 12-lead ECGs are needed in the supine and standing positions. The changes caused by exercise electrode placement can be kept to a minimum by keeping the arm electrodes off the chest, placing them on the shoulders, placing the leg electrodes below the umbilicus, and recording the baseline ECG supine. In this situation, the Mason-Likar modified exercise limb lead placement, if recorded supine, can serve as the resting ECG reference before an exercise test.

Few studies have correctly evaluated the relative yield or sensitivity and specificity of different electrode placements for exercise-induced ST-segment shifts. Using other leads in addition to V_5 will increase the sensitivity; however, the specificity is decreased. ST-segment changes isolated to the inferior leads are often false-positive responses. For clinical purposes, vectorcardiographic and body surface mapping lead systems do not appear to offer any advantage over simpler approaches.

The exercise protocol should be progressive with even increments in speed and grade whenever possible. Smaller, even, and more frequent work increments are preferable to larger, uneven, and less frequent increases, because the former yield a more accurate estimation of exercise capacity. The value of individualizing the exercise protocol rather than using the same protocol for every patient has recently been emphasized by many investigators. The optimum test duration is from 8 to 12 minutes; therefore the protocol workloads should be adjusted to permit this duration. Because ramp testing uses small increments, it permits a more accurate estimation of exercise capacity and can be individualized to yield a targeted test duration. As yet, however, only a few equipment companies manufacture a controller that performs such tests using a treadmill.

Target heart rates based on age should not be used because the relationship between maximum heart rate and age is poor and scatters widely around many different recommended regression lines. Such heart rate targets result in a sub-maximal test for some individuals, a maximal test for some others, and an unrealistic goal for even others. Blood pressure should be measured with a standard stethoscope and sphygmomanometer; the available automated devices cannot be relied on, particularly for detection of exertional hypotension. Borg scales are an excellent means of quantifying an individual's effort. Exercise capacity should not be reported in total time but rather as the oxygen uptake or MET equivalent of the workload achieved. This method permits the comparison of the results of many different exercise testing protocols. Hyperventilation should be avoided before testing. Subjects with and without disease may exhibit ST-segment changes with hyperventilation; hyperventilation to identify false-positive responders is no longer considered useful by most researchers. The postexercise period is a critical period diagnostically; therefore the patient should be placed in the supine position immediately after testing.

REFERENCES

1. Rochmis P, Blackburn H: Exercise tests: a survey of procedures, safety, and litigation experience in approximately 170,000 tests, *JAMA* 217:1061-1066, 1971.
2. Gibbons L et al: The safety of maximal exercise testing, *Circulation* 80:846-852, 1989.
3. Yang JC, Wesley RC, Froelicher VF: Ventricular tachycardia during routine treadmill testing, *Arch Intern Med* 151:349-353, 1991.
4. Irving JB, Bruce RA: Exertional hypotension and post exertional ventricular fibrillation in stress testing, *Am J Cardiol* 39:849-851, 1977.
5. Shepard RJ: Do risks of exercise justify costly caution? *Physician Sports Med* 5:58, 1977.
6. Cobb LA, Weaver WD: Exercise: a risk for sudden death in patients with coronary heart disease, *J Am Coll Cardiol* 7:215-219, 1986.
7. Schlant R et al: Clinical competence in exercise testing: a statement for physicians from the ACP/ACC/AHA Task Force on clinical privileges in cardiology, *Ann Intern Med* 107:588-589, 1987.
8. Milliken JA, Abdollah H, Burggraf GW: False-positive treadmill exercise tests due to computer signal averaging, *Am J Cardiol* 65:946-948, 1990.
9. Willems J et al: The diagnostic performance of computer programs for the interpretation of ECGs, *New Engl J Med* 325:1767-1773, 1991.
10. Balady GJ et al: Comparison of determinants of myocardial oxygen consumption during arm and leg exercise in normal persons, *Am J Cardiol* 57:1385-1387, 1986.
11. Balady GJ et al: Value of arm exercise testing in detecting coronary artery disease, *Am J Cardiol* 55:37-39, 1985.
12. Myers J, Froelicher VF: Optimizing the exercise test for pharmacological investigations, *Circulation* 82:1839-1846, 1990.
13. Hermansen L, Saltin B: Oxygen uptake during maximal treadmill and bicycle exercise, *J Appl Physiol* 26:31-37, 1969.
14. Buchfuhrer MJ et al: Optimizing the exercise protocol for cardiopulmonary assessment, *J Appl Physiol* 55:1558-1564, 1983.
15. Myers J et al: Comparison of the ramp versus standard exercise protocols, *J Am Coll Cardiol* 17:1334-1342, 1991.
16. Niederberger M et al: Disparities in ventilatory and circulatory responses to bicycle and treadmill exercise, *Br Heart J* 36:377, 1974.

17. Wickes JR et al: Comparison of the electrocardiographic changes induced by maximum exercise testing with treadmill and cycle ergometer, *Circulation* 57:1066-1069, 1978.
18. Balke B, Ware R: An experimental study of physical fitness of air force personnel, *US Armed Forces Med J* 10:675-688, 1959.
19. Astrand PO, Rodahl K: *Textbook of work physiology,* New York, 1986, McGraw-Hill.
20. Bruce RA: Exercise testing of patients with coronary heart disease, *Ann Clin Res* 3:323-330, 1971.
21. Ellestad MH et al: Maximal treadmill stress testing for cardiovascular evaluation, *Circulation* 39:517-522, 1969.
22. Stuart RJ, Ellestad MH: National survey of exercise stress testing facilities, *Chest* 77:94-97, 1980.
23. Sullivan M, McKirnan MD: Errors in predicting functional capacity for postmyocardial infarction patients using a modified Bruce protocol, *Am Heart J* 107:486-491, 1984.
24. Webster MWI, Sharpe DN: Exercise testing in angina pectoris: the importance of protocol design in clinical trials, *Am Heart J* 117:505-508, 1989.
25. Panza JA et al: Prediction of the frequency and duration of ambulatory myocardial ischemia in patients with stable coronary artery disease by determination of the ischemic threshold from exercise testing: importance of the exercise protocol, *J Am Coll Cardiol* 17:657-663, 1991.
26. Redwood DR et al: Importance of the design of an exercise protocol in the evaluation of patients with angina pectoris, *Circulation* 43:618-628, 1971.
27. Smokler PE et al: Reproducibility of a multi-stage near maximal treadmill test for exercise tolerance in angina pectoris, *Circulation* 48:346-351, 1973.
28. Lipkin DP et al: Factors determining symptoms in heart failure: comparison of fast and slow exercise tests, *Br Heart J* 55:439-445, 1986.
29. Goldman L et al: Comparative reproducibility and validity of systems for assessing cardiovascular function class: advantages of a new specific activity scale, *Circulation* 64:1227-1234, 1981.
30. Hlatky M et al: A brief, self-administered questionnaire to determine functional capacity (the Duke Activity Status Index), *Am J Cardiol* 64:651-654, 1989.
31. Borg G: Perceived exertion as an indicator of somatic stress, *Scand J Rehabil Med* 23:92-93, 1970.
32. Borg G, Holmgren A, Lindblad I: Quantitative evaluation of chest pain, *Acta Med Scand* 644:43-45, 1981.
33. Froelicher VF et al: A comparison of two-bipolar electrocardiographic leads to lead V_5, *Chest* 70:611, 1976.
34. Gamble P et al: A comparison of the standard 12-lead electrocardiogram to exercise electrode placements, *Chest* 85:616-622, 1984.
35. Kleiner JP, Nelson WP, Boland MJ: The 12-lead electrocardiogram in exercise testing, *Arch Intern Med* 138:1572-1573, 1978.
36. Rautaharju PM et al: The effect of modified limb positions on electrocardiographic wave amplitudes, *J Electrocardiol* 13:109-114, 1980.
37. Shapiro W, Berson AS, Pipberger HV: Differences between supine and sitting Frank-lead electrocardiograms, *J Electrocardiol* 9:303-308, 1976.
38. Sigler LH: Electrocardiographic changes occurring with alterations of posture from recumbent to standing positions, *Am Heart J* 15:146-152, 1938.
39. Dougherty JD: Change in the frontal QRS axis with changes in the anatomic positions of the heart, *J Electrocardiol* 3:299-311, 1970.
40. Bruce RA et al: Polarcardiographic responses to maximal exercise in healthy young adults, *Am Heart J* 83:206-212, 1972.

41. Mimbs JW, de Mello V, Roberts R: The effect of respiration on normal and abnormal Q-waves, *Am Heart J* 94:579-584, 1977.

42. Reikkinen H, Rautaharju P: Body position, electrode level, and respiration effects on the Frank lead electrocardiogram, *Circulation* 53(1):40-45, 1976.

43. Miranda CP et al: Usefulness of exercise-induced ST-segment depression in the inferior leads during exercise testing as a marker for coronary artery disease, *Am J Cardiol* 69:303-307, 1992.

44. Gutman RA et al: Delay of ST depression after maximal exercise by walking for two minutes, *Circulation* 42:229-233, 1970.

45. Lachterman B et al: "Recovery only" ST segment depression and the predictive accuracy of the exercise test, *Ann Intern Med* 112:11-16, 1990.

CHAPTER 2

Interpretation of Hemodynamic Responses to the Exercise Test

When interpreting the exercise test, it is important to consider each type of response separately. Each response has a different impact on making a diagnostic or clinical decision and must be considered with clinical information. A test should not be called *abnormal* (or *positive*) or *normal* (or *negative*), but rather the interpretation should specify which responses were abnormal or normal. Neither should the results be subjectively or objectively called *positive* or *negative*, but the particular responses should be recorded. The objective responses to exercise testing (exercise capacity, heart rate, blood pressure, electrocardiographic [ECG] changes, and dysrhythmias) and the subjective responses (patient appearance, the results of physical examination, and symptoms, particularly angina) require interpretation. The final report should be directed to the physician who ordered the test. It should contain information that helps in patient management and not vague "med-speak." Interpretation depends on the application for which the test is used and on the population tested.

EXERCISE PHYSIOLOGY

Two basic principles of exercise physiology are important to understand for interpretation of the exercise test. The first is a physiological principle: Total body oxygen uptake and myocardial oxygen uptake are distinct in their determinants and in the way they are measured or estimated (see box). Total body, or ventilatory, oxygen uptake (Vo_2) is the amount of oxygen extracted from inspired air as the body performs work. Myocardial oxygen uptake is the amount of oxygen consumed by the heart muscle. Accurate measurement of myocardial oxygen consumption requires the placement of catheters in a coronary artery and the coronary venous sinus to measure oxygen content. Its determinants include intramyocardial wall tension (left ventricular pressure end-diastolic volume), contractility, and heart rate. Myocardial oxygen uptake is best estimated by taking the product of the heart rate and systolic blood pressure (double product). This estimate is

---

TYPES OF OXYGEN CONSUMPTION OCCURRING WITH EXERCISE

Myocardial oxygen consumption $\cong$ Heart rate $\times$ systolic blood pressure
  (determinants include wall tension $\cong$ left ventricular pressure $\times$ volume;
  contractility; and heart rate)
Ventilatory oxygen consumption (V_{O_2}) $\cong$ External work performed, or cardiac
  output $\times$ AV_{O_2} difference*

*AV_{O_2} difference is approximately 15% to 17 vol% at maximal exercise; therefore V_{O_2} max is a noninvasive method for estimating cardiac output.

---

valuable clinically because exercise-induced angina often occurs at the same myocardial oxygen demand (double product), and thus it is useful for evaluating therapy. When the myocardial oxygen demand differs, the influence of other factors should be suspected, such as a recent meal, abnormal ambient temperature, or coronary artery spasm.

Key Point: An important basic principle of exercise physiology is that total body, or ventilatory oxygen consumption and myocardial oxygen consumption are distinct in their determinants and in the way they are measured or estimated. Although directly related to each other, this relationship can be altered (e.g., by training and beta-blockers).

The second principle is one of pathophysiology: Considerable interaction takes place between the various exercise test manifestations of abnormalities in myocardial perfusion and function. Not only are the ECG response and angina closely related to myocardial ischemia (coronary artery disease), but exercise capacity, systolic blood pressure, and heart rate responses to exercise also can be determined by myocardial ischemia, myocardial dysfunction, and responses in the periphery. Exercise-induced ischemia can cause cardiac dysfunction that results in exercise impairment and an abnormal systolic blood pressure response. Often it is difficult to separate the impact of ischemia from the impact of left ventricular dysfunction on exercise responses. The resulting interaction complicates the interpretation of the exercise test findings. The variables associated with perfusion and cardiac function abnormalities (i.e., metabolic equivalents [METs], maximum heart rate, and systolic blood pressure) have the greatest prognostic value.

    e severity of ischemia or the amount of myocardium in jeopardy is known clinically to be inversely related to the heart rate, blood pressure, and exercise level achieved. However, neither resting nor exercise ejection fraction (EF) correlates well with measured or estimated maximal VO_2 even in patients without signs or symptoms of ischemia.[1,2] Moreover, exercise-induced markers of ischemia do not correlate well with one another. Silent ischemia (i.e., when markers of ischemia are present without angina) does not appear to affect exercise capacity in patients with coronary heart disease.[3] Although cardiac output is generally considered the most important determinant of exercise capacity, studies suggest that in patients with heart disease, the periphery plays an important role in limiting exercise capacity.

EXERCISE CAPACITY OR FUNCTIONAL CAPACITY

The functional status of patients with heart disease is frequently classified by symptoms during daily activities. (New York Heart Association, Canadian, and Weber classifications are common examples.) However, there is no substitute for estimated or directly measured maximum Vo_2. Maximum Vo_2 (Vo_2 max) is the greatest amount of oxygen that a person can extract from inspired air while performing dynamic exercise involving a large part of the total body muscle mass. Because Vo_2 max is equal to the product of cardiac output and arterial venous oxygen (AVo_2) difference, it is a measure of the functional limits of the cardiovascular system. Maximum AVo_2 difference is physiologically limited to roughly 15 to 17 vol%. Thus maximum AVo_2 difference behaves more or less as a constant, making Vo_2 max an indirect estimate of maximum cardiac output.

Vo_2 max depends on many factors, including natural physical endowment, activity status, age, and gender, but it is the best index of exercise capacity and maximal cardiovascular function. As a rough reference, the Vo_2 max of the normal sedentary adult is approximately 30 ml/kg/min (8.5 METs), and the minimum level for physical fitness is 40 ml/kg/min (11 METs). Aerobic training can increase Vo_2 max by up to 25%, and bed rest lowers it. This increase depends on the initial level of fitness and age as well as the intensity, frequency, and length of training sessions. An individual performing aerobic training such as distance running can have a Vo_2 max as high as 60 to 90 ml/kg/min. For convenience, oxygen consumption is often expressed in multiples of basal resting requirements (METs). The MET is a unit of basal oxygen consumption equal to approximately 3.5 ml/kg/min. This value is the average oxygen requirement from inspired air necessary to maintain life in the resting state. The approximate MET costs for common activities are in Table 2-1.

Fig 2-1 illustrates the relationship of Vo_2 max to exercise habits and age.[4] Although the three activity levels have regression lines that fit the data as one would expect, there is much scatter around the lines, and the correlation coefficients are poor. This finding demonstrates the inaccuracy involved with trying to predict Vo_2 max from age and habitual physical activity. It is preferable to estimate an individual's Vo_2 max from the workload reached while performing an exercise test.

Key Point: A measurement of 5 METs is associated with a poor prognosis in patients under 65; it is the usual exercise limit in the period immediately after a myocardial infarction. A measurement of 10 METs is considered a degree of fitness, but in a patient with angina it is associated with no improvement in survival,

TABLE 2-1.

MET Demands for Most Common Activities

Activity	METs	Activity	METs
Mild		*Vigorous*	
Baking	2.0	Badminton	5.5
Billiards	2.4	Chopping wood	4.9
Bookbinding	2.2	Climbing hills	7.0
Canoeing (leisurely)	2.5	Cycling (moderate)	5.7
Conducting an orchestra	2.2	Dancing	6.0
Dancing, ballroom (slow)	2.9	Field hockey	7.7
Golf (with cart)	2.5	Ice skating	5.5
Horseback riding (walking)	2.3	Jogging (10-minute mile)	10
Playing a musical instrument	2.0	Karate or judo	6.5
Volleyball (noncompetitive)	2.9	Roller skating	6.5
Walking (2 mph)	2.5	Rope skipping	12
Writing	1.7	Skiing (water or downhill)	6.8
		Squash	12
Moderate		Surfing	6.0
Calisthenics (no weights)	4.0	Swimming (fast)	7.0
Croquet	3.0	Tennis (doubles)	6.0
Cycling (leisurely)	3.5		
Gardening (no lifting)	4.4		
Golf (without cart)	4.9		
Mowing lawn (power mower)	3.0		
Playing drums	3.8		
Sailing	3.0		
Swimming (slowly)	4.5		
Walking (3 mph)	3.3		
Walking (4 mph)	4.5		

From American Heart Association: *Exercise standards*, Dallas, 1990, The Association.

and consequently, either coronary artery bypass surgery (CABS) or medical management may be suggested. A measurement of 13 METs indicates a good prognosis in spite of any abnormal exercise test responses, and 24 METs can be achieved by well-trained aerobic athletes.

Exercise Capacity and Cardiac Function

Exercise capacity determined by exercise testing has been proposed as a means to estimate ventricular function. A direct relationship would appear to be supported by the fact that both resting EF and exercise capacity have prognostic value in patients with coronary heart disease. However, a marked discrepancy between resting ventricular function and exercise performance is frequently seen clinically. In addition, exercise capacity is poorly related to ventricular function in pa-

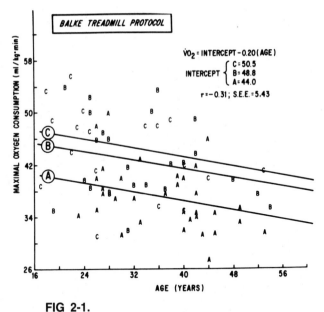

FIG 2-1.
Relationship of Vo$_2$ max to exercise habits and age.

tients with cardiomyopathies. Exercise-induced ischemia could limit exercise in spite of normal resting ventricular function; therefore patients with angina must be excluded, and silent ischemia must be considered when evaluating an interaction.

We investigated the relationship between resting ventricular function and exercise performance in patients with a wide range of resting EFs able to exercise to volitional fatigue.[5] A plot of resting EF versus measured Vo$_2$ max is shown in Fig. 2-2. This poor relationship ($r = 0.25$) confirms other studies among patients with chronic heart failure and coronary heart disease.[6-9]

The discrepancy between ventricular function and exercise capacity is now well known. Studies have used radionuclide, angiographic, and echocardiographic measures of ventricular size and function to document this finding in patients with heart disease. Correlations between exercise capacity and various indices of ventricular function have ranged from -0.10 to 0.24.[10] Increasing the heart rate and cardiac index appear to be the most important determinants of exercise capacity, but they often leave more than 50% of the variance in exercise capacity unexplained. The established clinical impression today is that good ventricular function does not guarantee normal exercise capacity and vice versa. Thus even in patients free of angina, exercise limitations or expectations should not be determined by ventricular function but rather by the patients' symptomatic responses to exercise.

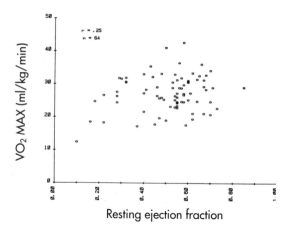

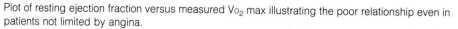

Resting ejection fraction

FIG 2-2.

Plot of resting ejection fraction versus measured Vo₂ max illustrating the poor relationship even in patients not limited by angina.

Key Point: Resting ventricular function and exercise capacity are important prognostic features of heart disease, but their association is not highly correlated in patients with stable disease. Abnormal ventricular function does not imply abnormal exercise capacity in clinical practice; therefore an exercise test must be performed to determine exercise capacity.

Use of Nomograms for Exercise Capacity

As experience with exercise testing has progressed, many protocols have been developed to best assess certain patient populations. Rapidly paced protocols may be suited to screening younger or active individuals (i.e., the Bruce and Ellestad protocols), whereas more moderate ones are adapted to older or deconditioned patients (i.e., the Naughton, Balke-Ware, and USAFSAM protocols). The main disadvantage to having so many techniques has been determining equivalent workloads between them. (For example, what does 5 minutes on a modified Bruce protocol mean in terms of a Balke-Ware protocol or of real-life activities such as hiking or grocery shopping?)

Vo₂ max can be reasonably estimated from the workload achieved in a given protocol. Because Vo₂ depends on age, gender, activity status, and disease status, tables that take these factors into account must be referred to so that accurate categorization of a certain MET value as either normal or abnormal can occur. A nomogram that makes it convenient to translate a MET level into a percentage of normal exercise capacity based on age and activity status for men follows: it is similar to that published by Bruce, Kusumi, and Hosmer[11] except that it considers METs instead of time as in the Bruce protocol.[12] The nomogram is based on a male referral population of 1388, after the exclusion of those with obvious disease, with a mean age of 57 (range 21 to 89). For those who could be so classified, a further subgrouping was made into sedentary (*N* = 253) and physically active (N = 346) groups. Activity status was classified by asking, "Do you perform 20 minutes or more of brisk walking 3 times a week, and/or do you regularly participate in an aerobic sport?"[13]

A separate nomogram was developed from 244 normal men who volunteered for maximal exercise testing with ventilatory gas exchange analysis. These subjects differed from the former in that they were not referred for any clinical reason and were a healthier, younger (mean age 45 ± 14 years, range 18 to 72) population. They were also classified into sedentary (N = 74) and active (N = 122) groups.

The predicted METs for age were calculated by the formulas obtained from the regression analysis using age as the independent variable. This calculation was done for the entire group, the sedentary group, and the active groups. A percentage of exercise capacity was obtained from the following equation:

$$\text{Exercise capacity} = \frac{\text{Observed MET level} \times 100}{\text{Predicted METs}}$$

Exercise capacity represents the actual percentage capacity for a given age based on METs performed, with 100% being the average for age.

Among patients tested for clinical reasons (referrals), regression analyses of METs against age for the entire group and for each of the two subgroups yielded the following equations:

All referrals: predicted METs = $(18.0 - 0.15)(\text{Age})$,
$(N = 1388)$, $\text{SEE}^* = 3.3$, $r = -0.46$, $p < 0.001$

Active: predicted METs = $(18.7 - 0.15)(\text{Age})$, $(N = 346)$,
$\text{SEE} = 3.0$, $r = -0.49$, $p < 0.001$

Sedentary: predicted METs = $(16.6 - 0.16)(\text{Age})$,
$(N = 253)$, $\text{SEE} = 3.2$, $r = -0.43$, $p < 0.001$

Analysis of variance (ANOVA) was performed for METs by the age grouping of less than 40, 40-49, 50-59, 60-69, 70-79, and 80-89 years ($p < 0.001$); respective box plots are illustrated in Fig 2-3, and the nomograms are presented as Figs 2-4 and 2-5.

Healthy volunteers were tested with ventilatory gas exchange analysis (*normals*). Regression analysis of METs against age for the normals and for active and sedentary subgroups yielded the following equations:

All (normal): predicted METs = $(14.7 - 0.11)(\text{Age})$,
$(N = 244)$, $\text{SEE} = 2.5$, $r = -0.53$, $p < 0.001$

Active: predicted METs = $(16.4 - 0.13)(\text{Age})$,
$(N = 122)$, $\text{SEE} = 2.5$, $r = -0.58$, $p < 0.001$

Sedentary: predicted METs = $(11.9 - 0.07)(\text{Age})$,
$(N = 74)$, $\text{SEE} = 1.8$, $r = -0.47$, $p < 0.001$

SEE, Standard error of the estimate.

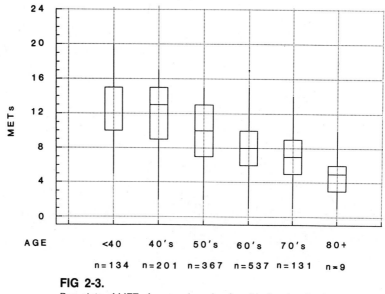

FIG 2-3.
Box plots of METs for age decades for all referral patients.

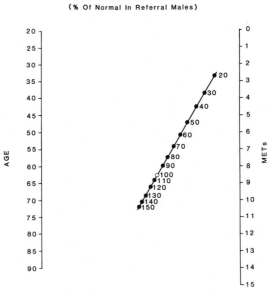

FIG 2-4.
Nomogram for all referral patients.

EXERCISE CAPACITY
(% Of Normal In Referral Males)

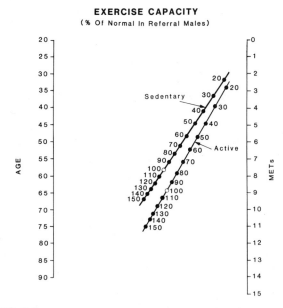

FIG 2-5.
Nomogram for referral patients classified as *active* or *sedentary*.

The nomograms for this group are presented in Figs 2-6 and 2-7.

The term *METs* is a more meaningful and useful expression of exercise capacity than the various conglomerations of protocol times and stages often used. Use of the term facilitates comparisons of data using different protocols and tailoring of protocols for particular patients. MET levels can be used for exercise prescription and for estimating levels of disability by using tables listing the MET demands of most common activities (Table 2-1).

Comparison With Other Populations

The regression analysis of this group of 1388 referred men from the Long Beach Veterans Administration (VA) differs from those developed by Froelicher, Allen, and Lancaster[14] in 1974 using United States Air Force (USAF) military personnel. Bruce, Kusumi, and Hosmer[11] derived their nomogram for functional capacity from 138 healthy men (mean age 49) and calculated the observed exercise capacity from the following equation:

$$\text{Predicted METs} = (13.7 - 0.08)(\text{Age}) \ (N = 138) \ \text{SEE} = 1.37$$

Their group consisted of healthy volunteers, like those in the USAF study, and the healthy volunteers from Long Beach, and all three populations were roughly the same age. Thus these equations yield approximately the same results for any given age. These results contrast with those of the population of patients who were referred to our hospital-based laboratory for evaluation of possible coronary artery disease.

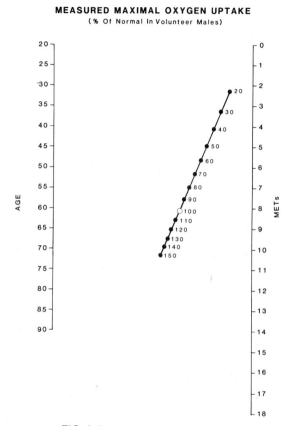

MEASURED MAXIMAL OXYGEN UPTAKE
(% Of Normal In Volunteer Males)

FIG 2-6.
Nomogram for all healthy volunteers.

When Dehn and Bruce[15] conducted a review of the literature regarding V_{O_2} max and its variations with age and activity, they derived a regression equation from a compilation of 17 previous studies encompassing 700 observations in healthy males of all ages: predicted METs = (16.2 − 0.11) (age). The results of previous studies by age decade are listed in Table 2-2 for comparison.

These nomograms are simple to use, requiring only values for age and observed MET levels to calculate the percentage for normal exercise capacity. For instance, after completing 6 minutes of a Bruce protocol (stage 2), a patient would have achieved an exercise capacity of 7 METs. If the patient were 55 years old, this would calculate to be an exercise capacity of 78% using the nomogram. Similarly, after completing 8 minutes of a Balke protocol, the same patient would also have achieved 7 METs and have an exercise capacity of 78%. Values obtained below 100% indicate exercise impairment relative to age group, whereas values above 100% indicate supranormal performance. Also, equations based on time in a protocol can be used to obtain particular MET levels. For example, for the Bruce protocol, METs = (1.11 + 0.016) (duration in seconds). Using treadmill speed and grade, METs = (mph × 26.8) × (0.1 + [grade × 0.018] + 3.5)/3.5.

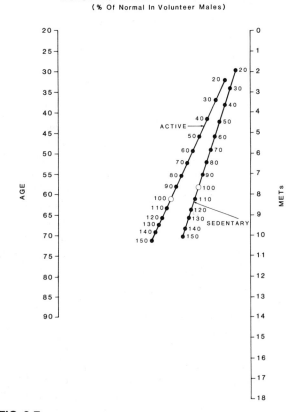

MEASURED MAXIMAL OXYGEN UPTAKE
(% Of Normal In Volunteer Males)

FIG 2-7.
Nomogram for healthy volunteers classified as *active* or *sedentary*.

TABLE 2-2.

MET Levels for Age Decades from Previous Studies

	Froelicher	Hossack	Pollock (Cooper's Clinic)	Morris (Referrals)
20-29	11 ± 2	13 ± 1	12 ± 2	—
30-39	10 ± 2	12 ± 2	12 ± 2	—
40-49	10 ± 2	11 ± 2	11 ± 2	11 ± 4
50-59	—	10 ± 2	10 ± 2	9 ± 4
60-69	—	8 ± 2	8 ± 2	8 ± 3
70-79	—	5 ± 1	8 ± 2	7 ± 3
80-89	—	—	—	5 ± 3

Using an ergometer workload, METs = ([2 × kpm/min + 300]/body weight in kilograms)/3.5. The total population nomograms are appropriate if activity status is unknown. The referral nomograms may be used for patients referred for testing for clinical reasons, and the normal nomograms may be more appropriate for individuals tested for screening or preexercise program evaluations.

Key Point: Nomograms facilitate the reporting of exercise capacity because they present the response as a percent relative to the normal for age, with 100% being normal for age.

MAXIMUM HEART RATE

The heart rate response to exercise is influenced by several factors including age, type of activity, body position, fitness, presence of heart disease, medications, blood volume, and environment. Of these, the most important is age because a decline in maximum heart rate occurs with increasing age.[16] This decline appears to result from intrinsic cardiac changes rather than neural influences. There is a great deal of variability around the regression line between maximum heart rate and age; thus age-related maximum heart rate is a relatively poor index of maximal effort. Maximum heart rate is unchanged or may be slightly reduced after a program of training. Resting heart rate is frequently reduced after training, which is due to enhanced parasympathetic tone.

Key Point: The heart rate response to maximal dynamic exercise depends on numerous factors but particularly age and health. Although a regression line of $(200 - 0.6)$ (age) is fairly reproducible, the scatter around this line is considerable (i.e., 1 standard deviation $= \pm 12$ beats/min). This makes age-predicted maximum heart rate relatively useless for clinical purposes. Such predictions are maximal for some individuals and submaximal for others.

Methods of Recording

The best way to measure heart rate is to use a standard ECG recorder and use the R-R intervals to calculate instantaneous heart rate. Methods using the arterial pulse or capillary blush technique are much more affected by artifact than ECG techniques. Some investigators have used averaging over the last minute of exercise or in immediate recovery; both methods are inaccurate. Heart rate drops quickly in recovery and can climb steeply even in the last seconds of exercise. Premature beats can affect averaging and must be eliminated to obtain the actual heart rate. Cardiotachometers are available but may fail to trigger or may trigger inappropriately on T waves, artifact, or aberrant beats, thus yielding inaccurate results.

Factors Limiting Maximum Heart Rate

Several factors may affect the maximum heart rate (HRmax) during dynamic exercise (refer to the box on p. 41). HRmax declines with advancing years and is affected by gender. Height, weight, and even lean body weight apparently are not independent factors affecting HRmax. Sheffield et al[17] treadmill tested 100 asymp-

---

FACTORS AFFECTING THE MAXIMUM HEART RATE IN RESPONSE TO DYNAMIC EXERCISE

Age	Bed rest
Gender	Altitude
Level of fitness	Type of exercise
Cardiovascular disease	True maximal exertion

---

tomatic women 19 to 69 years old and concluded that the regression of HRmax based on age in women was about 5 beats/min lower than in men. Some investigators report a substantial decrease in HRmax in well-trained athletes. Perhaps blood volume changes and cardiac hypertrophy can explain this phenomenon. However, it has not been a consistent finding. Although this point remains unsettled, it is possible that training in early life may result in cardiac hypertrophy or dilation.

Age, Fitness, and Cardiovascular Disease

Many studies have reported HRmax during treadmill testing in a variety of patients. Regressions with age have varied, depending on the population studied and other factors. Table 2-3 and Fig. 2-8 summarize these studies of HRmax and

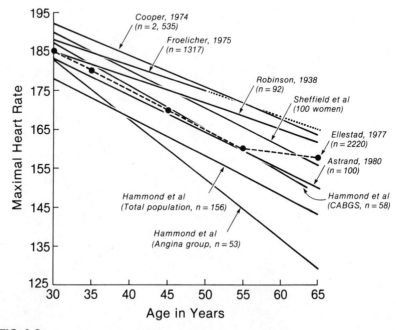

FIG 2-8.

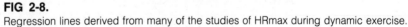
Regression lines derived from many of the studies of HRmax during dynamic exercise.

TABLE 2-3.
Summary of Studies of Maximum Heart Rate

Study	Number	Population Studied	Mean Age (SD or range)	Mean HR max (SD)	Regression line	Correlation Coefficient	Standard Error of the Estimate (beats/min)
Åstrand*	100	Asymptomatic men	50 (20-69)	166 ± 22	$y = 211 - 0.922$ (age)	NA	NA
Bruce	2091	Asymptomatic men	44 ± 8	181 ± 12	$y = 210 - 0.662$ (age)	-0.44	14
Cooper	2535	Asymptomatic men	43 (11-79)	181 ± 16	$y = 217 - 0.845$ (age)	NA	NA
Ellestad†	2583	Asymptomatic men	42 ± 7 (10-60)	173 ± 11	$y = 197 - 0.556$ (age)	NA	NA
Froelicher	1317	Asymptomatic men	38 ± 8 (28-54)	183	$y = 207 - 0.64$ (age)	-0.43	10
Lester	148	Asymptomatic men	43 (15-75)	187	$y = 205 - 0.411$ (age)	-0.58	NA
Robinson	92	Asymptomatic men	30 (6-76)	189	$y = 212 - 0.775$ (age)	NA	NA
Sheffield	95	Men with CHD	39 (19-69)	176 ± 14	$y = 216 - 0.88$ (age)	-0.58	11‡
Bruce	1295	Men with CHD	52 ± 8	148 ± 23	$y = 204 - 1.07$ (age)	-0.36	25‡
Hammond	156	Men with CHD	53 ± 9	157 ± 20	$y = 209 - 1.0$ (age)	-0.30	19
Morris	244	Asymptomatic men	45 (20-72)	167 ± 19	$y = 200 - 0.72$ (age)	-0.55	15
Morris	1388	Men referred for evaluation for CHD	57 (21-89)	144 ± 20	$y = 196 - 0.9$ (age)	-0.43	21

SD, Standard deviation; NA, not able to calculate from available data; CHD, coronary heart disease.
*Åstrand used bicycle ergometry; all other studies were performed on the treadmill.
†Data compiled from graphs in reference cited.
‡Calculated from available data.

are self-explanatory. To clarify the relationship between HRmax and age, Londeree and Moeschberger[18] performed a comprehensive review of the literature, compiling over 23,000 subjects of ages 5 to 81 years. A stepwise multiple regression revealed that age alone accounted for 75% of the variability; other factors added only about 5% and included mode of exercise, level of fitness, and continent of origin but not gender. The 95% confidence interval, even when accounting for these factors, was 45 beats/min (Fig. 2-9). Heart rates at maximal exercise were lower on bicycle ergometry than treadmill and lower still with swimming. Their analysis revealed that trained individuals had a significantly lower HRmax for their ages.

To evaluate the effect of the protocol used, the Bruce, Balke, and Taylor protocols were used to test 15 healthy men; each man performed one test per week for 9 weeks, repeating each protocol three times in randomized order.[19] The maximum heart rates achieved were reproducible within each protocol, and there were no significant differences in heart rate achieved among the three protocols. Graettinger et al[20] from our laboratory recently presented clinical, ECG, and functional determinants of HRmax. Despite controlling for age, activity status, gender, and hypertension, measures of cardiac size and function added little to the prediction of HRmax.

Older patients' motivation to exert themselves may also affect the HRmax. They may be restrained by poor muscle tone, pulmonary disease, claudication, orthopedic problems, and other noncardiac causes of limitation. The usual decline in HRmax with age is not as steep in people who are free from myocardial disease and stay active, but it still occurs.

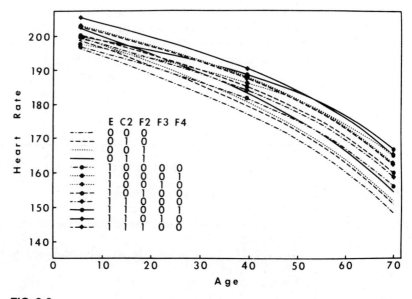

FIG 2-9.
Plot of Londeree and Moeschberger[18] summarizing studies on over 23,000 subjects.

Bed rest

Another factor that affects HRmax and that is important to clinical medicine is bed rest. Convertino et al[21] examined the cardiovascular responses to maximal exercise in a normal man after 10 days of bed rest. A significant increase in HRmax was found in tests after bed rest when compared with tests before bed rest.

Altitude

Altitude may affect the heart rate response to exercise. At sea level, atropine administration does not impair maximum heart rate, implying that parasympathetic withdrawal is complete at maximal exercise. HRmax decreases after prolonged hypoxia.

Measures of Maximal Effort

Various objective measurements have been used to confirm that a maximal effort was performed (see box). As maximal aerobic capacity is reached, the rate of oxygen consumption may plateau. A respiratory quotient (RQ) greater than 1.15 and a decrease or failure to increase oxygen uptake by 150 cc/min with increased workloads is the criterion for the plateau. However, in our experience a plateau is infrequently seen in continuous treadmill protocols and may actually be caused by holding onto the handrails, incomplete expired air collection, the criteria used for plateau, differences in the sampling interval, or the equipment.

The Borg scale has been developed to subjectively grade levels of exertion. This method is best applied to match levels of perceived exertion during comparison studies. The linear scale ranges from 6 (very, very light) to 20 (very, very hard), the nonlinear scale ranges from 0 to 10, and both correlate with the percentage of HRmax during exercise. RQ, or the ratio of carbon dioxide production to oxygen utilization, increases in proportion to exercise effort. Values of 1.15 are reached by most individuals at the point of maximal dynamic exercise. However, this quotient varies greatly, and its measurement requires gas exchange analysis during exercise. Lactic acid levels have also been used (i.e., greater than 7 or 8 mM), but they require mixed venous samples and also vary greatly between individuals.

INDICATORS OF MAXIMAL EFFORT

Patient appearance and breathing rate
Borg scale
Age-predicted heart rate and exercise capacity
Systolic blood pressure
Expired gas measurements: anaerobic threshold, respiratory quotient (RQ), plateau of V_{O_2}
Venous lactate concentration

Type of Dynamic Exercise

Although steps, escalators, ladders, and other devices are used, the three predominant types of exercise testing used clinically are the treadmill and supine and upright bicycle ergometry. The position and the type of exercise influence the heart rate responses. HRmax is consistent in a wide range of patients with various treadmill and upright ergometer protocols. Supine bicycle ergometry is used for radionuclide studies or for cardiac catheterization studies. Because of changes in venous return and filling pressures, the supine position results in lower resting heart rate and higher end-diastolic volumes.

Key Point: Dynamic exercise is preferred for testing because it can be graduated and controlled and puts a volume stress on the heart rather than a pressure stress. However, most activities usually combine isometric and dynamic exercise in varying degrees.

Chronotropic Incompetence or Heart Rate Impairment

Is exercise-induced angina or myocardial dysfunction the cause of chronotropic incompetence (CI)? Much of what has been called *chronotropic incompetence* is related to early termination of exercise related to angina pectoris.[22-25] Nevertheless, a significant number of patients are not limited by angina but have heart rate impairment (HRI). These patients also have significantly lower aerobic capacity than do age-matched patients with a normal heart rate response.

BLOOD PRESSURE RESPONSE

Systolic blood pressure should rise with increasing treadmill workload. Diastolic blood pressure usually remains about the same, but the fifth Korotkoff sound can sometimes be heard all the way to zero in healthy young subjects. Although a rising diastolic blood pressure can be associated with coronary heart disease, more likely it is a marker for labile hypertension, which leads to coronary disease. The highest systolic blood pressure should be achieved at maximal workload. When exercise is stopped, systolic blood pressure abruptly drops in 15% of the people tested because of peripheral pooling. To avoid fainting, patients should not be left standing on the treadmill. The systolic blood pressure usually normalizes on resuming the supine position during recovery but may remain below normal for several hours after the test. In spite of studies showing discrepancies between noninvasively and invasively measured blood pressure, the product of heart rate and systolic blood pressure, determined by cuff and auscultation, correlates with measured myocardial oxygen consumption during exercise. Usually, a patient's angina pectoris and abnormal ST-segment depression are precipitated at the same double product (systolic blood pressure multiplied by heart rate). This product is also an estimate of the maximal workload that the left ventricle can perform. The automated methods of measuring systolic blood pressure have not proved accurate. Although the available devices may correlate with manual methods, they have not yet been adequately validated, particularly for the detection of exertional hypotension.

Key Point: Systolic blood pressure rises to about twice its resting value during dynamic exercise, whereas diastolic blood pressure normally drops or stays the same.

Exertional Hypotension

Exercise-induced hypotension (EIH) has been demonstrated in most studies to predict a poor prognosis or a high probability of severe angiographic coronary artery disease. Although the prognosis of EIH has not been specifically examined in patients after myocardial infarction, an abnormal systolic blood pressure response indicates an increased risk for cardiac events in this population. In addition, EIH has been associated with cardiac complications during exercise testing and appears to be corrected by coronary artery bypass surgery.[26-28]

The normal blood pressure response to dynamic upright exercise consists of a progressive increase in systolic blood pressure, no change or a decrease in diastolic blood pressure, and a widening of the pulse pressure.[29] Even when tested to exhaustion, normal individuals do not exhibit a reduction in systolic blood pressure of any kind.[30] Normally, after exercise, there is a drop in both systolic and diastolic pressure. Exercise-induced decreases in systolic blood pressure can occur in patients with coronary artery disease, valvular heart disease,[31] cardiomyopathies, and arrhythmias. Occasionally, patients without clinically significant heart disease exhibit EIH during exercise because of antihypertensive therapy, including beta-blockers; because of prolonged strenuous exercise; or because of vasovagal responses. It can also occur in normal women. Pathophysiologically, EIH could result from chronic ventricular dysfunction, exercise-induced ischemia causing left ventricular dysfunction, or papillary muscle dysfunction and mitral regurgitation. Rich et al[32] described a patient in whom EIH was a result of right ventricular ischemia.

Numerous studies have addressed the diagnostic and prognostic implications of EIH. Their important findings regarding definition, prevalence, high-risk subgroups, intervention, and mortality are summarized in Table 2-4. One difficulty encountered in interpreting these previous studies is that although EIH has been consistently related to coronary artery disease and a poor prognosis, various criteria have been used to define it.[33] Irving and Bruce[34] reported on six men clinically diagnosed as having coronary heart disease, with postexertional ventricular fibrillation after maximal exercise testing, all of whom had exertional hypotension.

EIH is usually related to myocardial ischemia or myocardial infarction, is best

TABLE 2-4.

Summary of Studies Addressing Diagnostic and Prognostic Implications of Exercise-Induced Hypotension

Study	Definition	Prevalence of EIH	Prevalence of LM/3VD	Predictive Value of EIH for LM/3VD	Subgroups at High Risk	EIH Reversed by Revascularization	Mortality MED	Mortality CABG/PTCA
Dubach et al (1988)	SBP drop below rest	5% (94/2022)	45%	61%	No deaths in those with either ischemia or MI	18/22	12/95	0/22
Hammermeister (1983)	SBP drop below rest	7% (93/1241)	25%	50%	Angina, poor exercise capacity, LM/3VD with low EF	—	—	—
Weiner et al (1982)	SBP drop below rest	11% (47/436)	28%	55%	Ischemia, PVCs, poor exercise capacity	—	2/24	1/23
San Marco et al (1980)	Failure of SBP to rise 10 mm Hg in first minute or 20 mm Hg total drop	24% (90/378)	39%	70%	None found	—	—	—
Li et al (1979)	SBP equal to or drop below rest	23% (55/234)	100%	100%	—	33/37	—	—
Hakki et al (1986)	Decrease of SBP by 10 mm Hg	7% (127/1800)	—	—	3VD and LV dysfunction	—	—	—
Thomson and Keleman (1975)	SBP drop below rest	100% (17/17)	100%	100%	—	6/6	2/9	0/6
Levites et al (1978)	SBP drop below rest	3% (30/1105)	20%	20%	Women with false-positive results	—	—	—
Morris et al (1978)	Decrease of SBP by 10 mm Hg	5% (23/438)	24%	78%	None found	6/6	0/12	—
Mazzotta et al (1987)	Decrease of SBP by 5 mm Hg	20% (44/224)	—	—	None found	—	—	—
Gibbons et al (1987)	Decrease of SBP by 10 mm Hg	3% (27/820)	—	—	Older age, LM, 3VD, LV dysfunction	—	—	—

LM/3VD, Left main or three-vessel coronary artery disease; MED, medically treated; CABG/PTCA, patients treated with revascularization; SBP, systolic blood pressure; MI, myocardial infarction; EF, ejection fraction; PVC, premature ventricular contractions; LV, left ventricular.
From Dubach P et al: Circulation 78(6):1380-1387, 1988.

defined as a drop of systolic blood pressure during exercise below the standing preexercise value, and indicates a significantly increased risk for cardiac events. This increased risk is not found in those who did not have a prior myocardial infarction or signs or symptoms of ischemia during the exercise test. It is usually associated with three-vessel or left main coronary artery disease. Although EIH appears to be reversed by revascularization procedures, confirmation of whether these procedures have a beneficial effect on survival requires a randomized trial.

Key Points: (1) The definition of EIH is of crucial importance in the evaluation of the exercise test response. A drop in systolic blood pressure below preexercise standing values is the most ominous criterion, whereas a drop of 20 mm Hg or more without a fall below preexercise values has little if any predictive value. (2) EIH can result from left ventricular dysfunction (as reflected by myocardial infarction status) or ischemia. In patients in which EIH occurs without association with either of these two factors, EIH appears to be benign.

Exercise and Recovery Systolic Blood Pressure Ratio

Amon, Richards, and Crawford[35] have reported that the normal decline in systolic blood pressure during the recovery phase of treadmill exercise does not occur in some patients with coronary artery disease, whereas in others, recovery systolic blood pressure values exceed the peak exercise values.

Normal Heart Rate and Blood Pressure Values

The early emphasis placed on the exercise ECG tended to deemphasize other exercise responses. Measurements of these responses may improve the diagnostic value of exercise testing and may be useful for identifying the presence or the severity of coronary artery disease. The value of any measurement in providing diagnostic information from exercise testing depends on the accuracy and completeness with which a measurement has been made in healthy individuals (reference values) and the effectiveness with which certain limits of the measurement (discriminant values) separate healthy individuals from those subgroups with disease. The complete set of reference values in Fig 2-10 should help determine discriminant values for separating patient groups. Many exercise test responses do not have a Gaussian distribution and require that nonparametric statistical tests be used. Therefore discriminant values should be determined as percentiles rather than as standard deviations or confidence limits.

Using Hemodynamic Measurements to Estimate Myocardial Oxygen Consumption

Although heart rate and stroke volume are important determinants of maximum oxygen uptake and myocardial oxygen consumption, myocardial oxygen con-

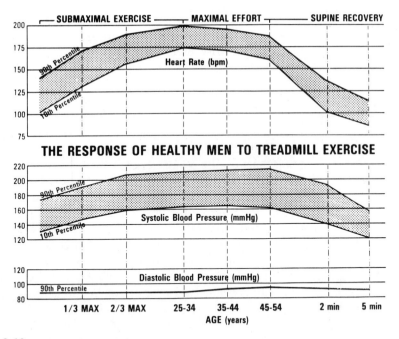

THE RESPONSE OF HEALTHY MEN TO TREADMILL EXERCISE

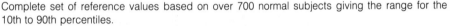

FIG 2-10.
Complete set of reference values based on over 700 normal subjects giving the range for the 10th to 90th percentiles.

sumption has other independent determinants. The relative metabolic loads of the entire body and the heart are determined separately and may not change in parallel with a given intervention. Although the heart receives only 4% of cardiac output at rest, it uses 10% of systemic oxygen uptake. The wide arteriovenous oxygen difference of 10% to 12 vol% at rest reflects the fact that oxygen in the blood passing through the coronary circulation is nearly maximally extracted. This value can be compared with the 4 vol% difference across the systemic circulation. When the myocardium requires a greater oxygen supply, coronary blood flow must be increased by coronary dilation. During exercise, coronary blood flow can increase through normal coronary arteries up to 5 times the normal resting flow.

The increased demand for myocardial oxygen consumption required for dynamic exercise is the key to the use of exercise testing as a diagnostic tool for coronary artery disease. Myocardial oxygen consumption cannot be directly measured in a practical manner, but its relative demand can be estimated from its determinants, such as heart rate, wall tension (left ventricular pressure and diastolic volume), contractility, and cardiac work. Although all of these factors increase during exercise, increased heart rate is especially detrimental in patients who have obstructive coronary disease. Increases in heart rate result in a shortening of the diastolic filling period, the time during which coronary blood flow is the greatest. In normal coronary arteries, dilation occurs. In obstructed vessels, however, dilation is limited and flow is decreased by the shortening of the diastolic filling period. This situation results in inadequate blood flow and inadequate oxygen delivery. However, changes in this threshold have been suggested to be caused by coronary artery spasm.[36]

SUMMARY

Because it can objectively demonstrate exercise capacity, exercise testing rather than functional classification is used for disability evaluation. No questionnaire or submaximal test or nonexercise stress test can give the same results as a symptom-limited exercise test. Age-predicted HRmax targets are relatively useless for clinical purposes, and it is surprising how much steeper the age-related decline in HRmax is in referred populations as compared with age-matched normal or volunteer populations. A consistent finding in studies of these populations has been a relatively poor correlation between HRmax and age. Correlation coefficients of -0.4 are usually found, with a standard error of the estimate from 10 to 25 beats per minute. In general, this correlation has not been tightened by considering activity status, weight, cardiac size, maximum respiratory quotient, or perceived exertion. Exertional hypotension, best defined as a drop in systolic blood pressure below standing rest, is very predictive of severe angiographic coronary artery disease and a poor prognosis. A failure of systolic blood pressure to rise is particularly worrisome after a myocardial infarction. Until automated devices are adequately validated, we strongly recommend that blood pressure be taken manually with a cuff and stethoscope.

The nomogram developed by Morris et al[12] greatly facilitates the description of exercise capacity relative to age and enables comparison among patients. Reporting exercise capacity as a percentage with 100% as normal for age has much to recommend it. Determining a patient's exercise capacity relative to age group peers is a useful means of assessing a patient's cardiovascular status. In addition, patients themselves seem to have a better understanding of this measurement. Thus it seems clear that using METs in interpreting the exercise test can improve communication among physicians and that calculating exercise capacity as a percentage of the norm relative to age group can do the same for dialogue between physicians and their patients.

REFERENCES

1. Myers J, Froelicher VF: Hemodynamic determinants of exercise capacity in chronic heart failure, *Ann Intern Med* 115:377-386, 1991.
2. McKirnan MD et al: Treadmill performance and cardiac function in selected patients with coronary heart disease, *J Am Coll Cardiol* 3:253-261, 1984.
3. Hammond HK, Kelly TL, Froelicher VF: Noninvasive testing in the evaluation of myocardial ischemia: agreement among tests, *J Am Coll Cardiol* 5:59-69, 1985.
4. Froelicher VF et al: Prediction of maximal oxygen consumption: comparison of the Bruce and Balke treadmill protocols, *Chest* 68:331-336, 1975.

5. McKirnan D et al: Treadmill performance and cardial function in selected patients with coronary heart disease, *J Am Coll Cardiol* 3:253-261, 1984.

6. Ehsani AA et al: The effects of left ventricular systolic function on maximal aerobic exercise capacity in asymptomatic patients with coronary artery disease, *Circulation* 70:552-560, 1984.

7. Weber KT et al: Oxygen utilization and ventilation during exercise in patients with chronic cardiac failure, *Circulation* 65:1213-1222, 1982.

8. Litchfield RL et al: Normal exercise capacity in patients with severe left ventricular dysfunction: compensatory mechanisms, *Circulation* 66:129-134, 1982.

9. Higginbotham MB et al: Determinants of variable exercise performance among patients with severe left ventricular dysfunction, *Am J Cardiol* 51:52-60, 1983.

10. Myers J, Froelicher VF: Hemodynamic determinants of exercise capacity in chronic heart failure, *Ann Intern Med* 115:377-386, 1991.

11. Bruce RA, Kusumi F, Hosmer D: Maximal oxygen intake and nomographic assessment of functional aerobic impairment in cardiovascular disease, *Am Heart J* 85:546-562, 1973.

12. Morris C et al: Nomogram for exercise capacity using METs and age, *J Am Coll Cardiol* 22:175-182, 1993.

13. Morris CK et al: The prognostic value of exercise capacity: a review of the literature, *Am Heart J* 122:1423-1430, 1991.

14. Froelicher VF, Allen M, Lancaster MC: Maximal treadmill testing of normal USAF aircrewmen, *Aerospace Med* 45:310-315, 1974.

15. Dehn MM, Bruce RA: Longitudinal variations in maximal oxygen intake with age and activity, *J Appl Physiol* 33:805-807, 1972.

16. Hammond K, Froelicher VF: Normal and abnormal heart rate responses to exercise, *Progress Cardiovasc Dis* 27:271-296, 1985.

17. Sheffield LT et al: Maximal heart rate and treadmill performance of healthy women in relation to age, *Circulation* 57:79-84, 1978.

18. Londeree BR, Moeschberger ML: Influence of age and other factors on maximal heart rate, *J Cardiac Rehab* 4:44-49, 1984.

19. Froelicher VF et al: A comparison of three maximal treadmill exercise protocols, *J Appl Physiol* 36:720-725, 1974.

20. Graettinger W et al: Influence of LV chamber size on maximal heart rate, *Circulation* 84:187-192, 1991.

21. Convertino V et al: Cardiovascular responses to exercise in middle-aged men after 10 days of bedrest, *Circulation* 65:134-140, 1982.

22. Ellestad MH, Wan MKC: Predictive implications of stress testing: follow-up of 2700 subjects after maximal treadmill stress testing, *Circulation* 51:363-369, 1975.

23. McNeer JF et al: The role of the exercise test in the evaluation of patients for ischemic heart disease, *Circulation* 57:64-70, 1978.

24. Bruce RA et al: Separation of effects of cardiovascular disease and age on ventricular function with maximal exercise, *Am J Cardiol* 34:757-763, 1974.

25. Hammond HK, Kelly TL, Froelicher V: Radionuclide imaging correlatives of heart rate impairment during maximal exercise testing, *J Am Coll Cardiol* 2(5):826-833, 1983.

26. Morris SN et al: Incidence of significance of decreases in systolic blood pressure during graded treadmill exercise testing, *Am J Cardiol* 41:221-226, 1978.

27. Thomson PD, Kelemen MH: Hypotension accompanying the onset of exertional angina, *Circulation* 52:28-32, 1975.

28. Li W, Riggins R, Anderson R: Reversal of exertional hypotension after coronary bypass grafting, *Am J Cardiol* 44:607-611, 1979.

29. Wolthuis RA et al: The response of healthy men to treadmill exercise, *Circulation* 55:153-157, 1977.
30. Saltin B, Sternberg J: Circulatory response to prolonged severe exercise, *J Appl Physiol* 19:833-838, 1964.
31. Atwood JE et al: Exercise and the heart: exercise testing in patients with aortic stenosis, *Chest* 93:1083-1087, 1988.
32. Rich MW et al: Exercise-induced hypotension as a manifestation of right ventricular ischemia, *Am Heart J* 115:184-186, 1988.
33. Weiner DA et al: Decrease in systolic blood pressure during exercise testing: reproducibility, response to coronary bypass surgery and prognostic significance, *Am J Cardiol* 49:1627-1631, 1982.
34. Irving JB, Bruce RA: Exertional hypotension and postexertional ventricular fibrillation in stress testing, *Am J Cardiol* 39(6):849-851, 1977.
35. Amon KW, Richards KL, Crawford MH: Usefulness of the postexercise response of systolic blood pressure in the diagnosis of coronary artery disease, *Circulation* 70:951-956, 1984.
36. Waters DD, et al: Clinical and angiographic correlates of exercise-induced ST-segment elevation: increased detection with multiple ECG leads, *Circulation* 61:286, 1980.

CHAPTER 3

Interpretation of ECG Responses

ELECTROCARDIOGRAPHIC RESPONSE TO EXERCISE[1-4]

In this chapter, the response of the electrocardiogram (ECG) to exercise will be presented in the order that the components of the waveform present during exercise testing. These responses will be described using the results from the USAF-SAM Normal Exercise ECG Study. Computer techniques derived data from 40 low-risk normal subjects to provide measurements of amplitude, interval, and slope relative to treadmill time.[5] Fig 3-1 shows the waveforms produced using median values of the measurements of all 40 subjects for leads V_5, aV_F, and V_2. These figures demonstrate the specific waveform alterations that occur in response to supine rest, treadmill exercise at a heart rate of 120, maximal treadmill exercise, 1-minute recovery, and 5-minute recovery.

P Wave

The P wave usually has only minor changes during exercise, and the appearance of P-pulmonale or P-mitrale is rare and of questionable significance. However, atrial repolarization affects ST segments in the inferior leads (II, aV_F, and III) and is particularily noticeable when the PR interval is short.[6] The possibility that exaggerated atrial repolarization waves during exercise could produce ST-segment depression mimicking myocardial ischemia was studied by Sapin et al.[7] The P waves, PR segments, and ST segments were studied in leads II, III, aV_F, and V_4 to V_6 in 69 patients whose exercise ECGs suggested ischemia. All had normal ECGs at rest. The exercise test produce false positives in 25 patients. A total of 44 patients with a similar age and gender distribution, anginal chest pain, and at least one coronary stenosis served as a true positive control group. The false-positive group was characterized by markedly downsloping PR segments at peak exercise, longer exercise time and more rapid peak exercise heart rate than those of the true positive group, and absence of exercise-induced chest pain. The false-positive group also displayed significantly greater absolute P-wave amplitudes at peak exercise and greater augmentation of P-wave amplitude by exercise in all six ECG leads than were observed in the true positive group. Multivariate analysis revealed that

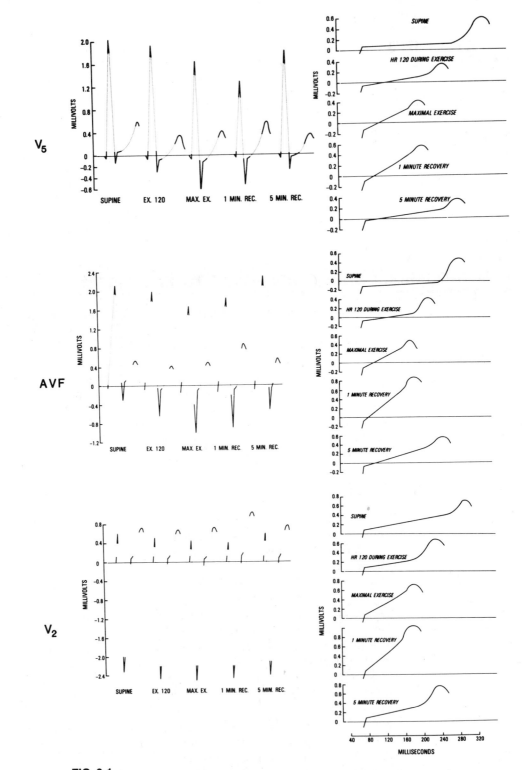

FIG 3-1.
Averaged waveforms produced using the median values of the measurements of 40 low-risk normal subjects.

exercise duration and downsloping PR segments in the inferior ECG leads were independent predictors of a false-positive test.

Q-Wave, R-Wave, and S-Wave Amplitudes

In leads V_5 and Y (II and aV_F), the Q wave shows very small changes from the resting values; however, it does become slightly more negative at maximal exercise. Measurable Q-wave changes were not noted in V_2.

Changes in median R-wave amplitude are not detected until near-maximal and maximal effort are approached. At maximal exercise and into 1-minute recovery, a sharp decrease in R-wave amplitude is observed in V_5. These changes are not seen in V_2. The lowest median R-wave values in II and aV_F occurred at maximal exercise, with R-wave amplitude increasing by the 1-minute recovery period. In V_5 the lowest R-wave amplitude was seen during 1-minute recovery. This quite different temporal response in the R waves in the lateral versus inferior leads is unexplained.

There is little change in S-wave amplitude in V_2. In the other leads, however, the S wave became greater in depth, or more negative, showing a greater deflection at maximal exercise, and then gradually returning to resting values in recovery. A decrease in the QS interval occurred, becoming shortest at maximal exercise. After 3 minutes of recovery, the QS interval returned to normal. A steadily decreasing RT-interval duration was observed as exercise increased. The shortest interval was seen at maximal exercise and during 1-minute recovery. Changes in this interval followed changes in heart rate.

As the R wave decreases in amplitude, the S wave increases in depth. The QS duration shortens minimally, but the RT duration decreases in a larger amount. QRS duration tends to decrease in normal subjects with exercise and increasing heart rates and to increase in patients with angina or left ventricular (LV) dysfunction.[15,16] There is too much overlap in QRS-duration responses to permit discrimination between them.

R-Wave Changes[8-10]

Mechanism of R-Wave Amplitude Changes

The cause of R-wave amplitude changes is debated. Brody's demonstration of a direct relationship between left ventricular volume and R-wave amplitude resulted in this being called the *Brody effect*.[11] However, there is other evidence against this concept.[12,13] The Brody hypothesis is contradicted by the fact that cardiac enlargement secondary to congestive heart failure may cause a decrease in R-wave amplitude. Further, if R-wave amplitude changes were strictly the result of changes in volume, R-wave amplitude would be expected to increase when a patient changes from a standing to supine position, since diastolic volume would increase. However, this change in R-wave amplitude does not necessarily occur. Axis shifts have also been implicated as the cause of changes in R-wave amplitude. However, the shift of the QRS- and ST-segment vectors toward the right and posteriorly is a normal response to exercise.

Study of Exercise-Induced R-Wave Changes Performed at the University of California at San Diego

Computer analysis of exercise ECGs has offered an opportunity to relate R-wave changes with ischemic ST-segment shifts.[14] In the University of California at San Diego (UCSD) study of exercise-induced R-wave changes, the ECG changes were recorded in three dimensions, enabling optimal representation of global myocardial electrical forces. Patients were separated into groups achieving maximum heart rates both higher and lower than the mean maximum heart rate of 161 beats per minute. Data on asymptomatic normal subjects showed that the R-wave amplitude typically increases from rest to submaximal exercise, perhaps to a heart rate of 140 beats per minute, then decreases to the maximal exercise endpoint (Fig 3-2). Therefore if a patient were limited by exercise intolerance, whether because of objective or subjective symptoms or signs, the R-wave amplitude would increase from rest to such an endpoint. Such patients may be demonstrating a normal R-wave response but be classified as *abnormal,* since the severity of disease causes a lower exercise tolerance and heart rate. Exercise-induced changes in R-wave amplitude have no independent predictive power but are associated with coronary artery disease (CAD) because such patients are often submaximally tested and an R-wave decrease normally occurs at maximal exercise.

Percentage of R-Wave Changes

Fig 3-2 illustrates the percentage change of R-wave amplitude for each individual compared with the R wave at supine rest in V_5 and Y (II and aV_F). At lower exercise heart rates, the great variability of R-wave response was apparent, and many normal individuals had significant increases in R-wave amplitude. Although most showed a decline at maximal exercise, some normal subjects had an increase, whereas others showed very little decrease. During 1-minute recovery there was a greater tendency toward a decline in lead V_5 but not inferiorly. Further into recovery, R-wave amplitude remained decreased in lead V_5 but increased inferiorly.

Key Point: A multitude of factors affect the R-wave amplitude response to exercise; the response does not have diagnostic significance.

ST-Slope, J-Junction Depression, and T-Wave Amplitude

Depression of the J junction and the tall-peaked T waves at maximal exercise and during 1-minute recovery can be an early sign of ischemia, but they are seen in normal subjects. Along with the J-junction depression, marked ST-segment up-sloping is seen. J-junction depression did not occur in V_2. The amplitude of the J junction in V_2 was changed very little through exercise but elevated slightly in recovery. It appears that the lead system affects the anterior-posterior presentation of the ST-segment vector more than anticipated. The J junction shifts either anteriorly or posteriorly in normal patients. The J junction was depressed in all other

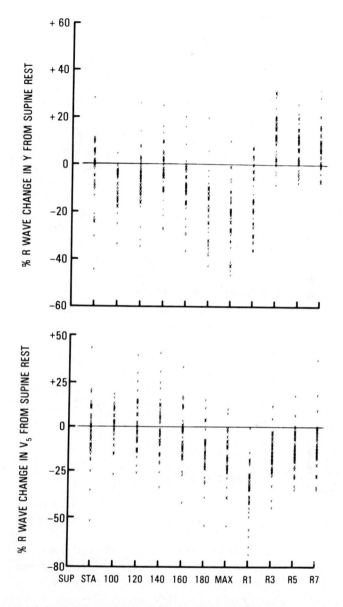

FIG 3-2.
R-wave changes relative to heart rate during progressive treadmill exercise in a group of low-risk normal subjects. This figure illustrates the percent change of R-wave amplitude for each individual compared with the R wave at supine rest in V_5 and Y.

leads to a maximum depression at maximal exercise; then in recovery it gradually returned toward but not to preexercise values. There was very little difference between the three left precordial leads. A dramatic increase in ST-segment slope was observed in all leads and was greatest during 1-minute recovery. These changes returned toward pretest values during later recovery.

J-Junction Depression

Mirvis, Ramanathan, and Wilson[17] studied junctional depression during exercise using left precordial isopotential mapping. During exercise, junctional depression was maximum along the left lower sternal border. In the early portion of the ST segment, they found a minimum isopotential along the lower left sternal border that was continuous with terminal QRS forces in intensity and location. The late portion of the ST segment had a minimum isopotential located in the same area as that observed at rest (i.e., the upper left sternal border). These observations suggested that junctional depression was the result of competition between normal repolarization and delayed terminal depolarization forces. Junctional depression is the result of negative potentials over the left lower sternal border during early repolarization. These negative potentials responsible for physiological junctional depression could be caused by delayed activation of basal areas of the left and right ventricles, which leads to accentuated depolarization-repolarization overlap.

ABNORMAL ST-SEGMENT CHANGES

Epicardial electrode mapping usually records ST-segment elevation over areas of severe ischemia and ST-segment depression over areas of lesser ischemia. ST-segment depression viewed from an electrode overlying normal epicardium is the reciprocal of the injury effect occurring in the endocardium. ST-segment elevation seen from the same electrode indicates transmural injury or, less frequently, epicardial injury. On the surface ECG, exercise-induced myocardial ischemia can result in one of three ST-segment manifestations: elevation, normalization, or depression.

ST-Segment Elevation

Variant angina with its associated ST-segment elevation was first described by Prinzmetal et al[18] in 1959 as being secondary to coronary artery spasm. Although cardiac catheterization showed that many of these patients had normal coronary arteries, subsequent studies showed that approximately half had significant fixed lesions as well.[19-21] Patients with variant angina can also have typical ST-segment depression during exercise testing.[22] Weiner et al[23] have reported on four patients with Prinzmetal angina who only developed ST-segment depression in recovery after treadmill tests.

Prevalence of Exercise-Induced ST-Segment Elevation

The most common ECG abnormality seen in the exercise laboratory is ST-segment depression, whereas ST-segment elevation is relatively rare. Table 3-1 summarizes studies of exercise-induced ST elevation. Its prevalence depends on the population tested, but it occurs more frequently in patients who have had Q-wave myocardial infarctions (MIs).[24-36]

TABLE 3-1.

Studies of Exercise-Induced ST-Segment Elevation During Standard Clinical Testing

Study	Size of Population Tested	Type of Population	Percent of Population With Prior MI	Number of Leads Measured for Elevation	Criteria for Elevation	Prevalence of Abnormal Elevation (%)	Percentage of Prior MI in Patients With Elevation
Bruce (1988)	3050	Angina	47	11	1 mm	4	83
Bruce (1974)	1136	CHD	47	CB_5	>0 mV	5	57
Sriwattanakomen (1980)	1620	All referred	—	11	1 mm	4	47
Longhurst (1979)	6040	All referred	—	12 + XYZ	0.5 mm	8	79
Chahine (1976)	840	VAMC	—	V_5, V_6	1 mm	4	86
Dunn (1981)	190	No anterior Q waves	0	aV_L and V_1	—	24	
Stiles (1980)	650	541 patients with ST depression versus 109 with ST elevation	10	11	1 mm	4	61
Waters (1980)	720	Mixed	1	12 ± CM_5	—	7	76

MI, Myocardial infarction; *CHD,* coronary heart disease; *VAMC,* Veterans Affairs Medical Center.
From Nosratian FJ, Froelicher VF: *Am J Cardiol* 63:986-987, 1989.

Methods of Measuring ST-Segment Elevation

ST-segment depression is measured from the isoelectric baseline; however, when ST-segment depression is present at rest, the amount of additional depression is measured. ST-segment elevation is always considered from the baseline ST level. Whether the elevation occurs over or adjacent to Q waves or in non–Q-wave areas is important. Unfortunately, many studies do not provide the methods of measurement or the conditions of the underlying ECG. The box lists some of the factors that should be considered when assessing studies of ST-segment elevation. Multiple causes for ST-segment elevation during treadmill testing have been suggested. These include LV aneurysm, variant angina, severe ischemic heart disease, and LV wall motion abnormalities. LV aneurysm after myocardial infarction is the

---

SOME FACTORS THAT SHOULD BE CONSIDERED WHEN ST-SEGMENT ELEVATION STUDIES ARE ASSESSED

Population tested (prevalence of MI patients, patients with varient angina or spasm)
Baseline (resting) ECG
ECG leads monitored
Leads in which elevation occurs relative to Q waves
Criteria for elevation
Methods of ST-shift detection (visual or computerized)
Accompanying ST-segment depression (reciprocal or not)

most frequent cause of ST-segment elevation on the resting ECG and occurs over Q waves or in ECG leads adjacent to Q waves. Early repolarization is a normal resting pattern of ST-segment elevation that occurs in normal individuals who do not have diagnostic Q waves. The ST level with early repolarization normally sinks to the isoelectric line with an increase in heart rate.

Key Point: Early repolarization is a term for ST-segment elevation seen in the normal resting ECG. An increase in heart rate causes it to drop to the isoelectric line. Only when the ST segment is depressed below the isoelectric line is ischemia the likely cause.

Ischemia or Wall Motion Abnormality?

There is controversy regarding whether ischemia or wall motion abnormality is the major cause of ST-segment elevation.[37-45] Studies of the issue are summarized in Table 3-1. In patients with ST-segment elevation during exercise when no abnormal Q wave is seen on the baseline ECG, there is a very high likelihood of a significant proximal narrowing in the coronary artery supplying the area where it occurs. It is also likely to be associated with serious dysrythmias. When elevation occurs in an ECG with abnormal Q waves, it is usually due to a wall motion abnormality, and the elevation can conceal ST-segment depression related to ischemia. Fig 3-3 is an example of ST-segment elevation in a normal baseline ECG (patient had a tight left anterior descending artery lesion that responded to percutaneous transluminal coronary angioplasty), and Fig 3-4 illustrates such a patient with normal angiographic findings (whose condition responded nicely to calcium channel blockers). Fig 3-5 shows the typical ST-segment elevation over Q waves that occurs after an MI. This patient is unusual in that the elevation occurs in multiple areas.

Key Point: ST-segment elevation normally occurs over diagnostic Q waves. Any ST-segment elevation on a normal ECG (other than in aV_R or V_1) indicates transmural ischemia, is very arrythmogenic, and localizes the ischemia.

ST-Segment Normalization, or Absence of Change

Another manifestation of ischemia can be the normalization, or absence of change, of the ST segment because of cancellation effects. ECG abnormalities at rest, including T-wave inversion and ST-segment depression, return to normal during attacks of angina and during exercise in some patients with ischemic heart disease. This cancellation effect is a rare occurrence, but it should be considered. The ST segment and T wave represent the uncancelled portion of ventricular repolarization. Because ventricular geometry can be roughly approximated as a hollow ellipsoid open at one end, the widespread cancellation of the relatively slow-dispersing electrical forces during repolarization is understandable. Patients with

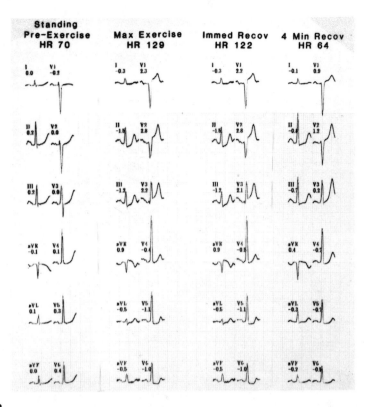

FIG 3-3.
Example of ST-segment elevation caused by a fixed lesion in a patient with a normal resting ECG.

severe CAD would be most likely to have cancellation occur, although they have the highest prevalence of abnormal tests. Manvi and Ellestad[27] reported that 20% of their patients with dyskinesia and CAD had normal tests, and Chahine, Raizner, and Ishimori[26] reported that in about 25% of their patients with dyskinesia and CAD, ST segments were normalized or minimally elevated during exercise. Nobel et al[46] reported normalization of inverted T waves and depressed ST segments in 11 patients during exercise-induced angina. Exercise testing failing to produce ST-segment depression or elevation in a patient with known CAD could be caused by two or more severely ischemic myocardial segments cancelling ST-segment vectors. Sweet and Sheffield[47] reported on a patient with minor ST-segment depression and T-wave inversion in lead V_5 whose ECG normalized, or "improved," during treadmill testing; he had an acute infarction 10 minutes after the test. This normalization of ST-segment depression should thus be considered ST-segment elevation.

Lavie et al[48] from the Mayo Clinic studied 84 consecutive patients with resting T-wave inversion. Radionuclide angiography revealed significant new wall-motion abnormalities in 13 of 47 patients (28%) with persistent T-wave inversion and in

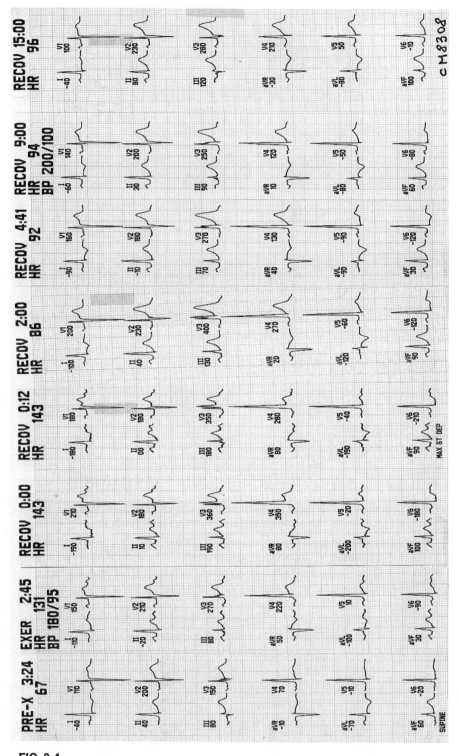

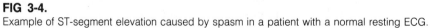

FIG 3-4.
Example of ST-segment elevation caused by spasm in a patient with a normal resting ECG.

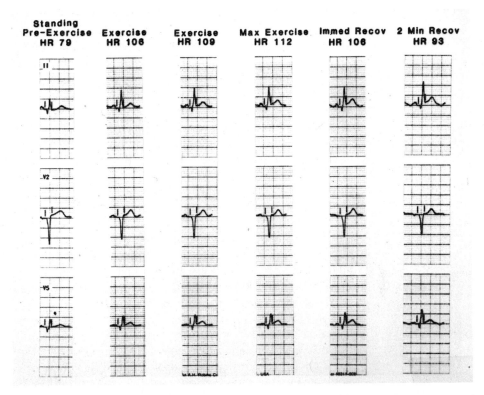

FIG 3-5.
Example of ST-segment elevation in a patient with an ECG exhibiting Q waves.

23 of 37 patients (62%) with T-wave pseudonormalization during exercise. The response of the ejection fraction to exercise was better in patients with persistent T-wave inversion than in those with pseudonormalization. Mechanical evidence of ischemia was seen in 14 of the 23 patients (61%) with T-wave pseudonormalization but without ST-segment depression. In patients with resting T-wave inversions, pseudonormalization was slightly more sensitive but less specific than a positive exercise test for predicting significant new wall-motion abnormalities or decreases in the ejection fraction with exercise. Pseudonormalization is not extremely useful alone, and in fact we only identify it when chest pain consistent with angina occurs as well.

The prevalence of normalization in which surface ST-segment changes are cancelled by multiple ischemic ST-segment vectors is not known. The patient's inability to give an adequate effort is a more likely explanation for the majority of false-negative exercise tests in patients with multivessel CAD. In patients with single-vessel disease, the decreased sensitivity of exercise testing is most likely due to insufficient myocardial ischemia to cause surface ECG changes.

ST-Segment Depression

The most common manifestation of exercise-induced myocardial ischemia is ST-segment depression. The standard criterion for this type of abnormal response is either horizontal or downward sloping ST-segment depression of 0.1 mV or more for 60 msec. The response appears to be a result of generalized subendocardial ischemia. A "steal" phenomena is likely from ischemic areas because of the effect of extensive collateralization in the subendocardium. ST-segment depression does not localize the area of ischemia to help indicate which coronary artery is occluded. The normal ST-segment vector response to tachycardia and to exercise is a shift rightward and upward. The degree of this shift appears to vary a fair amount biologically. Most normal individuals have early repolarization at rest, which shifts with exercise to the isoelectric PR-segment line in the inferior, lateral, and anterior leads with exercise. This shift can be further influenced by ischemia and myocardial scars. When the later portions of the ST segment are affected, flattening, or downward depression, can be recorded. Local effects and the direction of the spatial changes during repolarization cause the ST segment to have a different appearance at the many surface sites that can be monitored. The more leads with these apparent ischemic shifts, the more severe the disease.

The probability and severity of CAD are directly related to the amount of J-junction depression and are inversely related to the slope of the ST segment. Downsloping ST-segment depression is more serious than horizontal depression, and both are more serious than upsloping depression. However, patients with upsloping ST-segment depression, especially when the slope is less than 1 mV/sec, probably are at increased risk. If a slowly ascending slope is used as a criterion for abnormality, then the specificity of exercise testing will be decreased (more false positives will result), although the test will become more sensitive. One electrode can show upsloping ST-segment depression, whereas an adjacent electrode shows horizontal or downsloping depression. If an apparently borderline ST segment with an inadequate slope is recorded in a single precordial lead in a patient highly suspected of having CAD, multiple precordial leads should be scanned before the exercise test is called *normal.* An upsloping depressed ST segment may be the precursor of an abnormal ST-segment depression in the recovery period or at higher heart rates during greater workloads. It is preferable to call a test with an inadequate ST-segment slope but with ST-segment depression a *borderline response,* and added emphasis should be placed on other clinical and exercise parameters. Examples of the various criteria for ischemic ST depression are shown in Fig 3-6.

Key Point: The probability for ischemia and the likelihood of its severity are directly related to the amount of abnormal ST-segment depression and inversely related to the slope. (That is, downsloping ST-segment depression is the most and · upsloping is the least serious.)

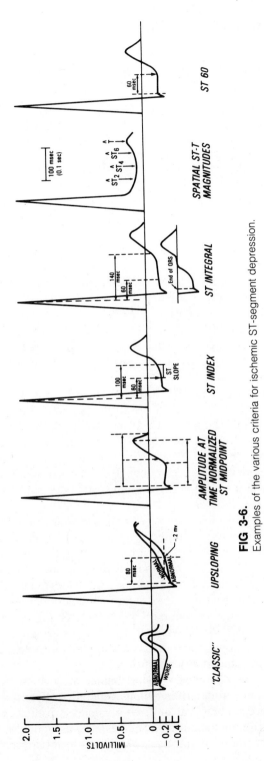

FIG 3-6.
Examples of the various criteria for ischemic ST-segment depression.

ST-Segment Depression in Recovery

Because of technical limitations, the first diagnostic use of the exercise ECG involved observations made only after exercise. After ECG techniques that made accurate ECG recording possible during activity were developed, the emphasis in testing shifted to changes occurring during the exercise period itself. The diagnostic accuracy of ST-segment changes limited to the period after exercise has been controversial. It has been proposed that such changes are more likely to represent false-positive responses[49] or to result from coronary artery spasm.[50] To facilitate imaging as soon as possible during recovery, studies[51] comparing nuclear procedures with the exercise ECG often do not even include an ECG evaluation done after exercise. Most exercise test scores only consider ST-segment changes occurring during exercise and exclude changes occurring during recovery alone. Although a cooldown walk is known to obscure ST shifts during recovery,[52] it has been recommended for safety reasons.

To study this issue, Lachterman et al[53] divided abnormal responders into exclusive groups: *exercise only, recovery only,* and *abnormal in both exercise and recovery.* In addition, there was a designation of *all abnormal* for all of the above or those abnormal at any time. *Abnormal in exercise* designated those that were abnormal during exercise (i.e., *exercise only* plus *abnormal in both exercise and recovery*), as if the ECG was monitored only during exercise, and *abnormal in recovery* designated those that were abnormal in recovery (i.e., *recovery only* plus *abnormal in both exercise and recovery*), as if the ECG was monitored only during recovery.

Of the 271 patients, 107 had no coronary lesion with a 75% or greater narrowing, 119 had single- or dual-vessel disease, and 45 had either left main or triple-vessel disease. The mean age of the total population was 59 years. Table 3-2 describes the observed patterns of ST-segment responses. Of the 271 patients, 138 (51%) had abnormal ST-segment responses; 20 (7%) had abnormal ST-segment responses during recovery only, 16 (6%) had abnormal ST-segment responses during exercise only, and 102 (38%) had abnormal ST-segment responses during exercise and recovery.

As shown in Table 3-2, there are few meaningful differences among the clinical features associated with the five patterns of ST-segment depression. Those with a normal response were the youngest. As expected, angina during the test was significantly more common in those with ST-segment depression than in those without, but over half of the patients with ST-segment depression exhibited silent ischemia. Differences in maximum ST-segment depression during and after exercise were consistent with the criteria for each group. In the recovery-only group, the mean value for ST-segment depression during exercise was 1.3 mm, but the slopes were upward in those with 1 mm or more depression, and none were abnormal by standard criteria during exercise.

There was a tendency toward higher mean hemodynamic parameters in the exercise-only group. These values generally reflected a greater exercise capacity and were even higher than those obtained in patients with a normal exercise response. The number of diseased vessels was significantly lower for those with a normal response and for those abnormal during exercise only. The recovery-only

TABLE 3-2.

Clinical and Exercise Variables in the Long Beach VAMC Study of the Performance of Temporal Patterns of ST-Segment Depression for Predicting Angiographic CAD

		Abnormal Responses					
	Normal Responses (133 Patients)	Exercise or Recovery (138 Patients)	Exercise Without Recovery (118 Patients)	Recovery Without Exercise (122 Patients)	Exercise and Recovery (102 Patients)	Exercise Only (16 Patients)	Recovery Only (20 Patients)
Age (years)	58 ± 9	61 ± 8	61 ± 8	61 ± 7	61 ± 7	62 ± 9	62 ± 7
Drugs used (%)							
Beta-blocker	19	23	22	24	23	19	30
Digoxin	14	10	12	10	12	13	0
Chest pain at presentation (%)							
Typical	42	61	63	62	63	56	50
Atypical	35	26	23	25	22	31	45
None or noncardiac	23	13	14	13	15	13	5
Chest pain during exercise (%)	21	53	53	52	53	56	50 ($p < 0.01$)
ST-segment depression (mm)							
Exercise	0.3 ± 0.7	2.1 ± 1.0	2.3 ± 0.9	2.2 ± 1.0	2.4 ± 1.0	1.7 ± 0.6	1.3 ± 0.8
Recovery	0.3 ± 0.6	1.9 ± 1.0	2.0 ± 1.0	2.1 ± 0.9	2.2 ± 0.9	0.7 ± 0.6	1.6 ± 0.6
Hemodynamic values							
METs	7 ± 3	7 ± 3	7 ± 3	7 ± 3	7 ± 3	8 ± 3	7 ± 3
Maximum heart rate (beats/min)	129 ± 24	129 ± 19	128 ± 18	129 ± 18	128 ± 17	132 ± 22	135 ± 22
Maximum systolic blood pressure (mm Hg)	171 ± 30	167 ± 28	166 ± 28	167 ± 28	165 ± 28	167 ± 30	173 ± 27
Maximum double product ($\times 10^3$)	22 ± 6	22 ± 5	21 ± 5	22 ± 5	21 ± 5	22 ± 6	24 ± 6
Cardiac catheterization values							
Vessels with ≥75% stenosis	1.5	1.7	1.7	1.8	1.8	1.0	1.5 ($p < 0.001$)
Ejection fraction (%)	67	66	66	65	65	72	67

patients had the highest maximum heart rate, systolic pressure, and double product despite the lowest exercise capacity. These findings support the conclusion that recovery-only changes are not associated with submaximal effort but are associated with exercise intolerance related to other factors such as poor physical conditioning.

Table 3-3 lists the performance of several temporal patterns of ST-segment depression for predicting coronary disease. As would be expected, the sensitivities become low for patterns that do not occur frequently. For comparison among patterns, the predictive value is the most important aspect to consider because it is the percent of all patients with the pattern who have coronary disease. All of the patterns have comparable predictive values, demonstrating that none is more likely to be associated with false-positive responses. The exercise-only group had a higher predictive value for any disease and a lower predictive value for left main or triple-vessel disease, which was consistent with the smaller mean vessel

TABLE 3-3.

Sensitivity, Specificity, and Positive Predictive Value for Temporal Patterns of Exercise-Induced ST-Segment Depression in Patients with CAD or Three-Vessel and Left Main Coronary Artery Disease[53]

Abnormal Responses	Any Significant Coronary Disease			Three-Vessel or Left Main Artery Disease		
	Sensitivity	Specificity	Predictive Value*	Sensitivity	Specificity	Predictive Value*
Exercise or recovery (138 patients)	67	74	80 (73-86)	80	55	26 (19-33)
Exercise without recovery considered (118 patients)	57	77	79 (71-86)	73	62	28 (20-36)
Recovery without exercise considered (122 patients)	61	79	82 (75-89)	73	61	27 (19-35)
Exercise and recovery (102 patients)	51	82	81 (74-89)	67	68	29 (21-38)
Exercise only (16 patients)	6	94	63 (35-85)	6	94	19 (4-46)
Recovery only (20 patients)	10	97	85 (62-97)	6	94	15 (3-38)

*95% confidence interval.

score and higher hemodynamic parameters found in this group. The all-abnormal group was significantly more sensitive than the abnormal-in-exercise group and retained its predictive value.

Other Studies Evaluating Recovery-Only ST-Segment Depression

The Program of Surgical Control of Hyperlipidemia (POSCH) data were used for one analysis of recovery-only changes, since baseline evaluation included treadmill exercise testing and coronary angiography. Karnegis et al[54] investigated hemodynamic, angiographic, and ECG variables in subjects whose diagnostic ECG changes appeared during exercise rather than during recovery. They concluded that the same clinical significance should be attributed to abnormal ST-segment responses that occur during recovery and that ECG, hemodynamic, and cardiac catheterization variables do not distinguish among subjects who exhibit these two different temporal responses.

Savage et al[55] evaluated 2000 exercise tests and identified 62 patients (3.2%) who developed 1 mm or more of either horizontal or downsloping ST-segment depression in the recovery period despite a normal ST-segment response during exercise. They concluded that isolated postexercise ST-segment depression was usually associated with CAD, that it often indicated multivessel disease, and that men were more likely to have abnormal thallium scans.

Froelicher et al[56] considered patterns of ST-segment depression in two groups of asymptomatic men undergoing screening exercise testing; one group consisted of men who underwent coronary angiography and the other of men who were followed for 5 years for cardiac events. ST-segment interpretation was the same as in the study by Lachterman et al.[53] As is shown in Table 3-4, recovery-only ST-segment depression had a similar predictive value as other patterns.

Ellestad[57] commented on patients who do not have ST-segment depression with or immediately after exercise but who develop changes 3 to 8 minutes later. In a follow-up of 308 subjects, he found this response to be a definite but weak predictor of subsequent coronary events. He contrasts this group to a normal group who has ST-segment depression at rest, returns to normal with exercise, and again develops ST-segment depression late in recovery.

Key Point: Abnormal ST-segment depression occurring only in recovery provides clinically useful information and is not more likely to represent a false-positive response. When considered with changes in exercise, changes in recovery increase the sensitivity of the exercise test without a decline in predictive value. A cooldown walk should be avoided after exercise testing, and exercise test scores and nuclear testing should consider recovery ST-segment measurements. Avoidance of a cooldown walk has not resulted in an increased complication rate.

R-Wave Amplitude Adjustment of ST-Segment Depression

The degree of exercise-induced ST-segment depression can be influenced by R-wave amplitude, which perhaps should be normalized to a standard voltage. If normalized, the average gain-factor correction of R-wave amplitude should be approximately 25 mm (i.e., the average R-wave voltage in V_5). Although others have found such R-wave adjustment to be helpful,[58,59] we have not found that it improves the diagnostic performance of the exercise test.

Exercise-Induced ST-Segment Depression Not Resulting From Coronary Artery Disease

The box lists some of the conditions that can result in false-positive responses. In a population with a high prevalence of heart disease other than CAD, an abnormal exercise test would be as diagnostic for that disease as it would be for CAD in

TABLE 3-4.

Analysis of the Predictive Value of Various Patterns of ST Depression from Screening Asymptomatic Aircrewmen*[56]

ST-Depression Occurrence Time	140 Men with Abnormal Treadmill Response in a Follow-Up Study			111 Men with Abnormal Treadmill Response in an Angiographic Study	
	Occurrence Rate (%)	Risk Ratio†	Predictive Value (%)	Occurrence Rate (%)	Predictive Value (%)
Exercise only	9	7	23	11	8
Recovery only	36	4	12	42	28
Exercise and recovery	55	12	25	47	39
All abnormal responders	100	14	20	100	30

*Recovery-only ST-segment depression had a predictive value similar to that of other patterns.
†Relative risk for cardiac events during follow-up observation compared with that for normal subjects.

SOME FACTORS THAT CAN RESULT IN FALSE-POSITIVE RESPONSES

Valvular heart disease	Left ventricular hypertrophy
Congenital heart disease	Wolff-Parkinson-White syndrome
Cardiomyopathies	Preexcitation variants
Pericardial disorders	Mitral valve prolapse syndrome
Drug administration	Vasoregulatory abnormality
Electrolyte abnormalities	Hyperventilation repolarization abnormalities
Nonfasting state	Hypertension
Anemia	Excessive double product
Sudden excessive exercise	Improper lead systems
Inadequate recording equipment	Incorrect criteria
Bundle branch block	
Improper interpretation	

---

populations with a high prevalence of CAD. Digitalis and other drugs can cause repolarization abnormalities in normal individuals during exercise testing. Patients who have had abnormal responses and who have anemia, have electrolyte level abnormalities, or are on medications should be retested when these conditions are altered. Meals and even glucose ingestion can alter the ST segment and T wave in the resting ECG and can cause a false-positive response. To avoid this problem, all ECG studies should be performed after at least a 4-hour fast. This requirement is also important because of the hemodynamic stress put on the cardiovascular system by eating—after eating, exercise capacity is decreased and angina occurs sooner.

T-WAVE CHANGES

A gradual decrease in T-wave amplitude was observed in all leads during early exercise. At maximal exercise the T wave began to increase, and at 1-minute recovery the amplitude was equivalent to resting values, except in leads II, aV_F, and V_2, where the T-wave amplitude was greater than at rest. However, there was a great deal of overlap.

U-WAVE CHANGES

In a study by Gerson, Morris, and McHenry,[60] 248 patients, 36 of whom had exercise-induced U-wave inversion, underwent exercise testing using leads cC_5 and V_L. Of 71 patients with significant left anterior descending or left main disease and no prior MI, 35% had U-wave inversion compared with only 4% of 57 patients without left anterior descending or left main disease and only 1% of 82 patients who had no CAD. U-wave inversion was diagnosed if a discrete negative deflection within the TP segment relative to the PR segment occurred during or after exercise. Inverted U waves were not diagnosed if the exercise heart rate increased to such a level that the QT interval could not be accurately measured.

OTHER FACTORS

Other factors that affect the ST-segment response to exercise include gender, digoxin, and bundle branch block.

Gender

Gender has an effect on the exercise ECG that is not explained by hormones alone. Giving estrogen to men does not increase the rate of false-positive responses. The lower specificity of exercise-induced ST-segment depression in women could result from hemodynamic or hemoglobin concentration differences. Table 3-5 summarizes the studies[61] that have evaluated the exercise ECG in women.

Robert, Melin, and Detry[62] assessed whether the diagnostic value of exercise testing could be enhanced for women by using multivariate analysis of exercise data. Between 1978 and 1984, 135 infarct-free women underwent exercise testing and coronary angiography. In this first group, maximal exercise variables were submitted to a stepwise logistic analysis. Workload, heart rate, and ST_{60} in lead X were selected to build a diagnostic model. The model was tested in a second group of 115 catheterized women (significant CAD in 47%) and of 76 volunteers. In both groups, sensitivity was better with logistic analysis (66% and 70%) than with the conventional analysis (68% and 59%) or with the previously described

TABLE 3-5.

Studies Evaluating the Diagnostic Value of the Exercise ECG in Women

Principal Investigator	Year	No.	Sensitivity (%)	Specificity (%)
Caru	1978	168	73	74
Cahen	1978	100	88	92
Sketch	1975	56	50	78
Detry	1977	45	89	63
Linhart	1974	98	71	78
Lesbre	1978	150	66	77
Broustet	1978	84	50	70
Barolsky	1979	92	60	68
Weiner	1979	580	76	64
Guiteras val	1982	112	79	66
Manca	1979	508	88	73
Bengtsson	1981	194	—	85
Morise	1993	234	—	—
Robert	1992	135	68	85

analysis (57% and 44%), and for many there was no loss of specificity (85% and 93%). Receiver-operator characteristic curves also showed a better diagnostic accuracy with the present model. The study concluded that for women, logistic analysis of exercise variables improves the diagnostic value of exercise testing.

Digoxin

Sundqvist, Atterhog, and Jogestrand[63] studied the effect of digoxin on the ECG at rest and during and after exercise in 11 healthy subjects. Exercise was performed on a heart rate–controlled bicycle ergometer with stepwise increased loads up to a heart rate of 170 beats per minute. The subjects were studied after administration of digoxin at two dose levels and after withdrawal of digoxin. Administration of digoxin, even at the small dose, induced significant ST-T–segment depression at rest and during exercise. The ST-T–segment changes were numerically small and dose dependent. There was usually junctional depression and no downsloping, but six individuals had as much as 1 mm of ST-segment depression. The most pronounced ST-segment depression occurred at a heart rate of 110 to 130 beats per minute. At higher heart rates the ST-segment depression was less pronounced but still statistically significant. During the first minutes after exercise, no significant digitalis-induced ST-T–segment depression was seen. This type of reaction is not usually seen in myocardial ischemia. Fourteen days after withdrawal of the drug there were no significant digitalis-induced ST-T–segment changes.

Left Bundle Branch Block

Whinnery, Froelicher, and Stuart[64] reported on 31 asymptomatic men who serially developed left bundle branch block (LBBB) and who were studied with maximal treadmill testing and coronary angiography. They demonstrated that there can be a marked degree of exercise-induced ST-segment depression in addition to that found at rest in healthy men with LBBB. No difference was found between the ST-segment response to exercise in those with or those without significant CAD. Thus the ST-segment response to exercise testing cannot be used to make diagnostic decisions on patients with LBBB. Fig 3-7 shows how LBBB can respond to exercise with further ST-segment depression.

Key Point: In patients with LBBB, the ST-segment response to exercise testing cannot be used to diagnose ischemia.

Right Bundle Branch Block

Whinnery, Froelicher, and Stuart[65] also reported on the response to maximal treadmill testing of 40 asymptomatic men with acquired right bundle branch block (RBBB). There was no exercise-induced ST-segment depression in the inferior and lateral leads. Exercise-induced ST-segment depression in the anterior precordial leads was frequently noted in patients with RBBB. This depression was

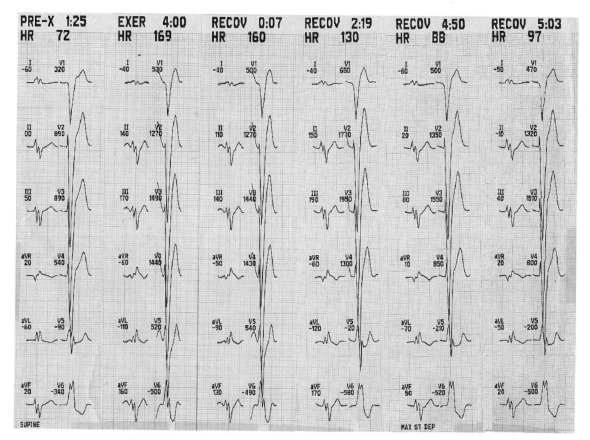

FIG 3-7.
Example of exercise-induced ST-segment depression in lateral leads in patient with LBBB without evidence of ischemia.

most apparent in the right precordial leads with an rSR, or a notched R wave. Because these leads often show a downsloping ST segment at rest, such a finding is not indicative of myocardial ischemia. Fig 3-8 shows ST-segment depression in lateral leads in patients with angina, and Fig 3-9 shows no ST-segment depression in lateral leads in a patient without coronary heart disease but with ST-segment depression anteriorly.

Key Point: In patients with RBBB, exercise-induced ST-segment depression in the lateral leads (V_4, V_5, and V_6) indicates ischemia but depression in the anterior precordial leads (V_1, V_2, and V_3) does not.

Rate-Dependent Bundle Branch Block

Vasey et al[66] reviewed the records of 2584 consecutive patients who underwent treadmill testing and coronary angiography to determine the relationship be-

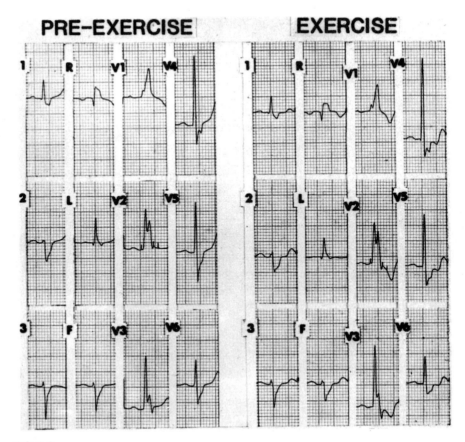

PRE-EXERCISE   EXERCISE

FIG 3-8.
Example of exercise-induced ST-segment depression in lateral leads in patient with RBBB with CAD and ischemia.

tween exercise-induced acceleration-dependent LBBB and the presence of CAD. Rate-dependent LBBB during exercise was identified in 28 patients (1.1%), who were categorized according to their symptoms: classic angina pectoris, atypical chest pain, symptomatic dysrhythmias, and asymptomatic dysrhythmias. Asymptomatic individuals were screened for silent CAD. CAD was present in 7 of 10 patients whose symptoms included classic angina pectoris, but 12 of 13 patients whose symptoms included atypical chest pain had normal coronary arteries. All 10 patients in whom LBBB developed at a heart rate of 125 beats per minute or higher were free of CAD, whereas 9 of 18 patients in whom LBBB developed at a heart rate of less than 125 beats per minute had CAD. Normal coronary arteries were present in three patients with angina symptoms and for whom both chest pain and LBBB developed during exercise. They concluded the following: (1) patients with atypical chest pain and rate-dependent LBBB are significantly less likely to have CAD than patients with symptoms of classic angina; (2) the onset of LBBB at a heart rate of 125 beats per minute or higher is highly correlated with the

PRE-EXERCISE   EXERCISE

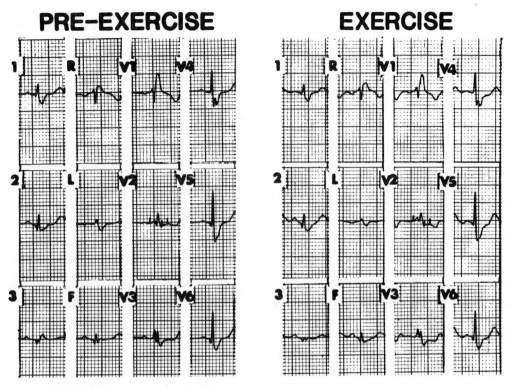

FIG 3-9.
Example of exercise-induced ST-segment depression in anterior leads in patient with RBBB without evidence of ischemia.

presence of normal coronary arteries, regardless of the patient's symptoms; and (3) patients with angina in whom chest pain and LBBB develop during exercise may have normal coronary arteries. Rate-dependent RBBB appears to be more benign than rate-dependent LBBB.

Key Point: Rate-dependent intraventricular blocks occurring during exercise often precede the appearance of chronic blocks present at rest.

Other Causes

Individuals with left ventricular hypertrophy and strain pattern on their resting ECGs are at high risk for CAD. Healthy individuals with Wolff-Parkinson-White syndrome can have exercise-induced ST-segment depression. Some individuals with preexcitation, a short PR interval, or a normal QRS complex may have a false-positive exercise test. Patients with mitral valve prolapse can have abnormal exercise tests but normal coronary angiograms. In individuals with this condition, false-positive responses are apparently more common, occurring in approximately 25% of cases.

Individuals with vasoregulatory asthenia, orthostatic or vasoregulatory abnormalities, and hyperventilation repolarization changes can have abnormal exercise-induced ST-segment changes without CAD. Such changes are unusual and have rarely been responsible for false-positive tests. Orthostatic and hyperventilation changes have been associated with mitral valve prolapse. When they occur with exercise-induced ST-segment changes, the interpretation of ischemia should be avoided, and the clinician must rely on other parameters to make a diagnosis.

Persons with hypertension or an excessive double product (systolic blood pressure × heart rate) during exercise could hypothetically have a physiological imbalance between myocardial oxygen supply and demand. An excessive number of false positives has not been found, however, in hypertensive patients. Barnard et al[67] demonstrated that a sudden high workload of treadmill exercise can yield ST-segment depression in healthy individuals on this basis. Foster et al[68] could not reproduce the ST-segment depression with sudden strenuous bicycle exercise even though the ejection fraction dropped in their normal subjects. A recorder with an inadequate frequency response can artifactually induce ST-segment depression in normal subjects or show upsloping depression when horizontal depression is present.

These conditions can be avoided and should not be the major causes of false-positive responses in a good exercise testing laboratory. The most common cause of a false-positive test should be the normal variant in a patient who has a physiological ST-segment vector that is similar to that produced by ischemia.

ST-SEGMENT SHIFT LOCATION AND ISCHEMIA

Many clinicians use the ST-segment shifts observed in different leads to imply ischemia in underlying areas of myocardium. However, validating the localization of ischemia with coronary angiography has several limitations. First, collaterals may adequately perfuse areas of the heart served by an obstructed artery. Second, coronary angiography cannot quantify the degree to which an infarcted area of the heart remains ischemic. Finally, the validity of relating anatomical lesions visualized at rest to exercise-induced changes in the ECG, both of which only infer ischemia, is questionable. These limitations partially explain the difficulty correlating ECG alterations with the specific number or location of coronary angiographic obstructions. With the advent of coronary artery bypass surgery, precise localization of critical ischemia has assumed more than academic interest. Localization could help direct surgical intervention to the site of jeopardized myocardium or to the source of angina pectoris, for example. Such localization is achieved, in fact, by thallium scintigraphy.

Abouantoun et al[69] studied 54 patients with stable coronary heart disease, all with exercise-induced thallium scintigraphic defects. None of the scintigraphic ischemic sites or angiographic diseased areas could be specifically identified by exercise-induced ST-vector shifts.

Fuchs et al[70] evaluated the use of the 12-lead ECG for localizing the site of CAD in 134 patients with angiographically documented single-vessel coronary disease. They reviewed 10 years of cardiac catheterization at Johns Hopkins Hospital to select patients who had ECGs recorded during MI, spontaneous rest angina, or treadmill exercise. Q-wave location correctly identified the location of the coronary lesion in 98% of the cases, ST-segment elevation in 91%, T-wave inversion in 84%, and ST-segment depression in only 60%. No response could separate right from left circumflex CAD. ST-segment elevation was recorded in 20 of 56 patients who underwent exercise testing. An association was found only between elevation in limb lead III and right CAD.

Simoons and Withagen[28] studied the exercise-induced spatial ST-segment vector shifts in 34 patients who had coronary angiography and thallium exercise scans because of clinical chest pain. They found that in patients with exercise thallium ischemia defects, the ST-segment vectors were posteriorly oriented in 15 of 22, and in those without ischemia defects, they were anteriorly oriented in 9 of 12. However, they could find no systematic difference between the ST-segment vector directions of patients with anteroseptal perfusion defects and of patients with posterolateral perfusion defects. These studies have been corroborated by the excellent angiographic study by Mark et al.[33]

Localized transmural ischemia results in generalized subendocardial ischemia that slows electrical conduction, changing the action potentials, as is seen in MI. The ST-segment changes registered during exercise partially depend on the location of scar tissue. ST-segment elevation or depression, or various combinations of ST-segment shifts, do not localize ischemia to myocardial areas or the arteries inferred by these areas. For instance, ST-segment shifts in leads II and aV_F do not necessarily indicate inferior ischemia (or right CAD), nor do shifts in V_5 indicate lateral ischemia (or left CAD).

Key Point: ST-segment depression is due to global subendocardial ischemia and does not localize on the surface ECG. The ST-segment vector is directed up the long axis of the ventricle.

SUBJECTIVE RESPONSES

Careful observation of the patient's appearance is necessary for the safe performance of an exercise test and is helpful in the clinical assessment of a patient. Patients who exaggerate their limitations or symptoms and those unwilling to cooperate are usually easy to identify. A drop in skin temperature during exercise can indicate an inadequate cardiac output with secondary vasoconstriction and can be an indication that a patient should not be encouraged to perform a higher workload. Neurological manifestations such as lightheadedness or vertigo can also be indications of an inadequate cardiac output.

Findings on physical examination can be helpful, but their sensitivity and specificity have not been demonstrated. Gallop sounds, a mitral regurgitant murmur, or a precordial bulge could be the result of left ventricular dysfunction. An S_3 can sometimes be heard in normals after exercise, but a new S_4 brought out by exercise may be specific for coronary heart disease. The physical findings of congestive heart failure, including rales and neck vein distention, should be rarely encountered in patients referred for exercise testing. However, some exercise testing laboratories use the sitting position for the recovery period to avoid problems with the patient who develops orthopnea. It is preferable to have patients lie supine after exercise testing but to allow those who develop orthopnea to sit up. Also, severe angina or ominous dysrhythmias after exercise can be lessened by allowing the patient to sit up. Attempts have been made to make the findings of the physical examination less subjective by using phonocardiography, apexcardiography, and cardiokymography.

Chest Pain

Weiner et al[71] reported on 281 consecutive patients studied with treadmill testing and coronary angiography with the following responses: 76 patients with ST-segment depression and treadmill test–induced chest pain, 85 patients with ST-segment depression and no chest pain, 40 patients with treadmill test–induced chest pain who had no ST-segment changes, and 80 patients with neither chest pain nor ST-segment changes. They found that 91% of the first group, 65% of the second group, 72% of the third group, and only 35% of the fourth group had significant angiographically determined CAD. Cole and Ellestad[72] followed 95 patients with abnormal treadmill tests. By the fifth follow-up year, the incidence of CAD was 73% in those with chest pain and abnormal ST-segment responses, compared with 43% in those who only had abnormal ST-segment responses. The mortality rate was also twice as high in those with ST-segment changes and chest pain induced by the treadmill test. Ischemic chest pain and ST-segment depression induced by the exercise test predicts the presence of CAD, and when they occur together, they are even more predictive of CAD than either alone. It is important, though, that a careful description of the pain be obtained from the patient to ascertain that it is typical rather than noncardiac pain.

OBSERVER AGREEMENT IN INTERPRETATION

The complexity of not only the human body but also the human mind has created in medicine measurements that when applied to medical diagnosis lead to observations with large variability (e.g., ST-segment displacement measurements). The inherently subjective nature of these medical observations requires questioning the results of most diagnostic methods—not only in terms of accuracy or validity but also in terms of agreement between different interpreters for a given test. Attempts at describing or assessing agreement have been complex and variable, as evidenced in the literature by the numerous terms used: *agreement, variability, consistency, within-observer correlation coefficients of disagreement,* and many others. Agreement is classified by two subgroupings: *intraobserver,* referring to agreement of the individual observer with himself or herself on two separate occasions, and *interobserver,* referring to agreement among two or more individuals.

Blackburn and the Technical Group on Exercise ECG[73] had 14 observers (from seven separate institutions) interpret 38 individual exercise ECG tests as *normal, abnormal,* or *borderline.* Five readers repeated the readings. In only 9 of the 38 exercise ECGs (24%) was there complete agreement among the 14 readers, and only 22 ECGs (58%) were read in agreement. This low value may be a result of the fact that Blackburn's study did not allow observers to make a dichotomous decision and instead made the borderline interpretation an option. In terms of intraobserver agreement, there was a wide range from 58% to 92% for a dichotomous decision. Blackburn attributed this wide variation in both interobserver and intraobserver agreement to the absence of defined criteria, technical problems such as noise, and differences in opinion about ST-segment upsloping. Computer analysis and strict criteria such as that of the Minnesota code have been recommended as means for increasing agreement in exercise ECG interpretation.

REPRODUCIBILITY OF TREADMILL TEST RESPONSES

Sullivan et al[74] studied 14 male patients with exercise test–induced angina and ST-segment depression with treadmill testing on 3 consecutive days to evaluate the reproducibility of certain treadmill variables. Computerized ST-segment analysis and expired gas analysis, including anaerobic threshold, were evaluated for reproducibility using an intraclass correlation coefficient analysis (ICC). The ICC is a generalization of the Pearson product-moment correlation, which is not affected by the addition or multiplication of a given number of observations and provides a better indication of reproducibility than does the coefficient of variation. Oxygen uptake had a higher reliability coefficient ($r = 0.88$) and a smaller 90% confidence interval when compared with treadmill time ($r = 0.70$), which was consistent with a better correlation. The double product and heart rate were highly reproducible ($r = 0.90$ and $r = 0.94$, respectively). In addition, the 90% confidence interval for both double product and heart rate was small. The ST_{60} displacement in lead X and the lead of greatest displacement were very reproducible ($r = 0.83$).

INTERPRETATION OF EXERCISE TEST–INDUCED DYSRHYTHMIAS

Exercise-induced supraventricular dysrhythmias are unusual and have not been related to CAD. Exercise-induced premature ventricular contractions (PVCs) are of major concern, however. They occur in approximately a third of asymptomatic men who perform a maximal treadmill test, and their prevalence is directly related to age. PVCs occur most frequently at maximal exercise and often are not reproduced on repeat testing. A subgroup of healthy men (approximately 2%)

will have severe exercise-induced ventricular dysrhythmias. This group will have 3 times the normal risk of developing CAD, but only about 10% of them will actually do so. Only 7% of those who develop CAD will have had so-called ominous ventricular dysrhythmias, and their PVCs will often occur at lower heart rates than they do in healthy subjects.

Busby, Shefrin, and Fleg[75] studied 1160 subjects ages 21 to 96 years who underwent maximal exercise treadmill testing an average of 2.4 times. Eighty (6.9%) developed frequent ($\geq$10% of beats in any 1 minute) or repetitive ($\geq$3 beats in a row) ventricular ectopic beats on at least one test. These 80 individuals were significantly older than the group without such dysrhythmia (63.8 $\pm$ 12.5 versus 50.0 $\pm$ 16.1 years). A striking age-related increase in the prevalence of frequent or repetitive exercise-induced ventricular ectopic beats was seen in men but not in women. ECG abnormalities at rest, exercise-induced ST-segment depression, thallium perfusion defects, duration of treadmill exercise, maximum heart rate, systolic blood pressure, and rate-pressure product did not differ between these 80 study subjects with frequent exercise-induced ventricular ectopic beats and a control group matched for age and gender. Furthermore, for the study and control groups, the incidence (10% versus 12.5%) of cardiac events (angina pectoris, nonfatal MI, cardiac syncope, or cardiac death) as well as of noncardiac mortality (each 7.5%) was found to be similar over a mean follow-up period of 5.6 years. No study subjects required antidysrhythmic drugs during this period. Thus frequent or repetitive exercise-induced ventricular ectopic beats in these predominantly older, asymptomatic individuals without apparent heart disease do not predict increased cardiac morbidity or mortality and therefore do not require specific therapy.

Dysrhythmias suppressed by acute exercise do not rule out the presence of CAD. In general, exercise-induced dysrhythmias must be interpreted in relation to the medical condition of the individuals in whom they occur. Exercise-induced ST-segment depression is related to subendocardial ischemia and is less arrythmogenic than ST-segment elevation (not over Q waves), which is associated with transmural ischemia. The presence of PVCs on the resting ECG should be used to classify patients as to their exercise response. The methods of recording and capturing PVCs greatly affect the prevalence data. Numerous prognostic studies have not demonstrated an independent risk associated with PVCs.[76-79]

Key Point: Ventricular dysrhythmias in general do not have the same significance in the exercise laboratory as they do in the coronary care unit. In the exercize laboratory, they are usually ominous only when occuring in patients with histories of sudden death, cardiomyopathy, valvular heart disease, and severe ischemia.

Exercise Testing to Evaluate ST-Segment Depression During Supraventricular Tachycardia

To detect coronary artery disease and myocardial ischemia, Petsas, Anastassiades, and Antonopoulos[80] used exercise testing to study 16 patients who had manifested ST-segment depression during episodes of paroxysmal supraventricular tachycardia (PSVT). No ST-segment depression was observed during exercise testing in 15 of the 16 patients tested. PSVT associated with ST-segment depression occurred during exercise testing in three cases. The ST-segment depression was immediately apparent, remained constant throughout the supraventricular tachycardia, and was almost instantly abolished following conversion to sinus rhythm. Patients with heart rates greater than 250 beats per minute during PSVT had marked ST-segment depression with the tachycardia. These results suggest that CAD and myocardial ischemia are not involved in the genesis of ST-segment depression during PSVT. Tachycardia may cause ST-segment depression by altering the slope of phase two of the ventricular action potential. Retrograde atrial activation may also induce ST-segment shifts in some cases.

Ventricular Tachycardia During Exercise Testing

Fleg and Lakatta[81] studied the prevalence of ventricular tachycardia (VT) associated with maximal treadmill exercise in 597 male and 325 female volunteers from the Baltimore Longitudinal Study on Aging who were ages 21 to 96 years and without apparent heart disease. Ten subjects, seven men and three women, with exercise-induced VT were identified, representing 1.1% of those tested; only one was younger than 65 years. All episodes of VT were asymptomatic and nonsustained. In 9 of 10 subjects, VT developed at or near peak exercise. The longest run of VT was 56 beats; multiple runs of VT were present in four subjects. Two subjects had exercise-induced ST-segment depression, but subsequent exercise thallium results were negative in each. Compared with a group of age- and gender-matched control subjects, those with asymptomatic, nonsustained VT displayed no difference in exercise duration, maximum heart rate, or the prevalence of coronary risk factors of exercise-induced ischemia as measured by the ECG and thallium scintigraphy. Over a mean follow-up period of 2 years, no subject developed symptoms of heart disease or experienced syncope or sudden death. Exercise-induced VT in apparently healthy subjects occured mainly in the elderly, was limited to short, asymptomatic runs of 3 to 6 beats usually near peak exercise, and did not predict increased cardiovascular morbidity or mortality rates over a 2-year follow-up.

Exercise Test–Induced Ventricular Tachycardia Study

The Long Beach Veterans Affairs Medical Center (LBVAMC) conducted a retrospective review of 3351 patients who had undergone routine clinical exercise testing between September 1984 and June 1989; 55 patients with exercise-induced VT were identified.[82] Mean follow-up was 26 months (ranging from 2 to 58 months). Fifty patients had nonsustained VT during exercise testing, and one of these patients died due to congestive heart failure during the follow-up period. Five patients had sustained VT during exercise testing, and one died suddenly seven months after the test. VT was reproduced in only 2 of the 29 patients who underwent repeated exercise testing. Nonsustained VT was defined as greater or equal to three consecutive ventricular ectopic beats. Sustained VT was defined as VT longer than 30 seconds or requiring intervention.

A total of 58 episodes of exercise-induced VT occurred in 55 patients. The patients had a mean age of 62 years, with a range of 39 to 76. Of the 55 patients, 50 had exercise-induced nonsustained VT (ranging from 3 to 21 beats). The mean (±1 SD) and median numbers of consecutive ventricular ectopic beats per episode were 4.5 (±3.6) and 3. Thirty of the patients with nonsustained exercise-induced VT exhibited only three consecutive ventricular ectopic beats. Of the 50 episodes of nonsustained ventricular tachycardia, 26 episodes occurred during exercise and 24 occurred in recovery; only 10 occurred at peak exercise and led to cessation of the exercise test. Five patients had exercise-induced sustained VT, two during exercise and three during recovery. Of these five patients, only two required intervention; one was given lidocaine intravenously, and one was cardioverted because of hypotension. The only other episode of serious ventricular dysrhythmia during this period occurred in a patient without prior cardiac history who developed ventricular fibrillation during exercise, which required electrical defibrillation.

The major findings of this study (Fig 3-10) are that the occurrence of nonsustained exercise-induced VT during routine treadmill testing is not associated with complications during testing or with increased cardiovascular mortality within 2 years after testing. In the study, the prevalence and reproducibility of exercise-induced VT were low (1.2% and 6.9%), despite a high prevalence of structural heart disease (mostly CAD) in the study population. The annual mortality rate among patients with exercise-induced VT was 1.7%, compared with 2.4% in the study population (171 deaths in 3351 patients). Thus exercise-induced VT during treadmill testing did not portend a worsened prognosis even among patients with

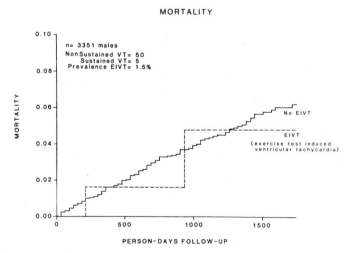

FIG 3-10.
Kaplan-Meier survival curve illustrating mortality with VT during standard treadmill testing in a referred clinical population.[82]

CAD. The number of patients with sustained ventricular tachycardia was small (five), and the patients were treated.

Mokotoff, Quinones, and Miller[83] selectively examined 26 of 45 consecutive patients with VT during exercise testing, 18 of whom had organic heart disease (mostly CAD). Half of the patients exhibited the minimum of three consecutive ventricular ectopic beats. Condini et al[84] described 47 patients with VT during exercise testing (a prevalence of 0.8% in 5730 treadmill tests). A total of 40 of 47 patients had heart disease, mostly CAD. VT was brief and self-terminated in all but one instance. No follow-up data were provided. Milanes et al[85] reported a 4.0% incidence of VT in 900 treadmill tests performed in patients with CAD, compared with a 0.07% incidence in 1700 tests among patients without CAD. They reported a 4-year mortality rate of 38% for patients with ventricular fibrillation or VT of four beats or more. Within this combined group for ventricular fibrillation and VT, 79% had an abnormal ST-segment response as well.

During exercise, transmural ischemia as indicated by ST-segment elevation is generally arrhythmogenic, whereas subendocardial ischemia associated with ST-segment depression is not. None of the patients with nonsustained VT had ST-segment elevation with their exercise test, and 20 had abnormal ST-segment depression. Of five patients with sustained VT, none had ST-segment elevation, and two had abnormal ST-segment depression before the onset of VT. Detry et al[86] reported on six patients without MI specifically referred to them for spontaneous angina, which is associated with ST-segment elevation. During exercise testing, five exhibited elevation, three of whom developed VT and one who developed ventricular fibrillation. We have subsequently seen one such patient who developed ST-segment elevation and then VT (20 beats) at maximal exercise.

SUMMARY

The interpretation of the exercise test is not a simple skill but requires the understanding of physiology and pathophysiology. Not all members of the medical profession can adequately interpret an exercise test. Certification is extremely important now that this technology is rapidly spreading beyond the subspeciality of cardiology. Training and experience are required for ECG testing as they are in other diagnostic procedures. In part for these reasons, the American College of Physicians has recently published guidelines on clinical competence for physicians performing exercise testing.[87] All of the results of the test must be considered. Attempts should be made to make the interpretation reliable by using good methods and following the suggestions in this chapter. When properly interpreted, the exercise test is one of the most important diagnostic and clinically helpful tests in medicine.

Observer agreement is best when using dichotomous interpretations and worst (most variable) when using more complex descriptions, such as those involved in specifying location or overlapping areas. Several possible ways to improve reliability include the following: (1) simple dichotomous decisions, (2) standardized report forms such as the one recommended by the American College of Physicians, (3) multiple observers or one very experienced reader, (4) multiple "blinded," or unbiased, interpretations, and (5) computer analysis. Computer analysis of the exercise ECG and measurement of gas-exchange variables can be highly reproducible. However, as long as human judgment with all its complexities remains the basis for the final interpretation, there will always be some variation.

ST-segment depression is a representation of global subendocardial ischemia, with a vector direction determined largely by the placement of the heart in the chest. ST-segment depression does not localize coronary artery lesions. ST-segment depression in the inferior leads (II, and aV$_F$) is most often due to the atrial repolarization wave, which begins in the PR segment and can extend to the beginning of the ST segment. Severe transmural ischemia, resulting in wall-motion abnormalities, causes a shift of the vector in the direction of the wall motion abnormality. However, preexisting areas of wall-motion abnormality (e.g., a scar) usually indicated by a Q wave, also cause such a shift, resulting in ST-segment elevation without ischemia. When the resting ECG shows Q waves of an old MI, ST-segment elevation is due to ischemia, wall-motion abnormalities, or both, whereas accompanying ST-segment depression can be caused by a second area of ischemia or reciprocal changes. When the resting ECG is normal, however, ST-segment elevation is due to severe ischemia (a spasm or a critical lesion), although accompanying ST-segment depression is reciprocal. Such ST-segment elevation is uncommon and very arrhythmogenic, and it localizes. Exercise-induced R-wave and S-wave amplitude changes do not correlate with changes in LV volume, ejection fraction, or ischemia. The consensus of many studies is that such changes do not have diagnostic value. ST-segment depression limited to the recovery period does not generally represent a false-positive response. Inclusion of analysis during this period increases the diagnostic yield of the exercise test. However, exercise test scores have not been adequately validated and should be used with caution. Performing exercise ECG analysis with scintigraphy or performing a cooldown walk can falsely lower the sensitivity of the exercise ECG because these techniques obscure ST-segment changes occurring in recovery. Downsloping ST-segment changes in recovery and prolongation of depression can also falsely improve test performance.

As with resting ventricular dysrhythmias, the significance of exercise-induced ventricular arrhythmias is related to the disease processes with which they are associated (e.g., history of syncope, sudden death, physical examination with a large heart, murmurs, ECG showing a prolonged QT segment, preexcitation, or Q waves). If there are no signs or symptoms of associated diseases, exercise-induced ventricular dysrhythmias can usually be ignored. Because exercise-induced ventricular dysrythmias most likely are not independently predictive of death in most patients with coronary disease, a better prediction can be obtained from other variables. Nonsustained VT is uncommon during routine clinical treadmill testing, is well tolerated, and is associated with a relatively good prognosis. Outcome is primarily determined by concomitant clinical features such as ventricular function, ischemia, and the presence or absence of symptoms. Treatment should be directed toward these signs and symptoms rather than the episode of dysrhythmia.

The same exercise test responses can have different meanings from one population or clinical subset to another; therefore interpretation depends on the application of the test.

REFERENCES

1. Simonson E: Electrocardiographic stress tolerance tests, *Progr Cardiovasc Dis* 13:269-292, 1970.
2. Blomqvist G: The Frank lead exercise electrocardiogram, *Acta Med Scand* 179:1-98, 1965.
3. Rautaharju PM et al: Waveform patterns in frank-lead rest and exercise electrocardiograms of healthy elderly men, *Circulation* 48:541-548, 1973.
4. Simoons ML, Hugenholtz PG: Gradual changes of ECG waveform during and after exercise in normal subjects, *Circulation* 52:570-577, 1975.
5. Wolthuis RA et al: Normal electrocardiographic waveform characteristics during treadmill exercise testing, *Circulation* 60:1028-1035, 1979.
6. Riff DP, Carleton RA: Effect of exercise on the atrial recovery wave, *Am Heart J* 82:759-763, 1971.
7. Sapin PM et al: Identification of false positive exercise tests with use of electrocardiographic criteria: a possible role for atrial repolarization waves, *J Am Coll Cardiol* 18:127-135, 1991.
8. Kentala E, Luurela O: Response of R wave amplitude to posterior changes and to exercise, *Ann Clin Res* 7:258-263, 1975.
9. Bonoris PE et al: Evaluation of R wave amplitude changes versus ST segment depression in stress testing, *Circulation* 57:904-910, 1978.
10. Eenige van MJ et al: Diagnostic incapacity of exercise-induced QRS wave amplitude changes to detect coronary artery disease and left ventricular dysfunction, *Euro Heart J* 3:9-16, 1982.
11. Brody DA: A theoretical analysis of intracavitary blood mass influence on the heart-lead relationship, *Circ Res* 54:731-738, 1956.
12. Levken J et al: Influence of left ventricular dimensions on endocardial and epicardial QRS amplitude and ST segment elevations during acute myocardial ischemia, *Circulation* 61:679-689, 1980.
13. Battler A, Froelicher V, Pfisterer M: Relationship of QRS amplitude changes during exercise to left ventricular function and volumes and the diagnosis of coronary disease. *Circulation* 60:1004-1013, 1979.
14. Myers J et al: Spatial R wave amplitude during exercise: relation with left ventricular ischemia and function, *J Am Coll Cardiol* 6:603-608, 1985.
15. Ahnve S et al: Computer analysis of exercise-induced changes in QRS duration in patients with angina pectoris and in normal subjects, *Am Heart J* 111(5):903-908, 1986.
16. Goldberger AL, Bhargava V: Effect of exercise on QRS duration in healthy men: a computer ECG analysis, *J Appl Physiol* 54(4):1083-1088, 1983.
17. Mirvis DM, Ramanathan KB, Wilson JL: Regional blood flow correlates of ST segment depression in tachycardia-induced myocardial ischemia, *Circulation* 2:363-373, 1986.
18. Prinzmetal M et al: Angina pectoris: a variant form of angina pectoris, *Am J Med* 27:375, 1959.
19. Endo M, Kanda I, Hosoda H: Prinzmetal's variant form of angina pectoris: re-evaluation of mechanisms, *Circulation* 52:33, 1975.

20. Shubrooks SJ, Bete JM, Hutter AM: Variant angina pectoris: clinical and anatomic spectrum and results of coronary bypass surgery, *Am J Cardiol* 36:142, 1975.

21. Higgins CB et al: Clinical and arteriographic features of Prinzmetal's variant angina: documentation of etiologic factors, *Am J Cardiol* 37:831, 1976.

22. Maseri A, Severi S, DeNes M: Variant angina: one aspect of continuous spectrum of vasospastic myocardial ischemia, *Am J Cardiol* 42:1019, 1978.

23. Weiner DA et al: ST segment elevation during recovery from exercise, *Chest* 74:133, 1978.

24. Fortuin NJ, Freisinger GC: Exercise-induced ST segment elevation: clinical, electrocardiographic and arteriographic studies in twelve patients, *Am J Med* 49:459, 1970.

25. Hegge FN, Tuna N, Burchell HB: Coronary arteriographic findings in patients with axis shifts or ST segment elevations on exercise testing, *Am Heart J* 86:603, 1973.

26. Chahine RA, Raizner AE, Ishimori T: The clinical significance of exercise-induced ST-segment elevation, *Circulation* 54:209, 1976.

27. Manvi KN, Ellestad MH: Elevated ST segments with exercise in ventricular aneurysm, *J Electrocardiol* 5:317-323, 1972.

28. Simoons M, Withagen A: *Nuc Cardiology* 17:154-156, 1978.

29. Sriwattanakomen S et al: ST segment elevation during exercise: electrocardiographic and arteriographic correlation in 38 patients, *Am J Cardiol* 45:762-768, 1980.

30. Longhurst JC, Kraus WL: Exercise-induced ST elevation in patients without myocardial infarction, *Circulation* 60:616-622, 1979.

31. Dunn RF et al: Exercise-induced ST-segment elevation in leads V_1 or aV_L: a predictor of anterior myocardial ischemia and left anterior descending coronary artery disease, *Circulation* 63:1357-1363, 1981.

32. Braat SH et al: Value of lead V_{4R} in exercise testing to predict proximal stenosis of the right coronary artery, *J Am Coll Cardiol* 5:1308-1311, 1985.

33. Mark DB et al: Localizing coronary artery obstructions with the exercise treadmill test, *Ann Intern Med* 106:53-55, 1987.

34. Bruce RA, Fisher LD: Unusual prognostic significance of exercise-induced ST elevation in coronary patients, *J Electrocardiol* 84-88, 1987.

35. De Feyter PJ et al: Clinical significance of exercise-induced ST segment elevation, *Br Heart J* 46:84-92, 1981.

36. Bruce RA et al: ST segment elevation with exercise: a marker for poor ventricular function and poor prognosis: Coronary Artery Surgery Study (CASS) confirmation of Seattle Heart Watch results, *Circulation* 4:897-905, 1988.

37. Hegge FN, Tuna N, Burchell HB: Coronary arteriographic findings in patients with axis shifts or S-T-segment elevations on exercise-stress testing, *Am Heart J* 5:603-615, 1973.

38. Lahiri A et al: Exercise-induced ST-segment elevation in variant angina, *Am J Cardiol* 45:887-893, 1980.

39. Caplin JL, Banim SO: Chest pain and electrocardiographic ST-segment elevation occurring in the recovery phase after exercise in a patient with normal coronary arteries, *Clin Cardiol* 8:228-234, 1985.

40. Hill JA et al: Coronary artery spasm and its relationship to exercise in patients without severe coronary obstructive disease, *Clin Cardiol* 11:489-494, 1988.

41. Fox KM et al: Significance of exercise-induced ST-segment elevation in patients with previous myocardial infarction, *Am J Cardiol* 49:933, 1982 (abstract).

42. Gerwitz H et al: Role of myocardial ischemia in the genesis of exercise-induced ST segment elevation in previous anterior myocardial infarction, *Am J Cardiol* 51:1293-1300, 1983.

43. Stiles GL, Tosati RA, Wallace AG: Clinical relevance of exercise-induced ST-segment elevation, *Am J Cardiol* 46:931-940, 1980.
44. Shimokawa H et al: Variable exercise capacity in variant angina and greater exertional thallium-201 myocardial defect during vasospastic ischemic ST segment elevation than with ST depression, *Am Heart J* 103:142-150, 1982.
45. Auora R et al: The role of ischemia and ventricular asynergy in the genesis of exercise-induced ST elevation, *Clin Cardiol* 11:127-132, 1988.
46. Nobel RJ et al: Normalization of abnormal T waves in ischemia, *Arch Intern Med* 136:391-402, 1976.
47. Sweet RL, Sheffield LT: Myocardial infarction after exercise-induced electrocardiographic changes in a patient with variant angina pectoris, *Am J Cardiol* 33:813-821, 1974.
48. Lavie CJ et al: Significance of T-wave pseudonormalization during exercise: a radionuclide angiographic study, *Chest* 94:512-516, 1988.
49. McHenry PL, Morris SN: *Exercise electrocardiography: current state of the art.* In Schlant RC, Hurst JW, eds: *Advance in electrocardiography,* vol 2, New York, 1976, Grune & Stratton.
50. Maseri A et al: "Variant" angina: one aspect of a continuous spectrum of vasospastic myocardial ischemia, *Am J Cardiol* 42:1019-1025, 1978.
51. Detrano R et al: Factors affecting sensitivity and specificity of a diagnostic test: the exercise thallium scintigram, *Am J Med* 84:699-710, 1988.
52. Gutman RA, Bruce R: Delay of ST depression after maximal exercise by walking for 2 minutes, *Circulation* 42:229-336, 1970.
53. Lachterman B et al: Does incidence of "recovery only" ST segment depression affect the predictive accuracy of the exercise test? *Ann Intern Med* 112:11-16, 1980.
54. Karnegis JN et al: Comparison of exercise-positive with recovery-positive treadmill graded exercise tests, *Am J Cardiol* 60:544-547, 1987.
55. Savage MP et al: Usefulness of ST-segment depression as a sign of coronary artery disease when confined to the post exercise recovery period, *Am J Cardiol* 60:1405-1406, 1987.
56. Froelicher VF et al: Value of exercise testing for screening asymptomatic men for latent coronary artery disease, *Progr Cardiovasc Dis* 18:265-276, 1976.
57. Ellestad M: *Stress testing: principles and practice,* ed 3, Philadelphia, 1986, Davis.
58. Hollenberg M et al: Influence of R wave amplitude on exercise-induced ST depression: need for a "gain factor" correction when interpreting stress electrocardiograms, *Am J Cardiol* 56:13-17, 1985.
59. Hakki A et al: R wave amplitude: a new determinant of failure of patients with coronary heart disease to manifest ST segment depression during exercise, *J Am Coll Cardiol* 3:1155-1160, 1984.
60. Gerson MC, Morris SN, McHenry PL: Relation of exercise induced physiologic ST segment depression to R wave amplitude in normal subjects, *Am J Cardiol* 46:778-782, 1980.
61. Val P, Chaitman B, Waters D: *Circulation* 65:1465-1472, 1982.
62. Robert AR, Melin JA, Detry JM: Logistic discriminant analysis improves diagnostic accuracy of exercise testing for coronary artery disease in women, *Circulation* 83(4):1202-1209, 1991.
63. Sundqvist K, Atterhog JH, Jogestrand T: Effect of digoxin on the electrocardiogram at rest and during exercise in healthy subjects, *Am J Cardiol* 57:661-665, 1986.
64. Whinnery JE, Froelicher VF, Stuart AJ: The electrocardiographic response to maximal treadmill exercise in asymptomatic men with left bundle branch block, *Am Heart J* 94:316-322, 1977.

65. Whinnery JE, Froelicher VF, Stuart AJ: The electrocardiographic response to maximal treadmill exercise in asymptomatic men with right branch bundle block, *Chest* 71:335-343, 1977.

66. Vasey CG et al: Exercise-induced left bundle branch block and its relation to coronary artery disease, *Am J Cardiol* 56:892-895, 1985.

67. Barnard R et al: Ischemic response to sudden strenuous exercise in healthy men, *Circulation* 48:936-944, 1973.

68. Foster C et al: Effect of warm-up on left ventricular response to sudden strenuous exercise, *J Appl Physiol* 53:380-383, 1982.

69. Abouantoun S et al: Can areas of myocardial ischemia be localized by the exercise electrocardiogram? A correlative study with thallium-201 scintigraphy, *Am Heart J* 108:933-941, 1984.

70. Fuchs RM et al: Electrocardiographic localization of coronary artery narrowings: studies during myocardial ischemia and infarction in patients with one-vessel disease, *Circulation* 66:1168-1175, 1982.

71. Weiner DA et al: The predictive value of anginal chest pain as an indicator of coronary disease during exercise testing, *Am Heart J* 96:458-462, 1978.

72. Cole JP, Ellestad, MH: Significance of chest pain during treadmill exercise: correlation with coronary events, *Am J Cardiol* 41:227-232, 1978.

73. Blackburn H, the Technical Group on Exercise ECG: The exercise electrocardiogram: differences in interpretation, *Am J Cardiol* 31:871-880, 1968.

74. Sullivan M et al: The reproducibility of hemodynamic, electrocardiographic, and gas exchange data during treadmill exercise in patients with stable angina pectoris, *Chest* 86:375-382, 1984.

75. Busby MJ, Shefrin EA, Fleg JL: Prevalence and long-term significance of exercise-induced frequent or repetitive ventricular ectopic beats in apparently healthy volunteers, *J Am Coll Cardiol* 14:1659-1665, 1989.

76. Sami M et al: Significance of exercise-induced ventricular arrhythmia in stable coronary artery disease: a coronary artery surgery study project, *Am J Cardiol* 54:1182-1190, 1984.

77. Califf RM et al: Prognostic value of ventricular arrhythmias associated with treadmill exercise testing in patients studied with cardiac catheterization for suspected ischemic heart disease, *J Am Coll Cardiol* 2:1060-1067, 1983.

78. Weiner DA et al: Ventricular arrhythmias during exercise testing: mechanism, response to coronary bypass surgery and prognostic significance, *Am J Cardiol* 53:1553, 1984.

79. Marieb MA et al: Clinical relevance of exercise-induced ventricular arrhythmias in suspected coronary artery disease, *Am J Cardiol* 66:172-178, 1990.

80. Petsas AA, Anastassiades LC, Antonopoulos AG: Exercise testing for assessment of the significance of ST segment depression observed during episodes of paroxysmal supraventricular tachycardia, *Euro Heart J* 11:974-979, 1990.

81. Fleg JL, Lakatta EG: Prevalence and prognosis of exercise-induced nonsustained ventricular tachycardia in apparently healthy volunteers, *Am J Cardiol* 54:762-769, 1984.

82. Yang JC, Wesley RC, Froelicher VF: Ventricular tachycardia during routine treadmill testing: risk and prognosis, *Arch Internal Med* 151:347-353, 1991.

83. Mokotoff D, Quinones M, Miller R: Exercise-induced ventricular tachycardia, clinical features relating to chronic ventricular ectopy, and prognosis, *Chest* 77:10-16, 1980.

84. Condini M et al: Clinical significance and characteristics of exercise-induced ventricular tachycardia, *Cathet Cardiovasc Diagn* 7:227-234, 1981.

85. Milanes J et al: Exercise tests and ventricular tachycardia, *West J Med* 145:473-476, 1986.

86. Detry JR et al: Maximal exercise testing in patients with spontaneous angina pectoris associated with transient ST segment elevation: risks and electrocardiographic findings, *Br Heart J* 37:897-905, 1975.

87. Schlant RC, Friesinger GC, Leonard JL: Clinical competence in exercise testing, *Circulation* 5:1884-1888, 1990.

CHAPTER 4

Diagnostic Applications of Exercise Testing

The general clinical applications of exercise testing and some special applications are listed in the box. Four applications require extensive review: diagnostic exercise testing, prognostic exercise testing, exercise testing of patients after myocardial infarction (MI), and screening of apparently healthy individuals. These applications therefore will be covered separately in this and the following three chapters. Other less common uses will be touched on in Chapter 8.

DIAGNOSIS OF CHEST PAIN AND OTHER CARDIAC FINDINGS

To evaluate the diagnostic value of a test for a disease, a clinician must demonstrate how well the test distinguishes between individuals with and those without the disease. Evaluation of exercise testing as a diagnostic test for coronary artery disease (CAD) depends on the population tested, which must be divided into those with and those without CAD, by independent techniques such as coronary angiography and clinical follow-up for coronary events.

Limitations of Coronary Angiography

Coronary angiography usually underestimates the pathological severity of CAD and can even be interpreted as normal when in fact severe CAD is present. Such a false reading can be caused by total cutoff of an artery at its origin, by diffuse atherosclerotic narrowing of an artery, or by failure to use proper views to visualize proximal left coronary artery lesions. Another limitation of coronary angiography is that coronary artery spasm as a cause of ischemia may be missed because it is often transient. Also, coronary angiographic interpretation is subject to variability related to observer error, as has been previously described. Recent studies using Doppler flow techniques and videodensitometric techniques have shown a wide discrepancy between angiographic lesions and coronary flow reserve.[1] Exercise

---

CLINICAL APPLICATIONS OF EXERCISE TESTING

General Applications
Diagnosis: Is significant coronary artery disease present?
Prognosis: Who is high risk? Who needs intervention?
Functional assessment: Who is disabled? What activities can be done safely?
Treatment assessment: Is medication or intervention effective?

Special Applications
Postmyocardial infarction (see Chapter 6)
Cardiac rehabilitation
Screening (see Chapter 7)
Exercise prescription
Preoperation evaluation
Dysrhythmias
Unstable angina (once stabilized)
Intermittent claudication
Pulmonary disease
Cardiac transplantation

---

electrocardiography (ECG) was a good predictor of the physiological significance (assessed by coronary flow reserve) of a coronary stenosis but less so of angiographically classified disease.

Coronary Collaterals

The occurrence and influence of coronary collateral circulation were studied by Pellinen et al[2] using bicycle ergometry in a random sample of 286 patients with angiographically documented CAD. Collaterals appeared increasingly in all three main coronary arteries in proportion to the grade of obstruction. The presence or absence of collaterals had no obvious influence on ST-segment response during the exercise test. In patients with triple-vessel disease, peak work capacity was better when collaterals to the left anterior descending artery were present.

Limitations of Clinical Follow-up and Pathological Events

There are some important limitations to using clinical and pathological events to distinguish individuals with CAD from those without it. Coronary disease events and symptoms can be caused by relatively minor lesions. Thrombosis and hemorrhage into nonobstructive plaques can cause symptoms or even death. Spasm occurs proximal to relatively minor lesions. Pathological studies have shown that approximately 7% of persons dying from clinically diagnosed MI have insignificant or no coronary atheroma. Coronary angiographic studies have shown that some patients with classic angina pectoris and MI can have normal coronary angiograms.

Key Point: In spite of their limitations, coronary angiography and the observation of clinical syndromes and coronary events are at present the most practical means for distinguishing between patients with and without CAD.

Predictive Accuracy Definitions

Sensitivity and *specificity* are the terms used to define how reliably a test distinguishes individuals with disease from those without it. Sensitivity is the percentage of total times that a test gives an abnormal result when those with the disease are tested. Specificity is the percentage of total times that a test gives a normal result when those without the disease are tested. The meaning of *specific* is quite different from the colloquial use of the term. The methods for calculating these percentages are shown in the box.

A basic step in applying any testing procedure to separate individuals with normal results from those with disease is to determine a discriminant value measured by the test that best separates the two groups. The problem is that there is usually a considerable overlap of test values in the groups with and without disease. For example, Fig 4-1 illustrates two bell-shaped normal distribution curves: one for the test variable in a population with normal results and the other for this variable in a population with disease. Along the vertical axis is the number of patients, and along the horizontal axis could be the value for such measurements as Q-wave size, exercise-induced ST-segment depression, or creatine phosphokinase levels. Note that there is considerable overlap between the two curves. The optimal test would be able to achieve the most marked separation of these two bell-shaped curves, minimizing the overlap. Unfortunately, most of the tests currently used for the diagnosis of CAD, including the exercise test, have a considerable overlap in the range of measurements for the normal population and for those with heart disease. Therefore problems arise when a certain value, or cutoff point,

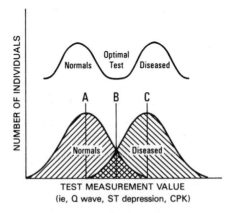

FIG 4-1.
Bell-shaped curves of the distribution of measurement values in patients with and without disease.

is used to separate these two groups (e.g., 0.1 mV of ST-segment depression, a 10 mm Hg drop in systolic blood pressure, less than 5 metabolic equivalents [METS] of exercise capacity, or three consecutive premature ventricular contractions). If the value is set far to the right (e.g., 0.2 mV of ST-segment depression), identifying nearly all those with normal results as free of disease and giving the test a high specificity, then a substantial number of those with the disease will be falsely identified as *normal*. If a value is chosen far to the left (e.g., 0.5-mm ST-segment depression), identifying nearly all those with disease as abnormal and giving the test a high sensitivity, then a substantial number of those without the disease will be falsely identified as abnormal. If a value is chosen that equally mislabels those without and those with disease, the test will have its highest predictive accuracy. However, there may be reasons for wanting to adjust a test to have a relatively higher sensitivity or relatively higher specificity than is possible when predictive accuracy is optimal. Remember that sensitivity and specificity are inversely related. That is, when sensitivity is the highest, specificity is the lowest and vice versa. Any test has a range of inversely related sensitivities and specificities that can be chosen by using a certain discriminant value, or cutoff point.

After a discriminant value that determines a test's specificity and sensitivity is chosen, the population tested must be considered. If the population is skewed toward individuals with a greater severity of disease, the test will have a higher sensitivity. For instance, the exercise test has a higher sensitivity in individuals with triple-vessel disease than in those with single-vessel disease. Also, a test can have a lower specificity if it is used in individuals more likely to give false-positive results. For instance, the exercise test has a lower specificity in individuals with mitral valve prolapse and in women.

Key Point: Sensitivity and specificity are inversely related, are affected by the population tested, and are determined by the choice of a discriminant value.

The sensitivity and specificity of exercise-induced ST-segment depression can be demonstrated by analyzing the results obtained when exercise testing and coronary angiography have been used to evaluate patients. The exercise test cutoff point of 0.1 mV of either horizontal or downsloping ST-segment depression had approximately an 84% specificity for angiographically significant CAD; that is, 84% of those without significant angiographic disease had a normal exercise test. These studies demonstrated a mean 66% sensitivity of exercise testing for angiographic CAD, with a range of 40% for single-vessel disease to 90% for triple-vessel disease. Sensitivity decreased for the milder degrees of CAD, but it is likely that some patients with single-vessel coronary disease do not have MI.

Two additional terms that help to define the diagnostic value of a test are its *relative risk* and *predictive value*. The box on p. 94 also shows how these terms are calculated. The *relative risk* is the relative chance of having disease if the test result is abnormal as compared with the chance of having disease if the test result is normal. The *predictive value* of an abnormal test result is the percentage of persons with an abnormal test result who have disease. Predictive value cannot be

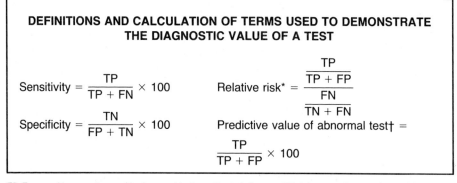

DEFINITIONS AND CALCULATION OF TERMS USED TO DEMONSTRATE
THE DIAGNOSTIC VALUE OF A TEST

$$\text{Sensitivity} = \frac{TP}{TP + FN} \times 100 \qquad \text{Relative risk*} = \frac{\dfrac{TP}{TP + FP}}{\dfrac{FN}{TN + FN}}$$

$$\text{Specificity} = \frac{TN}{FP + TN} \times 100 \qquad \text{Predictive value of abnormal test†} =$$

$$\frac{TP}{TP + FP} \times 100$$

TP, True positives, or those with abnormal test results and disease; *FN*, false negatives, or those with normal test results and with disease; *FP*, false positives, or those with abnormal test results and no disease; *TN*, true negatives, or those with normal test results and no disease.
*Relative risk, or risk ratio, is the relative rate of occurrence of a disease in the group with an abnormal test result compared with those with a normal test result.
†Predictive value of an abnormal response is the percentage of individuals with an abnormal test result who have disease.

estimated directly from a test's demonstrated specificity or sensitivity. Predictive value depends on the prevalence of disease in the population tested. Table 4-1 illustrates how a test with a 70% sensitivity and a 90% specificity performs in a population with a 5% prevalence of disease. Of 10,000 men, 5%, or 500 men, have disease. The middle column of the table lists the number of men with abnormal tests, and the far right column lists the number with normal tests. Because the test is 70% sensitive, 350 of those with disease will have abnormal tests and are true positives. The remaining 150 have normal tests and are false negatives. Because the test is 90% specific, 90% of the 9500 without disease are true negatives and the remainder are false positives. To calculate the predictive value, the number of true positives is divided by the number of those with an abnormal test. Table 4-1 also shows the performance of a test with the same 70% sensitivity and 90% specificity in a population with a 50% prevalence of disease. The predictive value of an abnormal response is directly related to the prevalence of the disease in the population tested. There are more false-positive responses when exercise testing is used in a population with a low prevalence of disease than when it is used in a population with a high prevalence of disease. This fact explains the greater number of false positives found when using the test as a screening procedure in an asymptomatic group as opposed to when using it as a diagnostic procedure in patients with symptoms most likely resulting from CAD. Also, in Table 4-1 are the calculations for a test with a sensitivity and specificity of 90% and for a test with a sensitivity of 90% and a specificity of 70%.

Key Point: Predictive value is determined by the prevalence of disease in the population tested. The best way to understand this relationship is to perform the calculations in Table 4-1 for yourself.

TABLE 4-1.

Test Performance Versus Predictive Value and Risk Ratio: a Model in a Population of 10,000

Disease Prevalence	Subjects	Number with Abnormal Test Results	Test Performance	Number with Normal Test Results
5%	500 diseased	450 (TP)	90% sensitivity	50 (FN)
		350 (TP)	70% sensitivity	150 (FN)
	9500 nondiseased	2850 (FP)	70% specificity	6650 (TN)
		950 (FP)	90% specificity	8550 (TN)
50%	5000 diseased	4500 (TP)	90% sensitivity	500 (FN)
		3500 (TP)	70% sensitivity	1500 (FN)
	5000 nondiseased	1500 (FP)	70% specificity	3500 (TN)
		500 (FP)	90% specificity	4500 (TN)

	Predictive Value of Abnormal Test		Risk Ratio*	
Disease Prevalence	5	50	5	50
Sensitivity/specificity				
70%/90%	27%	88%	27	3
90%/70%	14%	75%	14	5
90%/90%	32%	90%	64	9
66%/84%	18%	80%	9	3

TP, True-positive test result; FN, false-negative test result; FP, false-positive test result; TN, true-negative test result.

*Multiplied by that for normal subjects.

Range of Characteristic Curves

Plotting sensitivity versus specificity for a range of cutoff points provide an efficient way to compare test performances. Plots are particularly helpful when optimal cutoff points for discriminating patients with disease from those without disease are not established. An optimal cutoff point can be chosen along the plotted line. A straight diagonal line indicates that the measurement or test has no discriminating power for the disease being tested. The greater the area of the curve above the diagonal line, the greater its discriminating power. Range of characteristic (ROC) curves make it possible to determine and then choose the appropriate cutoff points for the desired sensitivity or specificity. An example of an ROC curve is given in Fig 4-2.

Probability Analysis and Bayes' Theorem

After the test result is known, the information most important to a clinician attempting to make a diagnosis is the probability of the patient having the disease. Such a probability cannot be accurately estimated from the test result and the diagnostic characteristics of only the test. It also requires knowledge before the test is administered of the probability of the patient having the disease. Bayesian analysis is one technique for determining this probability. Bayes' theorem states that

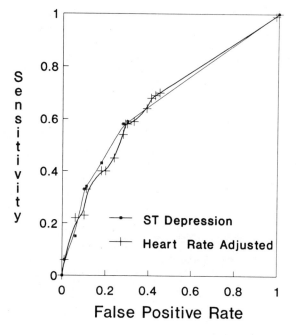

FIG 4-2.
ROC curve formed by plotting the sensitivity and specificity for a range of cutoff points.

the probability of a patient having the disease after a test is performed will be the product of the disease probability before the test and the probability that the test provided a true result.

The probability of a test result being true can be shown as the likelihood ratio, which is the ratio of true results to false results. The likelihood ratio is a direct indicator of the diagnostic value of a test: the higher it is, the greater the test's diagnostic value. In the case of an abnormal test result, the positive likelihood ratio equals the percent with disease with abnormal test sensitivity divided by the percent without disease with abnormal test specificity (calculated as *1-specificity*). In the case of a normal test result, the negative likelihood ratio equals the percent without disease with normal test specificity divided by the percent with disease with normal test sensitivity (calculated as *1-sensitivity*).

The following example shows how the ratio can be derived. Using conventional techniques of analyzing ST-segment depression with a cutoff point of 0.1 mV, the maximal or near-maximal exercise test has a sensitivity of approximately 66% and a specificity of 84%. Therefore the likelihood ratio for an abnormal test is calculated as follows:

$$\text{Positive likelihood ratio} = \frac{0.66}{1-0.84} = 4.125$$

The likelihood ratio for a normal test also follows:

$$\text{Negative likelihood ratio} = \frac{0.84}{1 - 0.66} = 2.47$$

Bayes' theorem may be expressed in the following fashion:

Posttest odds of disease = Pretest odds of disease × Likelihood ratio of results

The clinician often makes this calculation intuitively when he or she suspects as a false result the abnormal exercise test of a 30-year-old woman with chest pain (low prior odds or probability). The same abnormal response would be accepted as a true result in a 60-year-old man with angina who had a previous MI (high prior odds or probability).

Angiographic studies have been used to investigate the prevalence of significant CAD in patients with different chest pain syndromes. Because chest pain is the complaint in the majority of patients referred for a diagnostic exercise test, the nature of the pain would seem a practical basis for estimating the prior probability of CAD. Approximately 90% of the patients with true angina pectoris have significant angiographic coronary disease. In patients presenting with atypical angina pectoris, approximately 50% have significant angiographic coronary disease. *Atypical angina* refers to pain that has an unusual location, has prolonged duration, has inconsistent precipitating factors, or is unresponsive to nitroglycerin. Fig 4-3 demonstrates the calculation of the probability of CAD in such patients.

	PRE-TEST ODDS	LIKELIHOOD RATIO	POST-TEST ODDS	POST-TEST PROBABILITY
ANGINAL	9 : 1	ABNORMAL TEST (x4)	36:1	(36/37)=98%
		NORMAL TEST (x2.5)	9:2.5	(9/12)=75%
ATYPICAL ANGINA	1 : 1	ABNORMAL TEST (x4)	4:1	(4/5)=80%
		NORMAL TEST (x2.5)	1:2.5	(1/4)=25%
NON-ANGINAL	1 : 9	ABNORMAL TEST (x4)	4:9	(4/13)=31%
		NORMAL TEST (x2.5)	1:23	(1/24)=4%
ASYMPTOMATIC	1 : 19	ABNORMAL TEST (x4)	4:19	(4/23)=17%
		NORMAL TEST (x2.5)	1:48	(1/49)=2%

FIG 4-3.
Calculation of pretest and posttest probability of significant CAD based on pretest symptomatology and the likelihood ratio of the standard exercise test.

The 50-year-old male patient with typical angina pectoris has a 90% probability, or 9:1 chance, of having significant CAD. According to Bayes' theorem, an abnormal exercise test increases these odds from 9:1 to 63:1. Such an impressive change in odds, however, represents a relatively small increase in the probability of disease from 90% to 98%. Because such a patient still has a 78% probability of disease after a negative test, coronary angiography may yet be required to definitely rule out coronary disease. The greatest diagnostic impact of such probability calculations would be in patients with atypical angina. An abnormal test result would increase the odds from 1:1 to 4:1 and the probability of disease to 80%, for practical purposes, establishing the diagnosis. With a normal test, the probability of coronary disease would be reduced to 27%.

Key Point: Bayes' theorem is more helpful conceptually in clinical decision making than it is for actual probability calculation because of the wide confidence limits for predicting the presence or absence of disease.

Bayesian Versus Multivariate Analytical Techniques

To compare the relative accuracy of Bayesian analysis to discriminant function analysis, Detrano et al[3] analyzed 303 subjects referred for coronary angiography who also underwent exercise testing, thallium scintigraphy, and cinefluorosgraphy. Their results suggest that database discriminant function analysis, or multivariate anylasis, is more accurate than literature-based Bayesian analysis in predicting coronary disease based on clinical and noninvasive test results. The accuracy of the Bayesian method is questionable because it assumes independence from the population being tested and perhaps more importantly uses sensitivities and specificities derived from other patient populations with different testing protocols. Morise and Duval[4] have also presented work on this issue.

Methodological Problems with Diagnostic Studies

To determine why exercise testing remained controversial as a diagnostic test for CAD, Philbrick, Horwitz, and Feinstein undertook a methodological review of 33 studies published between 1976 and 1979 with each including at least 50 patients for a total of 7501 patients who had undergone both exercise tests and coronary angiography (Table 4-2). They found that seven methodological standards were necessary for reliable testing: (1) adequate identification of the groups selected for study, (2) adequate variety of anatomical lesions, (3) adequate analysis for relevant chest pain syndromes, (4) avoidance of a limited challenge group, (5) avoidance of workup bias, (6) avoidance of diagnostic review bias (allowing the result of the exercise test to influence the interpretation of the coronary angiogram), and (7) avoidance of test review bias (allowing when the result of the coronary angiogram to influence the interpretation of the exercise test). Of these seven methodological standards for research design, only the requirement for an

TABLE 4-2.

Angiographic Studies Evaluating the Diagnostic Value of Exercise Testing

Investigator	Year	No. of Patients	Sensitivity (%)	Specificity (%)
Hultgren	1967	55	66	100
Eliasch	1967	65	84	81
Demany	1967	75	64	49
Mason	1967	84	78	89
Kassenbaum	1968	68	47	97
Roitman	1970	100	73	82
Newton	1970	52	57	81
Fitzgibbon	1971	160	48	80
Cohn	1971	110	86	73
McConahay	1971	100	35	100
Ascoop	1971	96	59	94
Martin	1972	100	62	89
McHenry	1972	166	81	95
Kellerman	1973	74	54	96
Bartel	1974	465	65	92
Piessens	1974	70	65	83
Rios	1974	50	83	89
Sketch	1975	251	53	88
Borer	1975	89	49	41
Jelinek	1976	153	45	89
Goldschlager	1976	153	45	89
Santinga	1976	283	73	78
Detry	1977	98	55	85
Chaitman	1978	100	88	82
McNeer	1978	1222	53	91
Balnave	1978	70	81	100
Berman	1978	164	84	67
Weiner	1978	302	76	76
Chaitman	1979	200	84	72
Weiner	1979	2045	79	69
Aldrich	1979	181	40	92
Raffo	1979	100	91	96
Borer	1979	75	63	95
AVERAGES			66	84

Modified from Philbrick JT, Horwitz RI, Feinstein AR: *Am J Cardiol* 46:804, 1980.

adequate variety of anatomical lesions had received general compliance. Less than half of the studies had complied with any of the remaining six standards: adequate identification of the groups selected for study; adequate analysis for relevant chest pain syndromes; avoidance of a limited challenge group; and avoidance of bias due to workup, diagnostic review, or test review. Only one study had met as many as five standards.

These methodological problems help explain the wide range of sensitivity (35% to 88%) and specificity (41% to 100%) found for standard exercise testing. The variations could not be attributed to the usual explanations: the definition of anatomical abnormality, the technique of the exercise test, or the definition of an abnormal test. Determining the true value of exercise testing requires methodological improvements in patient selection, data collection, and data analysis. Another important but overlooked consideration is the need to exclude patients after MI. These patients most often have obstructive CAD and should not be included in diagnostic studies for detecting CAD; instead they can be included in studies to predict disease severity.

Two other problems in determining specificity are including enough individuals with normal results and defining *normal*. Should normal mean low-risk individuals or patients without significant angiographic disease?[6,7] If low-risk subjects are used, the problem of the test only presenting them with a limited challenge must be confronted. In addition, maximum heart rate is higher relative to age for low-risk subjects than for a patient group. As a result, heart rate appears to be a much more useful discriminator than it actually is in a clinical population.

A basic step in applying any test to distinguish patients without disease from those with disease is to determine a value measured by the test that best separates the two groups (i.e., the discriminant value, or cutoff point). Cutoff points cannot absolutely discriminate because those with and without disease have overlapping values. This overlap explains why sensitivity and specificity are inversely related: If you increase one by using a certain cutoff point, you decrease the other.

Gianrossi et al[8] recently used metaanalysis to investigate the variability of the reported diagnostic accuracy of the exercise ECG. A total of 147 consecutively published reports, involving 24,074 patients who underwent coronary angiography and exercise testing, were summarized and the results entered into a computer spreadsheet. Details regarding population characteristics and methods were entered, including publication year, number of ECG leads, exercise protocol, pre-exercise hyperventilation, definition of abnormal ST-segment response, exclusion of certain subgroups, and blinding of test interpretation. Wide variability in sensitivity and specificity was found: The mean sensitivity was 68% with a range of 23% to 100% and a standard deviation of 16%; the mean specificity was 77% with a range of 17% to 100% and a standard deviation of 17%.

Sensitivity was found to be significantly and independently related to the following study characteristics:

1. The method of dealing with equivocal or nondiagnostic tests: Sensitivity decreased when these tests were considered normal.
2. Comparison with a "better" test (e.g., thallium scintigraphy): The sensitivity of the exercise ECG was lower when the study compared it with another testing method being reported as "superior."
3. Exclusion of patients on digitalis: Exclusion of patients taking digitalis was associated with improved sensitivity.
4. Publication year: An increase in sensitivity and decrease in specificity were noted over the years the exercise test has been used. This phenomenon may result from the fact that as clinicians become more familiar with a test and increasingly trust its results, they allow its results to influence the decision to perform angiography.

Specificity was found to be significantly and independently related to four variables:

1. Treatment of upsloping ST-segment depression: When upsloping ST-segment depression was classified as abnormal, specificity was lowered significantly (73% versus 80%).
2. Exclusion or inclusion of subjects with prior MI: The exclusion of patients with prior MI was associated with a decreased specificity.
3. Exclusion or inclusion of patients with left bundle branch block: The specificity increased when patients with left bundle branch block were excluded.
4. Use of preexercise hyperventilation: This was associated with a decreased specificity.

Stepwise linear regression explained less than 35% of the variance in sensitivities and specificities reported in the 147 publications. This wide variability in the reported accuracy of the exercise ECG is not explained by the information available in the published reports. Though the variablity could be explained by unsuspected technical, methodological, or clinical variables that affect test performance by poorly understood mechanisms, it is more likely that the authors of the 147 reports did not disclose important information or did not consider the critical features known to affect test performance when performing and analyzing their studies.

Key Point: The wide variability in test performance makes it important that clinicians apply rigorous control of the methods they use for testing and analysis. ST-segment depression should be measured at the end of the QRS segment (ST∅ or J junction); upsloping ST-segment depression should be considered a borderline or negative result, and hyperventilation should not be performed before testing.

Guyatt[9] recommends that two criteria must be applied to judge the credibility and applicability of studies evaluating diagnostic tests. First, the evaluation must include clearly defined comparison groups, at least one of which is free of the disease of interest. The studies should include consecutive patients or randomly selected patients for whom the diagnosis is in doubt. Any diagnostic test appears to function well if obviously normal subjects are compared with those who obviously have the disease in question. In most cases, we do not need sophisticated testing to differentiate the normal population from the sick. Rather, we are interested in examining patients who are suspected but not known to have the disease of interest and in differentiating those who do from those who do not. If the patients enrolled in the study do not represent this "diagnostic dilemma" group, then the test may perform well in the study, but it may not perform well in clinical practice. In addition, patients who have had MI should not be included in studies attempting to distinguish those with disease from those without disease, although they may be included in studies to predict disease severity.

The second "believability" criterion requires an independent, "blind" comparison of the test with the performance of a "gold" standard. The gold standard should measure a clinically important state. For example, for CAD an invasive test, such as catheterization, is used as the gold standard rather than only chest pain. The gold standard result should not be available to those interpreting the test. Also, if the gold standard requires subjective interpretation (as would be the case even for coronary angiography), the interpreter should not know the test result. Blinding the interpreters of the test to the gold standard and vice versa minimizes the risk of bias.

If these two criteria are met, a study can be used as a basis for performing a test in clinical practice. To apply the test properly to patients, the following must be considered. Most tests merely indicate an increase or decrease in the probability of disease. To apply imperfect tests appropriately, the probability of disease must be estimated before the test is done (*pretest probability*), then this probability is revised according to the test result.

The clinician's estimate of pretest probability is based on the patient's history (including age, gender, and chest pain characteristics), the physical examination and initial testing, and the clinician's own experience with this type of problem. Although forming accurate estimates from examination and experience may sound difficult, it is what we implicitly do; we just do not usually make the estimates explicit. A lack of symptoms makes the pretest probability so low that a positive test result is most likely not to be associated with disease. Typical angina makes the pretest probability of disease so high that the test result does not affect diagnosis much. Atypical angina indicates a 50% chance of disease; therefore the test result affects the diagnosis. Thus the pretest probability determines interpretation of the test result. You can use the pretest probability from the chosen study as a guide, especially if the patients were randomly selected from a defined group or were in a consecutive series and if the clinical setting was similar to your own. Even then, the findings from the patient must be taken into account.

Sensitivity (the proportion of patients with disease in whom the test is positive) and specificity (the proportion of those without disease in whom the test is negative) must be taken into account. Calculating sensitivity and specificity is still the best way to use tests that yield yes/no results. For tests in which there are more than two possible results, a strongly positive result increases the probability more than a moderately positive result. Sensitivity and specificity can be presented in likelihood ratios, but a simple nomogram (Fig 4-4) can also be used to avoid calculations.[10]

SIGNIFICANCE AND EFFECT OF RESTING ST-SEGMENT DEPRESSION

Additional modalities to complement exercise testing have been developed to increase the diagnostic accuracy of exercise testing, especially for subsets of patients in whom standard exercise ECG is compromised such as those with resting ST-segment depression. (However, the additional expense of these modalities may limit their widespread applicability.) Resting ST-segment depression has been identified as a marker for adverse cardiac events in patients with and without

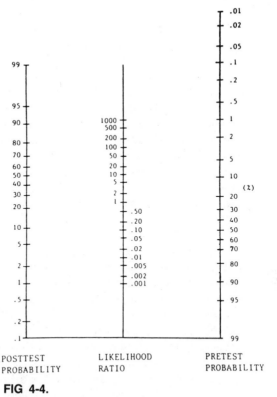

FIG 4-4.
Pretest and posttest nomogram.

known CAD.[11] In patients with resting ST-segment depression, the criterion of at least 2 mm of additional exercise-induced ST-segment depression has been a particularly useful marker for diagnosing coronary disease (a positive likelihood ratio of 3.4). Patients with resting ST-segment depression and a prior MI had a 2.5 times higher prevalence of severe CAD than patients without resting ST-segment depression (43% versus 17% prevalence, 95% confidence interval for observed difference [9% to 43%, $p < 0.001$]) and also had larger left ventricles after infarction. To identify severe CAD in postinfarction patients with persistent resting ST-segment depression, the criteria of at least 2 mm of additional exercise-induced ST-segment depression (a positive likelihood ratio of 3) and of the persistance of additional exercise-induced ST-segment depression at least 4 minutes into recovery (a positive likelihood ratio of 3.6) were better markers than the standard criterion of at least 1 mm of additional ST-segment depression (a positive likelihood ratio of 1.7). Receiver-operating characteristic curve analysis revealed that additional exercise-induced ST-segment depression continued to discriminate between those with or without any or severe coronary disease despite having baseline ST-segment depression at rest. After a cumulative follow-up of 4.4 years, patients with resting ST-segment depression with or without prior MI had a lower infarct-free survival rate than those without it. Therefore resting ST-segment depression not caused by left ventricular hypertrophy, conduction defects, or drug effects is a marker for a higher prevalence of severe CAD with a poor prognosis, and standard exercise testing continues to be diagnostically useful in these patients.

For diagnosing CAD in patients without a prior MI, the criteria of at least 2 mm of additional exercise-induced ST-segment depression and downsloping ST-segment depression during recovery were particularly effective. For the diagnosis of severe coronary disease in patients who had survived an MI, the criteria of at least 2 mm of additional exercise-induced ST-segment depression and prolonged recovery ST-segment depression were better markers than the standard criterion. Using other criteria, in addition to the standard criterion of at least 1 mm of additional ST-segment depression, appears to improve the diagnostic accuracy of standard exercise testing for this type of patient.[12-16] ST-segment depression persisting late into recovery is associated with severe disease.[17,18]

Key Point: Patients who had resting ST-segment depression on their baseline ECGs that was not caused by left ventricular hypertrophy, conduction defects, or drug effects have a higher prevalence of severe CAD and a poorer long-term prognosis than patients without resting ST-segment depression. Exercise-induced ST-segment depression therefore continues to have discriminatory power for the diagnosis of CAD in these patients. For the diagnosis of CAD in patients without a prior MI, the criteria of at least 2 mm of additional exercise-induced ST-segment depression and the appearance of downsloping ST-segment depression during recovery were particularly effective markers. For the diagnosis of severe coronary disease in patients who had survived an MI, the criteria of at least 2 mm of additional exercise-induced ST-segment depression and prolonged recovery ST-segment depression were better markers than the standard criterion.

ALTERNATE CRITERIA FOR PATIENTS ON DIGOXIN

Digoxin use at the time of exercise testing has been thought to invalidate the predictive value of exercise ECG as a marker for CAD. Therefore Miranda[19] performed an analysis to ascertain whether alternate methods of interpreting the exercise ECG could improve its clinical utility in patients receiving digoxin. The study found that men with resting ST-segment depression not due to conduction defects, left ventricular hypertrophy, or drug effects were more likely to have severe coronary disease and a poorer long-term prognosis than men without this abnormality on their baseline ECG. The exercise ECG therefore contains useful diagnostic information on patients who receive digoxin but only if criteria in addition to 1 mm of ST-segment depression are considered. A metaanalysis of 150 exercise testing studies over the past 22 years was performed by Detrano, Gianrossi, and Froelicher[16] to identify factors that affected the exercise test's diagnostic accuracy. There were 64 studies that included patients on digoxin during exercise testing and 21 studies that specifically excluded patients on digoxin; the mean sensitivity and specificity were both higher in the latter group of studies. A study by Meyers et al[15] also showed decreased diagnostic accuracy of exercise testing in patients on digoxin. These results support the argument of Sundqvist, Atterhog, and Jogestrand[20] that the standard criterion of 1 mm of exercise-induced ST-segment depression is inadequate for identifying CAD in the patient on digoxin. However, persistence of exercise-induced ST-segment depression at least 4 minutes into recovery and the development of downsloping ST-segment depression during recovery are reasonable markers for CAD in these same patients.

BETA-BLOCKER THERAPY

Herbert et al[21] have demonstrated that the ST-segment response and diagnostic testing are not affected by beta-blocker therapy. Their sample was composed of 200 middle-aged men referred for exercise testing to evaluate possible or definite CAD and subgrouped according to beta-blocker administration as initiated by their referring physician. They were tested using the standard ST criterion, and no differences in test performance were found between those treated with beta-blockers and those not treated. Therefore for routine exercise testing in the clinical setting, it appears unnecessary for physicians to accept the risk of stopping beta-blockers before testing when a patient is exhibiting possible symptoms of ischemia. Their results are illustrated in Fig 4-5.

INFERIOR LEAD ST-SEGMENT DEPRESSION

Miranda et al[22] found that exercise-induced ST-segment depression in inferior limb leads is a poor marker in and of itself for CAD. Precordial lead V_5 alone consistently outperformed the inferior lead and the combination of leads V_5 and II because lead II had such a high false-positive rate (Fig 4-6). Blackburn and Katigbak[23] studied 100 consecutive patients and found that lead V_5 alone detected 89% of ischemic ST-segment responses. Miller, Desser, and Lawson[24] evaluated 44 consecutive patients who had both abnormal exercise tests and perfusion defects on thallium-201 scintigraphy. Although 30 patients (68%) had ST-segment changes in the inferior leads, they also had concomitant ST-segment changes in leads V_4, V_5, or both, which lead to the conclusion that monitoring the inferior leads rarely provides additional diagnostic information. Mason et al[25] found that in 67 patients with angina who underwent exercise testing, 19 showed an abnormal ECG response in only one lead (a total of seven leads were monitored), but of these only 2 were isolated to lead II alone. Sketch et al[26] had seven patients manifest ST-segment depression in lead II only without concomitant ECG changes in lead V_5, but only three of these responses were true positives.

These studies support the argument that exercise-induced ST-segment depression in lead V_5 is an excellent marker for coronary disease and that inferior lead

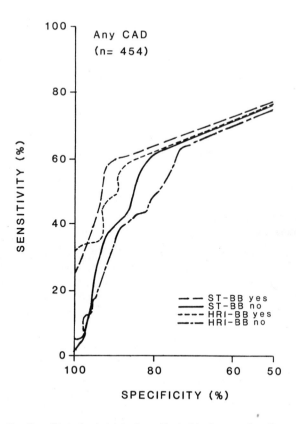

FIG 4-5.
ROC curve illustrating the effect of administration of beta-blockers on the diagnostic characteristics of the standard exercise ECG.

depression provides little additional diagnostic information. Riff and Carleton[27] studied patients with atrioventricular dissociation and demonstrated that atrial repolarization can cause J-junction depression in the inferior leads, which may produce the false-positive responses. Nevertheless, even though exercise-induced inferior lead ST-segment depression is not a reliable, independent marker for the diagnosis of CAD, when combined with segment depression in other leads, it is helpful for diagnosing severe ischemia, since the involvement of multiple leads has been associated with multivessel[28] and left main coronary disease.[29] However, it does not localize right coronary involvement.[30]

Key Point: In patients without prior MI and with normal resting ECGs, precordial lead V_5 alone is a reliable marker for CAD, and the monitoring of inferior limb leads adds little additional diagnostic information. Exercise-induced ST-segment depression confined to the inferior leads is of little value for the identification of coronary disease.

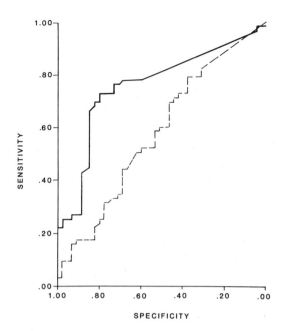

FIG 4-6.
ROC curve comparing ST-segment measurements in inferior leads (the dashed line is nearly straight, implying no separation) with those in lateral leads (*solid line*) for diagnosing significant angiographic CAD.

SUMMARY

In studies that took into account the number of coronary arteries involved, all found increasing sensitivity of the test as more vessels were involved. The most false negatives have been found among patients with single-vessel disease, particularly if the diseased vessel was not the left anterior descending artery. No matter what techniques are used, there is a reciprocal relationship between sensitivity and specificity. The more specific a test is (i.e., the more able it is to determine who is without disease), the less sensitive it is (i.e., the less able it is to determine who has disease) and vice versa. The values for sensitivity and specificity can be altered by adjusting the criterion used for determining an abnormal response. For instance, when the criterion for an abnormal exercise-induced ST-segment response is altered to a 0.2-mV depression, making it more specific for CAD, the sensitivity of the test will be reduced by half. For unknown reasons, the specificity of the ST-segment response is decreased when ST-segment depression is isolated to the inferior leads and when the test is used in women and in patients who have ST-segment depression at rest, left ventricular hypertrophy, vasoregulatory abnormalities, and mitral valve prolapse.

The standard criterion of 1 mm of exercise-induced ST-segment depression fails to distinguish between patients with or without CAD if they are taking digoxin at the time of exercise testing. However, persistence of exercise-induced

ST-segment depression at least 4 minutes into recovery and development of downsloping ST-segment depression during recovery are better markers for CAD in these same patients. Patients with a resting ST-segment depression on their baseline ECG not related to left ventricular hypertrophy, conduction defects, or drug effects have a higher prevalence of severe CAD and a poorer long-term prognosis than patients without resting ST-segment depression. Exercise-induced ST-segment depression continues to have discriminatory power for the diagnosis of CAD in these patients. For the diagnosis of CAD in patients without a prior MI, the criteria of at least 2 mm of additional exercise-induced ST-segment depression and downsloping ST-segment depression during recovery are particularly effective markers. For the diagnosis of severe coronary disease in patients who had survived a prior MI, the criteria of at least 2 mm of additional exercise-induced ST-segment depression and prolonged recovery ST-segment depression are better markers than the standard criterion. An understanding of predictive modeling (the effect of disease prevalence on positive predictive value) and Bayesian statistics (pretest and posttest probability and likelihood ratios) is important for the clinician. In addition, the rules by Philbrick, Horwitz, and Feinstein[5] and Guyatt[9] outlined are important for assessing new diagnostic techniques.

REFERENCES

1. Wilson RF et al: Accuracy of exercise electrocardiography in detecting physiologically significant coronary arterial lesions, *Circulation* 83:412-421, 1991.
2. Pellinen TJ et al: Coronary collateral circulation, *Clin Cardiol* 14:111-118, 1991.
3. Detrano R et al: Bayesian analysis versus discriminant function analysis: their relative utility in the diagnosis of coronary disease, *Circulation* 73:970-977, 1986.
4. Morise AP, Duval RD: Comparison of three Bayesian methods to estimate posttest probility in patients undergoing exercise stress testing, *Am J Cardiol* 64:1117-1122, 1989.
5. Philbrick JT, Horwitz RI, Feinstein AR: Methodologic problems of exercise testing for coronary artery disease: groups, analysis and bias, *Am J Cardiol* 46:807-816, 1980.
6. Rosanski A et al: The declining specificity of exercise radionuclide ventriculography, *New Engl J Med* 309:518-522, 1983.
7. Detrano R et al: Bayesian probility analysis: a prospective demonstration of its clinical utility in diagnosing coronary disease, *Circulation* 69:541-550, 1984.
8. Gianrossi R et al: Exercise-induced ST depression in the diagnosis of coronary artery disease: a metaanalysis, *Circulation* 80:87-98, 1989.
9. Guyatt GH: Readers' guide for articles evaluating diagnostic tests: what ACP Journal Club does for you and what you must do yourself, *ACP Journal Club* 115:A-16, 1991.
10. Fagan TJ: Nomogram for Bayes theorem, *New Engl J Med* 293:257-258, 1975.
11. Miranda CP, Lehmann KG, Froelicher VF: Correlation between resting ST segment depression, exercise testing, coronary angiography, and long-term prognosis, *Am Heart J* 122:1617-1626, 1991.
12. Kansal S, Roitman D, Sheffield LT: Stress testing with ST-segment depression at rest, *Circulation* 54:636-639, 1976.
13. Harris et al: Value and limitations of exercise testing in detecting coronary disease with normal and abnormal resting electrocardiograms, *Adv Cardiol* 22:11-15, 1978.

14. Roitman D, Jones WB, Sheffield LT: Comparison of submaximal exercise ECG test with coronary cineangiocardiogram, *Ann Intern Med* 72:641-647, 1970.

15. Meyers DG et al: The effect of baseline electrocardiographic abnormalities on the diagnostic accuracy of exercise-induced ST-segment changes, *Am Heart J* 119:272-276, 1990.

16. Detrano R, Gianrossi R, Froelicher VF: The diagnostic accuracy of the exercise electrocardiogram: a meta-analysis of 22 years of research, *Progr Cardiovasc Dis* 33:173-205, 1989.

17. Goldschlager N, Selzer A, Cohn K: Treadmill stress tests as indicators of presence and severity of coronary artery disease, *Ann Intern Med* 85:277-286, 1976.

18. Callaham PR, Thomas L, Ellestad MH: Prolonged ST-segment depression following exercise predicts significant proximal left coronary artery stenosis, *Circulation* 76(suppl IV):IV-253, 1987 (abstract).

19. Miranda C: Alternate criteria for interpretation of the examination for patients receiving digoxin, *Ann Intern Med,* in press.

20. Sundqvist K, Atterhog JH, Jogestrand T: Effect of digoxin on the electrocardiogram at rest and during exercise in healthy subjects, *Am J Cardiol* 57:661-665, 1986.

21. Herbert WG et al: Effect of β-blockade on the interpretation of the exercise ECG: ST level versus ST/HR index, *Am Heart J* 122:993-1000, 1991.

22. Miranda CP et al: Usefulness of exercise-induced ST-segment depression in the inferior leads during exercise testing as a marker for coronary artery disease, *Am J Cardiol* 69:303-308, 1992.

23. Blackburn H, Katigbak R: What electrocardiographic leads to take after exercise? *Am Heart J* 67:184-188, 1964.

24. Miller TD, Desser KB, Lawson M: How many electrocardiographic leads are required for exercise treadmill tests? *J Electrocardiol* 20:131-137, 1987.

25. Mason RE et al: Multiple-lead exercise electrocardiography: experience in 107 normal subjects and 67 patients with angina pectoris, and comparison with coronary cinearteriography in 84 patients, *Circulation* 36:517-525, 1967.

26. Sketch MH et al: Reliability of single-lead and multiple-lead electrocardiography during and after exercise, *Chest* 74:394-401, 1978.

27. Riff DP, Carleton RA: Effect of exercise on the atrial recovery wave, *Am Heart J* 81:759-763, 1971.

28. Weiner DA, McCabe CH, Ryan TJ: Prognostic assessment of patients with coronary artery disease by exercise testing, *Am Heart J* 105:749-755, 1983.

29. Weiner DA, McCabe CH, Ryan TJ: Identification of patients with left main and three vessel coronary disease with clinical and exercise test variables, *Am J Cardiol* 46:21-27, 1980.

30. Mark DB et al: Localizing coronary artery obstructions with the exercise treadmill test, *Ann Intern Med* 106:53-55, 1987.

CHAPTER 5

Prognostic Applications of the Exercise Test

RATIONALE

There are two principal reasons for estimating prognosis. The first reason is to provide accurate answers to patient's questions regarding the probable outcome of their illness. Most patients find this information useful in planning their affairs regarding work, recreational activities, personal estates, and finances. The second reason to estimate prognosis is to identify patients in whom interventions might improve outcome. The exercise test has been demonstrated to be of value for estimating prognosis not only in patients with stable symptoms but also in new patients, such as those with uncompleted infarcts due to thrombolytic therapy,[1] those with non–Q-wave myocardial infarctions (MIs),[2] and those who have had unstable angina.[3,4] A study evaluating the appropriateness of performing coronary angiography in clinical practice concluded that angiography was inappropriate nearly a fourth of the time, mainly because of failure to obtain an exercise test.[5] Since angiography is performed at rest and does not usually quantitate coronary blood flow,[6] the resulting patterns are static, although patients with certain known coronary pathoanatomical patterns are conferred a survival benefit from bypass surgery.[7] To deliver cost-effective health care, an effort has been made to use decision analysis based on clinical and exercise test variables to decide who should undergo cardiac catheterization.[8,9] This chapter will deal with estimating prognosis for patients with stable coronary artery disease (CAD); Chapter 6 will cover testing patients after MIs, and Chapter 7 will discuss screening asymptomatic individuals.

PATHOPHYSIOLOGY

The basic pathophysiological features of CAD that determine prognosis include the risk of arrhythmia, the amount of remaining myocardium (reflected by left ventricular [LV] function), and the amount of myocardium put in jeopardy by ischemia. Dysrhythmias are not independently predictive of CAD or prognosis but are closely related to LV abnormalities. What exercise test responses are due to myocardial ischemia or dysfunction? The exercise responses caused by ischemia include angina, ST-segment depression, and ST-segment elevation over electrocardiogram (ECG) areas without Q waves. Predicting the amount of ischemia (i.e., the amount of myocardium in jeopardy), however, is difficult. It appears to be inversely related to the double product at the onset of signs or symptoms of ischemia. The exercise responses caused by ischemia or LV dysfunction include chronotropic incompetence, or heart rate impairment;[10] a drop in systolic blood pressure;[11] and a poor exercise capacity.[12] The dual association of ischemia and LV dysfunction explains why they are so important in predicting prognosis. Exercise-induced dysrhythmias indicate electrical instability most often caused by LV dysfunction rather than ischemia (except for ST-segment elevation in a normal ECG that is very arrythmogenic) and do not appear to have independent predictive power.

The only exercise response specifically associated with LV dysfunction is ST-segment elevation over diagnostic Q waves. This response indicates that these patients have depressed LV function and possibly larger aneurysms and thus are at higher risk than those whose Q waves do not exhibit ST-segment elevation.[13,14]

Previous studies have shown that exercise capacity poorly correlates with LV function in patients without signs or symptoms of right-sided heart failure.[15] Exercise testing is not very helpful in identifying patients with moderate LV dysfunction. LV dysfunction is better recognized by a history of congestive heart failure (CHF) or by physical examination, resting ECG,[16] echocardiogram, or radionuclide ventriculography.

Can we decide who needs to undergo cardiac catheterization among patients with stable CAD? Making such a decision is easy when symptoms cannot be controlled, but otherwise it is often difficult to decide who should be considered for intervention to prolong life.

STATISTICAL METHODS

To determine which patients need cardiac catheterization, follow-up studies must be performed and the special statistical methods of survival analysis applied. Survival analysis consists of a group of univariate and multivariate mathematical techniques that use person-time units of exposure to calculate hazard or risk. The key difference between it and other statistical methods is that it takes into account when a patient is removed from exposure as a result of being lost to follow-up or removed from risk (e.g., by undergoing coronary artery bypass surgery [CABS] or percutaneous transluminal coronary angioplasty [PTCA] or as a result of the study being terminated). Comparisons are made between person-time units of survival and of exposure. For example, consider two groups of 100 patients; both have 10 deaths in a year of follow-up (a 10% mortality). However, in one group, all 10 die at the beginning of the year, and in the other group they all die at the end of the year. The former situation certainly would have a worse significance than the latter but only would be detected by appropriate survival analysis and not by simple proportion testing (because both had a 10% death rate).

The two most commonly used survival analysis techniques are the Kaplan-Meier survival curve for univariate analysis and the Cox proportional hazards model for multivariate analysis. Multivariate analysis is necessary because many of the variables interact. Variables can be univariately associated with death, but the association may be through other variables. For instance, digoxin use is associated with death through CHF, and exercise-induced ST-segment elevation is associated with death most often through the underlying Q waves.

This chapter will discuss studies that have used exercise testing in patients with stable coronary heart disease to predict the following:

1. Angiographic findings
2. Cardiovascular disease endpoints
3. Improved survival with coronary artery bypass surgery

In addition, a special group of follow-up studies that included variables from clinical assessment and the resting ECG, the exercise test, and cardiac catheterization will be considered separately. These studies utilized multivariate statistical models to determine which variables best predicted prognosis and permitted simple metaanalysis.

Predicting Angiographic Findings

To determine which clinical characteristics obtained by a physician during an initial clinical examination are important for estimating the likelihood of triple-vessel or left main CAD and to determine whether estimates based on these characteristics remain valid when applied prospectively and in different patient groups, Pryor et al[17] examined clinical characteristics predictive of severe disease in 6435 consecutive symptomatic patients referred for suspected CAD between 1969 and 1983. A total of 11 of 23 characteristics were important for estimating the likelihood of severe angiographic disease. These included type of chest pain, history of previous MI, age, sex, duration of chest pain symptoms, risk factors, carotid bruit, and chest pain frequency. A model using these characteristics accurately estimated the likelihood of severe disease in an independent sample of 2342 patients. The model also accurately estimated the prevalence of severe disease in large series of patients reported in the literature.

A similar study was performed by Hubbard et al[18] from the Mayo Clinic. Five variables were found to be predictive of severe disease: age, gender, diabetes, typical angina, and history of prior MI. An international cross-validation study was performed by Detrano et al,[19] who concluded that use of their algorithm could avert at least 10 angiograms on patients with less severe disease for every missed case of severe disease. These studies demonstrate that the clinician's initial evaluation can identify patients at high or low risk of anatomically severe CAD.

Table 5-1 summarizes some of the angiographic studies that have tried to predict left main CAD using exercise testing.[20-22] Different criteria have been used with varying results. *Predictive value* here refers to the percentage of those with

TABLE 5-1.

Studies Evaluating the Predictive Value and Sensitivity of the Exercise Test for Identifying Patients with Left Main Coronary Artery Disease

Principle Investigator	Year	No. With Left Main Disease (Total)	Criterion	Predictive Value (%)	Sensitivity (%)
Cheitlin	1975	11 (106)	0.2 mV depression	24	100
Goldschlager	1976	15 (410)	0.1 mV downsloping	8	67
McNeer	1978	108 (1472)	0.1 mV in stage I and II	23	47
Nixon	1979	26 (115)	Angina or 0.1 mV depression at low work load	19 26	96 54
Levites, Anderson	1978	11 (75)	0.2 mV depression abnormal in stage I	50 24	82 63
Morris	1978	18 (460)	Exertional hypotension	14	17
Sanmarco	1980	29 (378)	0.3 mV only	15	24
			Exertional hypotension	15	28
			Both	27	35
Blumenthal	1981	14 (40)	0.2 mV depression	38	100
			Anterior and inferior depression	57	93
			Exertional hypotension	75	21
Weiner	1981	35 (436)	Strongly positive	32	74
			Exertional hypotension	23	23

Predictive value, Percentage of those with abnormal response who have left main disease as defined by criteria; *sensitivity,* percentage of those with left main disease who have an abnormal response as defined by the investigators.

the abnormal criteria who actually had left main disease. Naturally, most of the false positives actually had CAD but less severe forms of it. *Sensitivity* here refers to the percentage of those with left main disease who are detected. Because these criteria have been refined over time, the study by Weiner[23] using the Coronary Artery Surgery study (CASS) data deserves further mention. Weiner defined a markedly positive exercise test response as shown in the box. This definition was based on a study of 436 consecutive patients referred for suspected or known CAD who were able to undergo exercise testing and coronary angiography. Patients with left main disease were distinguished as a group from patients with triple-vessel disease by an early onset and longer persistence of ST-segment de-

---

STRONGLY POSITIVE RESPONSE OF WEINER FROM CORONARY ARTERY SURGERY STUDY

More than 0.2 mV downsloping ST-segment depression
Involvement of five or more leads with ST-segment depression
Occurrence of ST-segment depression at less than 5 METs
Prolonged ST-segment depression late into recovery

pression and by a greater number of leads in which the depression occurred. A fall in systolic blood pressure (SBP) occurred in 23% of patients with left main disease versus 17% of those with triple-vessel disease and 6% of those with single- or double-vessel disease. As an indicator of left main or triple-vessel CAD, a fall in SBP had a predictive value of 66% and a sensitivity of 19%. The criterion of 0.2 mV or more of ST-segment depression occurred in 44% of such patients and had only a slightly lower predictive value (64%). Analysis of combined test variables disclosed that the development of 0.2 mV or more of downsloping ST-segment depression beginning at 4 metabolic equivalents (METs), persisting for at least 6 minutes into recovery and involving at least five ECG leads, had the greatest sensitivity (74%) and predictive value (32%) for left main coronary disease. This abnormal pattern identified left main or triple-vessel disease with a sensitivity of 49%, a specificity of 92%, and a predictive value of 74%.

It appears that individual clinical or exercise test variables are unable to detect left main coronary disease because of their low sensitivity or predictive value. However, a combination of the amount, pattern, and duration of ST-segment response was highly predictive and reasonably sensitive for left main or triple-vessel coronary disease. The question still remains of how to identify those with abnormal resting ejection fractions who will benefit the most with improved survival after CABS. Perhaps those with a normal resting ECG will not need surgery for increased longevity because of the associated high probability of normal ventricular function. Blumenthal et al[24] validated the ability of a strongly positive exercise test response to predict left main coronary disease even in patients with minimal or no angina.

Lee, Cook, and Goldman,[25] using excellent statistical methods and considering many clinical and exercise test variables, found only three variables to help predict left main disease: angina type, age, and the amount of exercise-induced ST-segment depression. Using a Bayesian approach, they found that the pretest likelihood of left main disease was best determined by the type of angina and by age. In spite of the many clinical markers considered, such as unstable angina and history of MI, only age and angina type were found best for predicting pretest probability of disease. The only exercise test variable that was found to then improve the posttest probability was the amount of ST-segment depression.

Metaanalytic Studies Predicting Angiographic Severity

To evaluate the variability in the reported accuracy of the exercise ECG for predicting severe coronary disease, Detrano et al[26] applied metaanalysis to 60 consecutively published reports comparing exercise-induced ST-segment depression with coronary angiographic findings. The 60 reports included 62 distinct study groups composed of 12,030 patients who underwent both tests. Technical and methodological factors were analyzed. Wide variability in sensitivity and specificity was found (mean sensitivity of 86% [range from 40% to 100%, standard deviation of 12%]; mean specificity of 53% [range from 17% to 100%, standard deviation of 16%]) for left main or triple-vessel disease. All three variables found to be significantly and independently related to sensitivity were methodological: the exclusion of patients with right bundle branch block, the comparison with another exercise test thought to be superior in accuracy, and the exclusion of patients taking digitalis. Exclusion of patients with right bundle branch block and comparison with a "better" exercise test were both significantly associated with sensitivity for the prediction of triple-vessel disease or left main CAD. Unfortunately, this study did not consider the effect of the criterion for changes in ST segment.

Hartz, Gammaitoni, and Young[27] did consider the effect of the ST criterion when they compiled results from the literature on the use of the exercise test to identify patients with severe CAD. Estimates of sensitivity and specificity were pooled to determine the ability of the exercise test to identify triple-vessel or left main CAD. The criterion of 1 mm of ST-segment depression averaged a sensitivity of 75% and a specificity of 66%, and the criterion of 2 mm averaged a sensitivity of 52% and a specificity of 86%. This large variability among the studies in the estimated sensitivity and specificity of a given criterion for severe CAD could not be explained by reported variations in study design.

Statistical Methods for Predicting Disease Severity

Controversy currently exists regarding the most appropriate statistical methods for predicting severe CAD. The most common methods used include Bayesian statistics and discriminant function analysis. The Bayesian approach, which considers pretest clinical variables, is a logical method in clinical practice and helps the clinician decide which tests are appropriate. However, most statisticians believe that discriminant function analysis permits a more robust prediction of disease. As previously noted, Lee, Cook, and Goldman,[25] using the Bayesian approach, found that the only pretest clinical variable with predictive power for left main disease was the type of chest pain and the only exercise test variable with predictive power was the amount of ST-segment depression. The results of the Lee study were controversial, though, since pretest factors such as prior MI and other exercise test variables, including exercise capacity and SBP response, are considered important predictors of severe disease. Therefore we decided to apply discriminant function analysis to determine whether similar results would be obtained.[28]

Discriminant function analysis revealed that the maximum amount of horizontal or downsloping ST-segment depression in exercise or recovery was the most powerful predictor of disease severity, with 2 mm ST-segment depression yielding a sensitivity of 55% and specificity of 80% for prediction of severe angiographic disease (either triple-vessel disease or left main disease). Patients with increasingly severe disease also demonstrated a greater frequency of abnormal hemodynamic responses to exercise.

Our findings suggested that the exercise test would best distinguish left main, or left main–equivalent, disease only when there was significant disease in the right coronary artery (i.e., similar to triple-vessel disease). Otherwise, the exercise responses would be similar to patients with double-vessel disease. Ribisl's study[29] showed, in fact, that left main disease produced responses significantly different from triple-vessel disease only when it was accompanied by a 70% or greater narrowing of the right coronary artery. Ribisl had studied 607 male patients to determine whether patterns and severity of CAD could be predicted using standard clinical and exercise test data and found that there were significant differences in

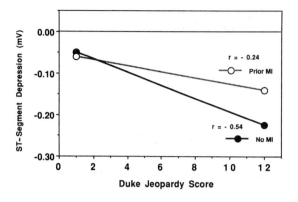

FIG 5-1.

Relationship of Duke Coronary Artery Jeopardy Score with ST-segment depression in patients with and without prior MI demonstrating that the correlation is better if patients with lesions supplying infarcted tissue are excluded from analysis.

clinical, hemodynamic, and ECG measurements among patients with progressively increasing disease severity determined by angiography.

Several related issues have also been studied: the correlation of ST-segment shift with a coronary jeopardy score, the impact of dividing the ST-segment shift by the change in heart rate (the ST/HR index), and the effect of beta-blockers on exercise test response. Fig 5-1 illustrates the correlation of the maximum amount of abnormal ST-segment depression during exercise or recovery with the Duke Coronary Artery Jeopardy Score. It shows that viable ischemic myocardium correlates better with ST-segment depression in patients with no MI than in patients with diseased vessels caused by dead myocardium (MI patients). Fig 5-2 illustrates that the exercise test does not function worse in patients treated with beta-blockers and that standard ST analysis outperforms the ST/HR index in either situation.[30] The ST/HR index findings are in agreement with those in the report of Bobbio et al,[31] which included data from 10 centers.

Predicting Cardiac Endpoints

Two of the many studies that predicted prognosis in chronic stable CAD are summarized in Table 5-2: the study from Duke University by McNeer et al[22] and the

TABLE 5-2.

Two Studies Using the Exercise Test to Predict Prognosis in Patients with Stable CAD

Investigator	Patients	Follow-Up Period	High Risk	Low Risk
McNeer	1472	1 year	>1 mm of ST-segment depression at <7 METs (higher if MHR <120)	No ST depression, >13 METs, or MHR >160
Weiner	4083	4 years	CHF or 1 mm of ST-segment depression at <5 METs	>13 METs

MHR, Maximum heart rate.

study from the CASS data by Weiner et al.[23] Both studied over 1000 patients and had at least a 1-year follow-up. In the Duke study, those at high risk had more than 1 mm of ST-segment depression at less than 7 METs; the risk was even higher if the maximum heart rate was less than 120. Those at low risk did not have ST-segment depression, were able to exceed 13 METs, or had a maximum heart rate of over 160. CASS patients at high risk had markers of CHF or ST-segment depression at a low workload (less than 5 METs). Patients able to exceed 13 METs were at low risk regardless of their other responses.

The study by Podrid, Graboys, and Lown[32] has placed some doubt on the use of exercise testing to identify high-risk patients. They contend that the prevailing view "that patients with marked amounts of ST depression have far advanced multivessel disease and that CABS is the only way to improve their outlook" is in error. In their select group of patients with normal ventricular function who were referred because of profound ST-segment depression, they did not find a bad prognosis. With a mean follow-up of 6 years, in 142 patients with CAD and severe ST-segment depression, there was only a 1.4% mortality and only 1.3% per year had CABS. This study shows that it is necessary to consider multiple variables when predicting the risk of ischemic heart disease. A relatively low-risk group can

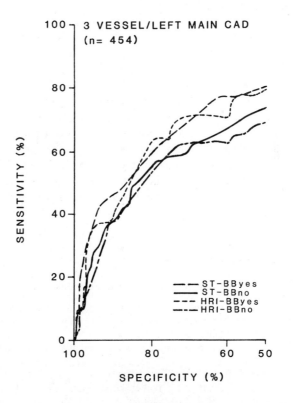

FIG 5-2.
Range of characteristics (ROC) curves of ST-segment depression and the ST/HR index in patients based on beta-blocker administration.

be found in any population identified by using one risk predictor and by excluding patients with other risk predictors.

Other studies have confirmed the prognostic value of exercise testing. Dagenais et al[33] analyzed the factors influencing the 5-year survival rate in 220 patients with at least 0.2 mV of ST-segment depression during exercise testing. They confirmed previous observations that survival was inversely proportional to the duration of exercise: All patients who achieved 10 METs survived, and the patient survival rate declined as exercise capacity declined.

Bruce, Fisher, and Hossack[34] analyzed the Seattle Heart Watch data, derived by applying noninvasive criteria to a test series in a later population sample, for exercise-enhanced risk assessment of events caused by coronary heart disease. The two exercise predictors of survival were duration of exercise and the ST-segment response.

Predicting Improved Survival with CABS

Which exercise test variables indicate those patients who would have an improved prognosis if they underwent CABS? The problem with the studies available is that the patients were not selected for surgery according to their exercise test results; instead, the analysis is retrospective.

Bruce et al[35] demonstrated noninvasive screening criteria for patients who had improved 4-year survival after CABS. They found that patients with cardiomegaly, with less than 5 METs exercise capacity, or with a maximum SBP of less than 130 would have a better outcome if treated with surgery than with medical therapy. When two or more of the above parameters were present, the patients were at the highest risk and exhibited the greatest differential for improved survival with bypass. Four-year survival in this group would be 94% for those who had surgery versus 67% for those who received medical management (in those who had 2 or more of the above factors). In the European surgery trial,[36] patients who had an exercise test response of 1.5 mm of ST-segment depression, baseline ST-segment depression, or claudication had improved survival with surgery. From the CASS study group,[37] in more than 5000 nonrandomized patients, the surgical benefit

TABLE 5-3.

Studies Evaluating Exercise Test Responses Indicate Improved Survival With Coronary Artery Bypass Surgery

Study	Markers of Improved Survival With Surgery
Seattle Heart Watch	Cardiomegaly, <5 METs or maximum SBP <130
European Surgery Trial	ST-segment depression at rest, 1.5 mm of ST-segment depression with exercise, or claudication
Coronary Artery Surgery Study (CASS)	1 mm of ST-segment depression at <5 METs; no difference in survival if 10 METs exceeded
Veterans Affairs Coronary Artery Bypass Surgery	Two or more of the following: 2 mm of ST-segment depression HR >140 at 6 METs Exercise-induced PVCs

for survival was greatest in patients with 1 mm of ST-segment depression at less than 5 METs. Among the patients with triple-vessel disease with this exercise test response, the 7-year survival was 50% in those medically managed versus 81% in those who underwent CABS. There was no difference in mortality in patients able to exceed 10 METs exercise capacity. From the Veterans Affairs (VA) randomized surgery trial, Hultgren et al[38] reported a 79% survival rate with CABS versus 42% for medical management in patients with two or more of the following: 2 mm or more of ST-segment depression, a heart rate of 140 or greater at 6 METs, or exercise-induced premature ventricular contractions (PVCs). The results from these four studies are summarized in Table 5-3.

SPECIAL FOLLOW-UP STUDIES OF STABLE CAD

Clinical evaluation, exercise testing, and coronary angiography are routinely used by physicians to decide whether interventions are needed in patients with CAD. Since the pioneering studies from the University of Alabama,[39,40] numerous investigators have studied the prognostic value of specific clinical, exercise test, and catheterization variables in patients with CAD. Implicitly underlying these studies has been the question of whether exercise testing and coronary angiography improve prediction sufficiently to merit their performance despite their expense and risk.

Using discriminant function analysis, Oberman et al[39] found that cardiac enlargement on chest x-ray films and histories of CHF were the two most predictive independent clinical variables for CAD and that angiography improved prediction of death. Although they did not consider exercise test results because of incomplete data, they did find that those unable to perform the test had a poorer prognosis. Ellestad and Wan[40] reported the predictive implications of maximal exercise testing in 2700 individuals followed from 6 months to 9 years. ST-segment depression and prior MI were associated with subsequent higher mortality.

Hammermeister, De Rouen, and Dodge[41] assessed 733 medically treated patients by going stepwise, first through clinical markers and then through the exercise test. CHF was the most important clinical variable, and maximum double product was the most important treadmill variable. Maximum SBP, heart rate, and exercise capacity were far less important. Gohlke et al[42] followed 1034 patients with CAD specifically to answer the following question: Does exercise testing provide additional prognostic information when angiographic information is available? They found that exercise workload, angina during the exercise test, and maximum heart rate independently predict risk of death. Brunelli, Cristofani, and L'Abbate[43] reported their findings in 1083 patients younger than 65 years of age who were followed for a mean of 66 months. They found that clinical markers stratified risk and that coronary angiography added prognostic information only in patients with moderately severe disease. Q-wave presence and history of infarction were the most important clinical predictors, although CHF was not considered. Exercise-induced ST-segment depression was not considered independently but rather was combined with angina and exercise capacity to create a marker associated with cardiovascular death. Weiner et al[44] analyzed 30 exercise test, coronary angiographic, and clinical variables in 4083 patients to identify predictors of mortality in medically treated patients with symptomatic CAD. Regression analysis demonstrated that seven variables were independent predictors of survival. A high-risk subgroup (annual mortality of about 5%) was designated, consisting of patients with either CHF or ST-segment depression and a final exercise stage in the Bruce protocol of 1 or less (5 METs or less). In a subgroup of 572 patients with triple-vessel disease and good LV function, the probability of survival at 4 years ranged from 53% for patients only able to achieve the first half of stage 1 to 100% for patients able to exercise into stage 5 (MET level of 10).

Several other large studies have examined the predictive value of exercise testing. Mark et al[45] studied 2842 consecutive patients who underwent cardiac catheterization and exercise testing and whose data were entered into the Duke computerized medical information system. Peduzzi et al[46] reported on the 7-year follow-up of 245 patients who had a baseline treadmill test and were treated by medical management. Lerman et al[47] reported on 190 patients with exercise test and coronary angiograms who were followed for 6 years. Wyns et al[48] evaluated the independent prognostic information provided by exercise testing by using the life-table method to calculate the survival rates of 372 men referred for coronary arteriography. A second study from Saint-Luc Hospital in Brussels excluded patients with a prior MI.[49] In a VA Medical Center, 588 male patients who underwent exercise testing and cardiac catheterization were followed to determine whether cardiovascular mortality could be predicted by clinical and exercise test data.[50]

These nine studies used multivariate survival analysis techniques, and the results are shown in Table 5-4. The variables chosen are listed in order of predictive power. Some investigators combined variables, whereas others did not consider key variables or excluded patients with certain clinical features (e.g., CHF or digoxin use). Nevertheless, two of the nine found a history of CHF, two found exercise SBP, and one found resting ST-segment depression associated with death (see box). In contrast to the Long Beach study,[50] though, three found exercise-induced ST-segment depression, and six of the nine found poor exercise capacity to be predictive of death. Unfortunately for comparison, the Duke study[45] did not provide the maximum SBP collected. Age is not chosen as a predictor by most of the studies because of the narrow age range for patients submitted to cardiac catheterization. Exertional hypotension has previously been examined in our population and in the other studies reviewed. This is the first time it was chosen as a predictor by a multivariable model, rather than just observed univariately.[50] The issue of whether the standing pretreadmill SBP is representative of the patient's usual blood pressure is still not resolved, though.

Because of the differences in the variables that have independent predictive power in the reported studies, their key characteristics are presented in Table 5-4. No obvious population, methodological, or test characteristics explain the different results. All studies had to deal with interventions that alter the natural history, but each excluded patients on the basis of these interventions, except for the earlier VA CABS study.[38]

METAANALYSIS OF PROGNOSIS IN STABLE CAD

Poor exercise capacity	6/9
CHF	3/9
ST-segment depression	
Resting	2/9
Exercise	3/9
Exercise SBP	3/9

Exercise test and catheterization *(9 suitable studies with follow-up after a MEDLINE search)*

The first explanation that comes to mind for the failure of ST-segment depression to predict prognosis in our study[50] and five of the other nine studies might be that the clinical process was highly effective in selecting high-risk patients with exercise-induced ST-segment depression for interventions. Ischemic exercise test variables clearly are related to ischemic events during follow-up (e.g., nonfatal MI, CABS, and PTCA). This relationship is logical but of little help in clinical decision making, since the clinician has no trouble in justifying these procedures for patients whose symptoms accelerate after adequate medical management, given the established symptomatic benefit from interventions. The problem lies in justifying intervention to improve survival for patients whose symptoms are satisfactorily managed medically. These studies show that simple clinical indicators can stratify these patients with stable CAD into high- or low-risk groups (see box). Cardiac catheterization is not needed to do so in the majority of such patients.

Workup Bias

All of these studies selected patients by requiring that they also undergo coronary angiography. To evaluate the effect of this selection process, the Duke group repeated their analysis in an outpatient population that did not undergo cardiac catheterization.[51] The same variables were chosen in their Cox proportional hazards model, and the same equation was derived. The first Duke study[45] had used inpatients, all of whom had a catheterization, but the later report only included outpatients evaluated before the decision for cardiac catheterization. Their score based on treadmill time, exercise-induced ST-segment depression, and treadmill angina performed as well for prognosis as it did in the first study. Therefore workup bias did not affect their prognostication model.

We similarly analyzed 2546 male patients who underwent noninvasive evaluation, including exercise testing, for CAD. In contrast to the Duke group, though, we included exercise SBP and clinical data in our model. Although a history of CHF and digoxin use were the most powerful variables in both VA studies, surprisingly, different exercise test variables had prognostic power. In the model from the first VA study,[26] in which patients were selected based on catheterization results, only exertional hypotension had predictive power, but in the model from the second VA study (only noninvasive clinical evaluation),[50] exercise-induced ST-

TABLE 5-4.

Population Descriptors, Including Clinical Variables and Results from Exercise Testing and Coronary Angiography in the Follow-Up Studies of Multivariate Prediction of Cardiac Events

Descriptors	LB VAMC (no cath)	LB VAMC	VA CABS	CASS	Duke
Clinical					
Years entered	1984-1990	1984-1990	1970-1974	1974-1979	1969-1981
Population size	2546	588	245	4083	2842
Age	59	59 (mean)	519 (mean)	50	49 (median)
Males	100%	100%	100%	80%	70%
CHF	5%	8%	9%	8%	4%
MI	23%	45%	54%	40%	29%
Q waves (at least one)	21%	37%	38%	22%	22%
Digoxin	8%	8%	NA	14%	11%
Beta-blockers	22%	35%	14%	40%	54%
Typical angina	21%	52%	100%	50%	47%
Exercise Test					
1-mm ST-segment depression (%)	22%	58%	72%	44%	35%
Angina	4%	35%	66%	80%	50%
MHR (beats/min)	137	124	125	138	134
Maximum SPB (mm Hg)	175	159	156	171	160
METs	8.4	6.6	5.7	NA	7
PVCs	5%	12%	19%	12%	6%
Cardiac Catheterization Findings					
Triple-vessel disease	NA	14%	55%	23%	22%
Left main artery disease	NA	7%	13%	7%	5%
No significant lesion	NA	26%	0%	34%	40%
Ejection fraction	NA	60 (mean)		57%	60 (median)
Significant lesion criteria	NA	70%	50%	70%	75%
Follow-up					
Years	5	5	7	5	5
CABS	2%	20%	24%	36%	24%
Annual cardiovascular mortality	1.5%	2.7%	NA	1.0%	1.6%
Annual total mortality	2.8%	3.5%	4.0%	1.6%	1.8%
Independent predictors of mortality by priority	CHF/ digoxin	CHF	E-I PVCs	CHF	E-I ST dep
	METs	SBP drop	MHR >140	Treadmill stage	Angina index
	Max SBP	Resting ST dep	E-I ST dep >2 mm	E-I ST dep	Treadmill time
	E-I ST dep				

LB, Long Beach; *VAMC*, Veterans Affairs Medical Center; *NA*, not applicable; *MHR*, maximal heart rate; *PVCs*, premature ventricular contractions; *E-I*, exercise-induced; *dep*, depression; *max*, maximal; *AP*, angina pectoris.

Italian	Belgian	Belgian (no MI)	German	Seattle	Buenos Aires
1976-1979	1972-1977	1978-1985	1975-1978	1971-1974	1972-1982
1083	372	470	1238	733	180
49 (mean)	48	52	50 (mean)	52 (mean)	51 (mean)
90%	100%	100%	90%	80%	96%
Excluded	1%		Excluded	13%	Excluded
42%	39%	Excluded	>50%	40%	64%
37%	39%	Excluded	50%	45%	
	0%	Excluded	8%	18%	
	0%				
95%	67%	75%	95%	86%	71%
42%	27%	54%	56%		65%
60%	49%	44%	61%		60%
130	148	140	118	145	128
171	NA	186	182	160	151
5.4	9	8	5	6.5	5.2
15%	2%	NA		18%	21%
5%	34%	26%	33%	12%	44%
5%	8%	8%	0%		8%
26%	18%	22%	0%	39%	0%
60	NA	65	60	60	
75%	50%	50%	50%	70%	75%
5.5	5	5	5	3.5	6
15%	28%	29%			9%
1.5%	1.8%	2.0%		2.6%	4.6%
2.0%	2.4%		2.4%	3.1%	
Q wave	Age	Age	Exercise capacity	CHF	Max SBP <130
Prior MI	Exercise capacity	Max exercise score (−2 to +2) (MHR, ST 60, AP, watts, ST slope)	Angina	Max double product Max SBP	ST elevation
Effort ischemia			MHR	Angina frequency	<4 METs Inappropriate dyspnea
Exercise capacity				Resting ST dep	

segment depression, exercise SBP, and exercise capacity had predictive power. In the first study, the workup bias inherent in choosing patients based on cardiac catheterization resulted in a sicker, older, more disabled group with a higher annual cardiac mortality (2.6% versus 1.5%). The second study included a population with a near-normal, age-adjusted exercise capacity, but the first study population had an average age-adjusted exercise capacity that was 75% of normal. A score was derived from the predictive variables by using the coefficients as weights: 5 × (CHF/dig [yes = 1, no = 0]) + (exercise-induced ST-segment depression in millimeters) + (change in SBP score) − (METs). Three groups were formed using the scores: <−2 (low-risk), −2 to +2 (moderate-risk), and >+2 (high-risk). The Kaplan-Meier survival curves are illustrated in Fig 5-3. This score enabled determination of a low-risk group (80% of the population) with an annual mortality of less than 1% over the first 3 years after the exercise test, a moderate-risk group (14% of the population) with a 4% annual mortality, and a high-risk group (6% of the population) with a 7% annual mortality over the 3 years after the exercise test. Fig 5-4 illustrates how the VA score outperformed the Duke score for prognosis of CAD in the VA population.

The total population, including those selected and not selected based on catheterization, is analogous to that seen by a clinician before deciding whether to catheterize. Univariate survival statistics were performed using Kaplan-Meier survival curves for two pointsteps of the score. From these curves, the average annual mortality for the 3 years after testing was calculated. The scores were then plotted against average annual cardiovascular mortality (Fig 5-5). Fig 5-6 is a histogram showing the distribution of patients for values of the score.

In patients selected based on catheterization, the mean VA prognostic score was −2.8 (±5), compared with −5.7 (±5) in the total population, and 53% ($N = $ 312) had a VA prognostic score of less than −2 associated with an annual mortal-

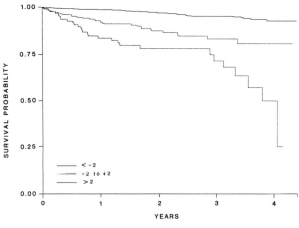

VA TM SCORE= 5 (CHF [0,1]) + EI ST DEPRESSION (millimeters) + CHANGE SBP SCORE (0-5) − METs

FIG 5-3.
The Kaplan-Meier survival curves for the VA prognostic score.

ity of less than 2%. Thus in over half of the patients selected based on catheterization, the catherization was unnecessary if performed to lessen their chance of cardiovascular death, since their prognosis was so good that no intervention could improve it. In the patients selected based on bypass surgery, the mean score was −0.5 (±5), which is associated with an estimated annual cardiovascular mortality rate of 5%, and 35% of these patients had a score less than −2.

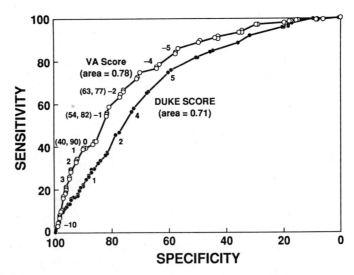

FIG 5-4.
ROC curve of the VA score and the Duke score for predicting cardiovascular death.

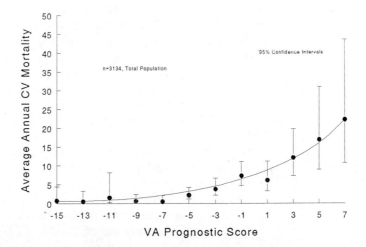

FIG 5-5.
Plot of the average cardiovascular mortality against the VA prognostic score, including 95% confidence intervals. Cardiovascular (CV) mortality = 0.0026(VA score)^3 + 0.103(VA score)^2 + 1.37(VA score) + 6.75.

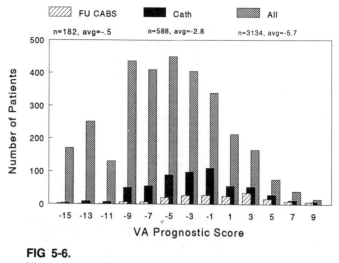

FIG 5-6.
Histograms of patients according to the VA prognostic score.

The disagreement among studies predicting prognosis indicates that workup bias can affect the decision to use invasive procedures. Cardiac death occurs along a spectrum of possibilities; there are patients with myocardial damage who die of CHF (or pump failure) and those with normal ventricles in whom ischemia precipitates death. The clinical and exercise test markers would be expected to be quite different for patients who die at the extremes of this spectrum. Although markers of myocardial damage (history of CHF and presence of Q waves) track the former, markers of ischemia (angina and ST-segment depression) better predict the latter. Still other markers, such as dysrhythmias, poor exercise capacity, and exertional hypotension, are associated with both. Further complicating prediction algorithms, *damage* markers predict short-term deaths, whereas *ischemic* markers predict deaths occurring 2 or more years later. Consequently, accurately associating clinical and exercise test markers with death becomes quite difficult. Differences in populations may favor one or the other type of mortality (pump failure versus ischemia), which may explain why ischemic variables are more predictive in one population and myocardial damage variables more predictive in another.

Enthusiasm for cardiac catheterization and revascularization may well have led to an acceptance of invasive measurements as superior to clinical variables for prognostication in patients with CAD. Although clinical variables were mentioned in early studies, key ones often were not considered, nor were they considered together or defined as accurately as they are today. In the drive toward technological advancement, it frequently was assumed that laboratory methods and images were more accurate and precise than simple clinical data. Also, the importance of clinical data could have been underestimated because of the nonavailability of modern survival analysis techniques. A further consideration is that the recently noted decline in mortality, indicated by vessel score, is not actually due to disease treatment but to patient selection (i.e., excluding patients with CHF because it is being diagnosed better).

Bypass surgery is associated, at best, with a 2% mortality; therefore patients with a score of less than −2 should be informed that their mortality in the next year would be higher with surgery than with medical management. These patients might not elect to have catheterization if they understood this situation. Regression equations based on clinical characteristics can be used to give a patient an individualized estimate of mortality with CABS, and the VA prognostic score can be used to estimate morality with medical management.

Current medical practice has taken a very aggressive approach toward managing atherosclerotic CAD, both in terms of diagnosis and therapy. In spite of decreasing cardiovascular mortality, over 380,000 bypass procedures were performed in 1990, compared with 180,000 in 1983 in the United States.[52] This increase is occurring in spite of the emergence of PTCA as a therapeutic option. Health care costs are increasing, and part of this increase is due to unnecessary procedures. The basics of medicine appear to be superseded by technology, and the reimbursement policy has favored this trend. However, evidence for the importance of the patient history and physical examination in the diagnostic process has reemerged. A recent study demonstrated that the history correctly leads to the diagnosis in over 80% of the usual patients who go to a general medicine clinic, with an additional 10% coming from the physical examination results.[53] Many studies have been published examining this issue and trying to explain why these procedures appear to be performed inappropriately. One explanation has been that financial incentives cause the problem. Our studies, carried out in a socialized medical system (i.e., the VA), also found an inappropriate number of procedures performed. This finding suggests that factors other than financial are involved. It appears that physicians have an exaggerated perception of the risk of stable CAD. Perhaps making the correct follow-up data available to them could alter practice.

A common clinical problem is justifying intervention to improve survival for patients whose symptoms are satisfactorily managed medically. In the VA population, a history of CHF or of digoxin administration and three exercise test responses are the most important predictors of cardiovascular death. On the basis of clinical and exercise test data, the annual cardiovascular mortality rate of patients with signs and symptoms of coronary heart disease can be estimated. Our simple equation could have a major impact on the appropriate use of cardiac catheterization. In our study, over half of the patients selected based on cardiac catheterization are exposed to a higher risk with the performance of CABS (assuming a 2% to 4% operative mortality) than with medical management. Cardiac catheterization is not needed for prognosis in the majority of such patients. Clinical judgment must be applied to decide whether intervention is likely to improve survival in high-risk patients. Variables available from the usual noninvasive workup of patients with known or suspected CAD can be used to estimate cardiovascular mortality. Exercise-induced ST-segment depression can be falsely excluded from predictive models because of workup bias. Specifically, the VA prognostic score can estimate the average annual cardiovascular mortality rate in male

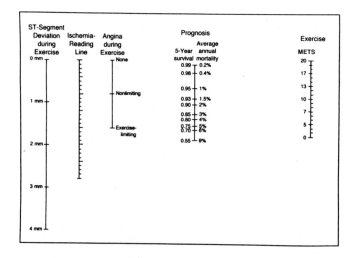

FIG 5-7.
The Duke nomogram estimates prognosis from the parameters of the Duke score in five steps. First, the observed amount of ST-segment depression is marked on the ST-segment deviation line. Second, the observed degree of angina is marked on the line for angina, and these two points are connected with a straight edge. Third, the point where this line intersects the ischemia-reading line is noted. Fourth, the observed exercise capacity in METs is marked on the line. Finally, the mark on the ischemia-reading line is connected to the mark on the MET line, and the estimated 5-year survival or average annual mortality rate is read from the point at which this line intersects the prognosis scale. For instance, even patients with 2 mm of ST-segment depression and angina occurring during the test will still have less than a 3% annual cardiovascular mortality rate if their exercise capacity is 7 METs or greater. (From Mark D et al: *N Engl J Med* 325:849-853, 1991.)

veterans being evaluated for stable CAD, obviating the need for cardiac catheterization in many of them. In the general population, particularly when women are included, the Duke score is recommended. These scores and their components are listed in the box. The Duke score is also represented in Fig 5-7.

PROGNOSTIC STUDIES OF SILENT ISCHEMIA DURING EXERCISE TESTING

The preoccupation of many physicians with silent ischemia (i.e., ST-segment depression without anginal symptoms) has occurred because of four clinical observations:

1. The increased risk of coronary events when screening asymptomatic men
2. The frequency of painless ST-segment depression during exercise testing in patients with coronary heart disease
3. Episodes of painless ST-segment depression noted during holter monitoring
4. The apparent high risk of painless ST-segment depression in patients with unstable ischemic syndromes

PROGNOSTIC SCORES

Duke score = METs − 5 × (mm E-I ST depression) − 4 × (TM AP index)
VA score = 5 × (CHF/dig) + mm E-I ST depression + Change in SBP score − METs
Treadmill angina pectoris (TM AP): 0 if no angina, 1 if angina occurred during test, 2 if angina was the reason for stopping
CHF/dig score: 0 if no history of CHF and patient not receiving digoxin, if history of CHF or patient receiving digoxin
Change in SBP score: from 0 for rise greater than 40 mm Hg to 5 for drop below rest (scored in increments of 10 mm Hg)

E-I, Exercise induced; *TM, treadmill; AP*, angina pectoris; *dig*, digoxin.

Its potential dangers include sudden death resulting from the lack of a warning mechanism and myocardial fibrosis leading to CHF. As with many other clinical syndromes, dividing it into subsets can be very helpful. The types of silent ischemia are:

Type I   Occurring in asymptomatic, apparently healthy individuals
Type II   Occurring in patients after an MI
Type III   Occurring in patients with known CAD

It was hypothesized that silent myocardial ischemia had a worse prognosis than angina pectoris because patients with it do not have an intact warning system. However, in studies of patients referred for diagnostic purposes or with stable coronary syndromes, silent myocardial ischemia detected by exercise testing has been associated with a lesser or similar prognosis as angina pectoris. Because exercise testing has advantages over ambulatory monitoring in terms of the leads monitored, chest pain description, and fidelity of the recording apparatus, confirmation of these findings would help resolve the controversy over the relative prognostic impact of silent myocardial ischemia. Exercise testing studies give one means of evaluating the risk of silent ischemia. Unfortunately, these exercise test studies do not evaluate patients with true silent ischemia. The patients are being tested because of some symptoms, usually angina; it is just that they do not have angina at the time of their tests. However, patients with true silent ischemia are rare. Therefore the following data from exercise test studies give us a good idea of how the usual patients seen in clinical practice with silent ischemia are likely to do.

To evaluate the significance of ischemic ST-segment depression without associated chest pain during exercise testing, data were analyzed for 2982 patients from the CASS registry who underwent coronary arteriography and exercise testing and were followed up for 7 years.[54] At Duke, Mark et al[55] evaluated the clinical correlates and long-term prognostic significance of silent ischemia during exercise. To evaluate whether patients with silent myocardial ischemia during exercise testing are at increased risk for developing a subsequent acute MI or sudden death, the data on 424 such patients with proven CAD from the CASS registry were analyzed.[56] Callaham[56a] et al performed a study to determine the effect of silent ischemia on prognosis in patients undergoing exercise testing. In addition, this data provided the opportunity to demonstrate whether differences between the prevalence of silent ischemia and its impact on prognosis could be explained by age or by MI and diabetes mellitus status. Fig 5-8 illustates how age affects the prevalence of silent ischemia. MI or diabetes status did not affect the prevalence of silent ischemia, whereas age clearly did.

Exercise Capacity and Silent Ischemia

In the Callaham study, maximal exercise capacity in METs was not found to be independently associated with mortality. However, patients able to attain an exercise capacity of 8 METs or greater during the exercise test had a 1% 2-year mortality. Conversely, patients unable to perform 5 METs had a 9% 2-year mortality, and patients unable to exceed 2 METs had a 13% 2-year mortality. Dangenais et al[56b] reported 6-year cumulative survival in 298 moderately treated patients with exercise-induced ST-segment depression equal to or greater than 2 mm. In those with silent myocardial ischemia, survival was 85%, whereas it was significantly lower (80%) in those with angina pectoris. Patients with silent myocardial ischemia reached a greater heart rate and higher MET level than those with painful ischemia. Cumulative survival was very much related to the MET level achieved. Those who reached 10 METs had very few deaths, whereas those with less than 5 METs had approximately a 50% survival. Thus silent myocardial ischemia during treadmill testing does not predict increased risk for death. It appears that the concern that patients with silent myocardial ischemia were at higher risk because of failure of their warning mechanism than their peers with angina is not substantiated.

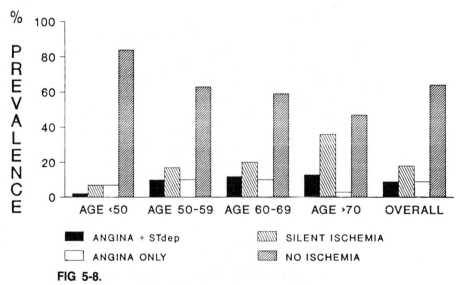

FIG 5-8.
The prevalence of silent ischemia during exercise testing according to age.

CASS: Diabetes Mellitus and Silent Ischemia

To evaluate the significance of ischemic ST-segment depression without anginal chest pain during exercise testing among patients with diabetes mellitus, Weiner et al[58] analyzed the data on 45 such patients from the CASS registry. Silent myocardial ischemia during exercise testing adversely affected survival, and coronary artery bypass graft surgery improved the survival of diabetic patients with silent myocardial ischemia and triple-vessel disease.

Angiographic Studies of Silent Ischemia

Visser et al[58] from the Netherlands studied 280 patients with anginal complaints, without prior MI, and with a positive exercise test. Miranda et al[59] performed a retrospective analysis of 416 male veterans referred for exercise testing who were selected based on cardiac catheterization. Exercise-induced ST-segment depression was a better marker for CAD than exercise test–induced angina, and symptomatic ischemia (ST-segment depression plus angina) was a better indicator of severe angiographic disease than silent ischemia. In the Program On the Surgical Control of Hyperlipidemia (POSCH), 838 subjects with hyperlipidemia who had one healed MI were studied and followed for 6 to 13 years with similar results.[60]

Table 5-5 reviews the angiographic studies of silent ischemia encompassing almost 6000 patients. It is obvious that patients with symptomatic ischemia had a higher prevalence of severe angiographic disease than did patients with silent ischemia.

SUMMARY

Why do the various prognostic studies fail to get the same results? Most likely the explanation lies in the fact that cardiac patients die for reasons ranging along a pathophysiological spectrum from CHF with little remaining myocardium to an ischemic-related event with ample remaining myocardium. Clinical and exercise test variables most likely associated with CHF deaths (CHF markers) include a history or symptoms of CHF, prior MI, Q waves, and other indicators of LV dysfunction. Variables most likely associated with ischemic deaths (ischemic markers) are angina and both rest and exercise ST-segment depression. Ischemic markers are associated with a later and lesser risk, whereas CHF or LV dysfunction markers are associated with a sooner and greater risk of death. A problem arises, however, because ischemic deaths occur later in follow-up and are more likely to occur in those lost to follow-up, whereas CHF deaths are more likely to occur early (within 2 years) and are more likely to be classified. Some variables can be associated with either extreme of cardiovascular death; these include exercise capacity, maximum heart rate, and maximum SBP. Their dual association may explain why they are reported most consistently in the available studies. Workup bias probably explains why exercise-induced ST-segment depression fails to be a predictor in most angiographic studies.

Rather than stressing the differences, though, it is better to stress the consistencies between studies. Risk can be assessed by considering simple clinical vari-

TABLE 5-5.

Studies of Silent Ischemia During Exercise Testing with Angiographic Correlation

Study	No. of patients	Exclusions	NOISCH MVD (%)	3V/LM (%)	APO MVD (%)	3V/LM (%)	SI MVD (%)	3V/LM (%)	STAP MVD (%)	3V/LM (%)
Amsterdam	92	CAD, coronary stenoses <70%, normal exercise test	—	—	62	—	77	—	82	—
Deligonul	390	CAD, coronary stenoses <50%, digoxin use, left bundle branch block, left main artery disease, left ventricular hypertrophy, failed PTCA	49	10	50	5	64	18	71	23
Erikssen	103	Coronary stenoses <50%, previously known CAD, "other" heart disease, hypertension, diabetes mellitus, malignancy, musculoskeletal disorders, any other advanced disease	50	—	45	—	45	—	75	—
Falcone	473	CAD, coronary stenoses <50%, digoxin use, left bundle branch block, CHF, valvular disease, variant angina, no exercise ST-segment depression	—	—	—	—	85	56/5	84	55/7
Mark	1698	CAD, coronary stenoses <75%, left bundle branch block, exercise ST-segment elevation, unstable angina, valvular disease, congenital heart disease, cardiac surgery	—	27	—	37	79	48/12	88	60/12
Miranda	200	Digoxin use, coronary stenoses <75%, left ventricular typertrophy, left bundle branch block, CABG or PTCA, women, prior MI, resting ST-segment depression	16	6	13	9	50	20	51	30
Miranda	216	Digoxin use, coronary stenoses <75%, left ventricular typertrophy, left bundle branch block, CABG or PTCA, women, resting ST-segment depression	36	10	33	9	58	23	64	32
Ouyang	60	Coronary stenoses <70%, no exercise ST-segment depression	—	—	—	—	74	29/11	81	54/6
Stern	480	CAD, coronary stenoses <70%, no exercise ST-segment depression, digoxin use, "baseline ECG changes," valvular disease, cardiomyopathy	—	—	—	—	66	33	72	36
Visser	280	CAD, coronary stenosis <50%, no exercise ST-segment depression, left ventricular typertrophy, left bundle branch block, CHF, valvular disease, cardiomyopathy, prior MI, congenital heart disease	—	—	—	—	38	13	74	38
Weiner	1583	CAD, coronary stenoses <70%	42	13	55	23	63	29	74	38
Weiner	302	Coronary stenoses <70%, digoxin use, left bundle branch block, left ventricular hypertrophy, valvular disease, patients without either exercise angina or ST-segment depression that did not achieve 85% of submaximum heart rate	21	—	67	—	51	—	94	—
TOTAL	5877	MEANS	36	13	46	17	63	31	76	41

NOISCH, Normal exercise test; *APO*, angina pectoris only during exercise test; *SI*, ST-segment depression only during exercise test; *STAP*, ST-segment depression and angina pectoris during exercise test; *MVD*, multivessel disease; *3D/LM*, triple-vessel/left main coronary artery disease.

ables. More than 5 METs of exercise capacity, no evidence or history of CHF or ventricular damage (e.g., no Q waves), no ST-segment depression, or only one of these clinical findings is associated with a very low risk. These patients are low risk in exercise programs and need not be considered candidates for CABS to prolong their life. High-risk patients can be identified by two or more of the clinical markers or by the scores. Exertional hypotension is particularly ominous. High-risk patients in exercise training programs should have lower goals and should be monitored. Such patients should also be considered candidates for CABS to lengthen their lives. Intervention may not always be feasible, but it should at least be considered.

The mathematical models for determining prognosis are usually more complex than those used for identifying severe angiographic disease. Diagnostic testing can use multivariate discriminant function analysis to determine the probability of severe angiographic disease. Prognostic testing must use survival analysis, which eliminates patients with uneven follow-up as a result of being lost to follow-up or of other cardiac events (e.g., CABS or PTCA) and must account for time-person units of exposure. Survival curves must be developed, and the Cox proportional hazards model is often preferred. How to test these models for confidence, accuracy, reproducibility, and power is controversial.

As shown by Stone et al,[61] the status of the right coronary artery greatly affects the hemodynamic and ST-segment segment responses to exercise testing in patients with multivessel coronary disease. Left main disease, or left main equivalents, cannot be distinguished from double-vessel disease when the right coronary is not diseased.

From this perspective, it is obvious that there is much information supporting the use of exercise testing as the first noninvasive step after the history, the physical examination, and the resting ECG in the prognostic evaluation of CAD patients. It accomplishes both purposes of prognostic testing: to provide information regarding the patient's status and to help make recommendations for optimal management. The exercise test results help clinicians make reasonable decisions for the selection of patients who should undergo coronary angiography. Perhaps some of the newer computerized ST-segment scoring techniques will enable an even more accurate prediction of high-risk patients. Because the exercise test can be performed in the doctor's office and provides valuable information for clinical management about activity levels, response to therapy, and disability, the exercise test is the reasonable first choice for prognostic assessment.

Simple clinical and exercise test scores can be used to decide which patients need interventions to improve their prognosis; these scores frequently obviate the need for cardiac catheterization. The VA score is recommended for the male veteran population and the Duke score for the general population, including women. Patients can be given estimates of their relative annual mortality with medical versus surgical therapy by using scores and case mix data.[62] However, quality of life issues cannot be resolved with such scores; these issues require an understanding physician and an informed patient. In general, physicians overestimate the danger of ischemia; perhaps if given accurate mortality estimates, the practice of medicine would be more conservative.

REFERENCES

1. Topol EJ et al: Exercise testing three days after onset of acute myocardial infarction, *Am J Cardiol* 60:958-962, 1987.
2. Benjamin ST et al: Usefulness of early exercise testing after non–Q-wave myocardial infarction in predicting prognosis, *Am J Cardiol* 57:738-744, 1986.
3. Butman S et al: Early exercise testing in unstable angina: angiographic correlation and prognostic value, *J Am Coll Cardiol* 1:638–645, 1983.
4. Swahn E et al: Predictive importance of clinical findings and a predischarge exercise test in patients with suspected unstable coronary artery disease, *Am J Cardiol* 59:208-214, 1987.
5. Chassin MR et al: How coronary angiography is used: clinical determinants of appropriateness, *JAMA* 258:2543-2547, 1987.
6. Marcus ML, Wilson FR, White CW: Methods of measurement of myocardial blood flow in patients: a critical review, *Circulation* 76:245-251, 1987.
7. Bolli R: Bypass surgery in patients with coronary artery disease: indications based on the multicenter randomized trials, *Chest* 92:760-764, 1987.
8. Pauker SG, Kassirer JP: Decision analysis, *New Engl J Med* 316(5):250-272, 1987.
9. Knoebel SB: What we can't explain can hurt us and our patients, *J Am Coll Cardiol* 10:879-881, 1987.
10. Hammong HK, Kelly TL, Froelicher VF: Radionuclide imaging correlatives of heart rate impairment during maximal exercise testing, *J Am Coll Cardiol* 2:826-833, 1983.
11. Dubach P et al: Exercise-induced hypotension in a veteran population: criteria, causes, and prognosis, *Circulation* 78:1380-1387, 1988.
12. Morris CK et al: The prognostic value of exercise capacity: a review of the literature, *Am Heart J* 122:1423-1430, 1991.
13. Stone PH et al: Prognostic significance of the treadmill exercise test performance 6 months after myocardial infarction, *J Am Coll Cardiol* 8:1007-1017, 1986.
14. Haines DE et al: Exercise-induced ST segment evaluation 2 weeks after uncomplicated myocardial infarction: contributing factors and prognostic significance, *J Am Coll Cardiol* 9:996-1003, 1987.
15. McKirnan MD et al: Treadmill performance and cardiac function in selected patients with coronary heart disease, *J Am Coll Cardiol* 3:253-261, 1984.
16. Bounous EP et al: Prognostic value of the simplified Selvester QRS score in patients with coronary artery disease, *J Am Coll Cardiol* 11:35-41, 1988.
17. Pryor DB et al: Estimating the likelihood of severe coronary artery disease, *Am J Med* 90:553-562, 1991.
18. Hubbard BL et al: Identification of severe coronary artery disease using simple clinical parameters, *Arch Intern Med* 152(2):309-312, 1992.
19. Detrano R et al: Algorithm to predict triple-vessel/left main coronary artery disease in patients without myocardial infarction: an international cross-validation, *Circulation* 83 (suppl III):89-96, 1991.
20. Cheitlin MD et al: Correlation of "critical" left coronary artery lesions with positive submaximal exercise tests in patients with chest pain, *Am Heart J* 89(3):305-310, 1975.
21. Goldschlager N, Selzer A, Cohn K: Treadmill stress tests as indicators of presence and severity of coronary artery disease, *Ann Intern Med* 85:277-286, 1976.
22. NcNeer JF et al: The role of the exercise test in the evaluation of patients for ischemic heart disease, *Circulation* 57:64-70, 1978.
23. Weiner DA, McCabe CH, Ryan TJ: Identification of patients with left main and three vessel coronary disease with clinical and exercise test variables, *Am J Cardiol* 46:21-27, 1981.

24. Blumenthal DS et al: The predictive value of a strongly positive stress test in patients with minimal symptoms, *Am J Med* 70:1005-1010, 1981.

25. Lee TH, Cook EF, Goldman L: Prospective evaluation of a clinical and exercise-test model for the prediction of left main coronary artery disease, *Med Decis Making* 6:136-144, 1986.

26. Detrano R: Exercise-induced ST segment depression in the diagnosis of multivessel coronary disease: a meta analysis, *J Am Coll Cardiol* 14:1501-1508, 1989.

27. Hartz A, Gammaitoni C, Young M: Quantitative analysis of the exercise tolerance test for determining the severity of coronary artery disease, *Int J Cardiol* 24:63-71, 1989.

28. Schlant RC et al: Guidelines for exercise testing: a report of the American College of Cardiology/American Heart Association Task Force on assessment of cardiovascular procedures (subcommittee on exercise testing), *J Am Coll Cardiol* 8(3):725-738, 1986.

29. Ribisl PM et al: Angiographic patterns and severe coronary artery disease, *Arch Intern Med* 152:1618-1624, 1992.

30. Herbert W et al: Effect of beta-blockade on the interpretation of the exercise ECG: ST level versus ST/HR index, *Am Heart J* 122(4):993-1000, 1991.

31. Bobbio M et al: Exercise-induced ST depression and ST/heart rate index to predict triple-vessel or left main coronary disease: a multi-center analysis, *J Am Coll Cardiol* 19:11-18, 1992.

32. Podrid PJ, Graboys T, Lown B: Prognosis of medically treated patients with coronary artery disease with profound ST segment depression during exercise testing, *New Engl J Med* 305:1111-1118, 1981.

33. Dagenais GR et al: Survival of patients with a strongly positive exercise electrocardiogram, *Circulation* 65:452-456, 1982.

34. Bruce RA, Fisher LD, Hossack KF: Validation of exercise-enhanced risk assessment of coronary heart disease events: longitudinal changes in incidence in Seattle community practice, *J Am Coll Cardiol* 5:875-881, 1985.

35. Bruce RA et al: Enhanced risk assessment for primary coronary heart disease events by maximal exercise testing: 10 years' experience of Seattle Heart Watch, *J Am Coll Cardiol* 2:565-573, 1983.

36. European Cooperative Group: Long-term results of prospective randomized study of coronary artery bypass surgery in stable angina pectoris, *Lancet* 1173-1180, 1982.

37. Weiner DA et al: The role of exercise testing in identifying patients with improved survival after coronary artery bypass surgery, *J Am Coll Cardiol* 8(4):741-748, 1986.

38. Hultgren HN et al: The 5-year effect of bypass surgery on relief of angina and exercise performance, *Circulation* 72:V79-V83, 1985.

39. Oberman A et al: Natural history of coronary artery disease, *Bull NY Acad Med* 48:1109-1125, 1972.

40. Ellestad M, Wan M: Prediction implications of stress testing, *Circulation* 51:363-369, 1975.

41. Hammermeister KE, De Rouen TA, Dodge HT: Variables predictive of survival in patients with coronary disease: selection by univariate and multivariate analyses from the clinical, electrocardiographic, exercise, arteriographic, and quantitative angiographic evaluation, *Circulation* 59:421-430, 1979.

42. Gohlke H et al: Exercise testing provides additional prognostic information in angiographically defined subgroups of patients with coronary artery disease, *Circulation* 68:979-985, 1983.

43. Brunelli C, Cristofani R, L'Abbate A, for the ODI Study Group: Long-term survival in medically treated patients with ischemic heart disease and prognostic importance of clinical and electrocardiographic data (Italian CNR Multicenter Prospective Study OD1), *Euro Heart J* 10:292-303, 1989.

44. Weiner DA et al: Prognostic importance of a clinical profile and exercise test in medically treated patients with coronary artery disease, *J Am Coll Cardiol* 3:772-779, 1984.
45. Mark DB et al: Exercise treadmill score for predicting prognosis in coronary artery disease, *Ann Intern Med* 106:793-800, 1987.
46. Peduzzi P et al: Prognostic value of baseline exercise tests, *Progr Cardiovasc Dis* 28:285-92, 1986.
47. Lerman J et al: Follow-up of patients after exercise test and catheterization, *Medicina (Buenos Aires)* 46:201-211, 1986.
48. Wyns W et al: Prognostic value of symptom limited exercise testing in men with a high prevalence of coronary artery disease, *Euro Heart J* 6:939-945, 1985.
49. Detry JM et al: Non-invasive data provide independent prognostic information in patients with chest pain without previous myocardial infarction: findings in male patients who have had cardiac catheterization, *Euro Heart J* 9:418-426, 1988.
50. Morrow K et al: Prediction of cardiovascular death in men undergoing noninvasive evaluation for CAD, *Ann Intern Med* 118:689-695, 1993.
51. Mark D et al: Prognostic value of a treadmill exercise score in outpatients with suspected coronary artery disease, *New Engl J Med* 325:849-853, 1991.
52. Graboys TB et al: Results of a second-opinion trial among patients recommended for coronary angiography, *JAMA* 268(18):2537-2540, 1992.
53. Peterson MC et al: Contributions of the history, physical examination, and laboratory investigation in making medical diagnoses, *West J Med* 156:163-165, 1992.
54. Weiner DA et al: Significance of silent myocardial ischemia during exercise testing in patients with coronary artery disease, *Am J Cardiol* 59:725-729, 1987.
55. Mark DB et al: Painless exercise ST deviation on the treadmill: long-term prognosis, *J Am Coll Cardiol* 14:885-892, 1989.
56. Weiner DA et al: Risk of developing an acute myocardial infarction or sudden coronary death in patients with exercise-induced silent myocardial ischemia: a report from the Coronary Artery Surgery Study (CASS) Registry, *Am J Cardiol* 62:1155-1158, 1988.
56a. Callaham P et al: Exercise-induced silent ischemia: age, diabetes mellitus, previous myocardial infarction and prognosis, *J Am Coll Cardiol* 14:1175-1180, 1989.
56b. Dangenais G et al: Survival with painless, strongly positive ECGs, *AM J Cardiol* 62:892–895, 1988.
57. Weiner DA et al: Significance of silent myocardial ischemia during exercise testing in patients with diabetes mellitus: a report from the Coronary Artery Surgery Study (CASS) Registry, *Am J Cardiol* 68:729-734, 1991.
58. Visser FC et al: Silent versus symptomatic myocardial ischemia during exercise testing: a comparison with coronary angiographic findings, *Int J Cardiol* 27:71-78, 1990.
59. Miranda C et al: Comparison of silent and symptomatic ischemia during exercise testing in men, *Ann Intern Med* 114:649-656, 1991.
60. Karnegis JN et al: Positive and negative exercise test results with and without exercise-induced angina in patients with one healed myocardial infarction: analysis of baseline variables and long-term prognosis, *Am Heart J* 122:701-708, 1991.
61. Stone PH, LaFollette L, Cohn P: Patterns of exercise treadmill test performance in patients with left main coronary disease: detection dependent on left coronary dominance or coexistent dominant right coronary artery, *Am Heart J* 104:13-19, 1982.
62. Parsonnet V, Dean D, Bernstein A: A method of uniform stratification of risk for evaluating the results in acquired adult heart disease, *Circulation* 79(suppl I):I-3-I-12, 1989.

CHAPTER 6

Exercise Testing of Patients Recovering From Myocardial Infarction

INTRODUCTION

The benefits of performing an exercise test in patients who have had a myocardial infarction (MI) are listed in the box. Submitting patients recovering from MI to exercise testing can expedite and optimize their discharge from the hospital and has been performed as early as 3 days after an infarct. Patients' responses to exercise, their work capacity, and their limiting factors at the time of discharge can be assessed by the exercise test. Exercise testing before discharge is important for giving patients guidelines for exercise at home, reassuring them of their physical status, and determining the risk of complications. Patients should not be given the impression that if they "fail" the test they will end up in the cardiac catheterization laboratory. Performing another test after 3 weeks or more provides a safe basis for advising patients to resume or increase their activity levels and return to work.

Safety of Exercise Testing Soon After Myocardial Infarction

The risk of death and major dysrhythmias from performing an exercise test soon after MI is very small. However, most exercise testing is performed on clinically selected patients with MI: those without major complications such as heart failure, severe dysrhythmias or ischemia, left ventricular (LV) dysfunction, or other severe diseases. The characteristics that place a patient with MI at higher risk are listed in the box. Risk is highest in those rejected for testing for these clinical reasons. Nevertheless, the exercise test can determine the possible risk the patient may incur with exercise. It is certainly safer that adverse reactions be observed in controlled circumstances. As a precaution, a heart rate limit of 140 beats per minute and a metabolic equivalent (MET) level of 7 is used as an arbitrary cutoff point for patients under 40 and 130 beats per minute and an MET level of 5 for patients over 40. Particularly for patients on beta-blockers, a Borg perceived-exertion level in the range of 16 is used to end the test. In addition, conservative clinical indications for stopping the test should be applied. The physician can gain

---

BENEFITS OF EXERCISE TESTING AFTER MI

Predischarge Submaximal Test
Setting safe exercise levels (exercise prescription)
Optimizing discharge
Altering medical therapy
Triaging for intensity of follow-up
Providing first step in rehabilitation (assurance and encouragement)
Reassuring spouse
Recognizing exercise-induced ischemia and dysrhythmias

Maximal Test for Return-to-Normal Activities

Determining limitations	Triaging for invasive studies
Prognosticating	Deciding on medications
Reassuring employers	Prescribing exercise
Determining level of disability	Continuing rehabilitation

**CHARACTERISTICS THAT LEAD TO CLASSIFICATION
OF AN MI AS COMPLICATED**

Congestive heart failure
Cardiogenic shock
Large MI as determined by creatine phosphokinase, electrocardiogram (ECG), or
   both
Pericarditis
Dangerous dysrhythmias and conduction problems (including atrial fibrillation and
   bundle branch block)
Concurrent illnesses
Pulmonary embolus
Continued ischemia (angina and ST-segment shifts)
Stroke or transient ischemic attack
Prior large MI

---

valuable information about the patient by being there during the test and interacting with the patient.

Effect on Patient and Spouse Confidence

Taylor et al[1] evaluated the effects of involving the spouse in the exercise test on both patient and spouse confidence levels. For treadmill tests 3 weeks after uncomplicated acute MIs, they compared 10 wives who did not observe the test, 10 who observed the test, and 10 who observed and performed the test themselves. Perceived confidence levels in their husbands' physical and cardiac capabilities were significantly greater among wives who also performed the test than in the other two groups. In a similar study, Ewart et al[2] demonstrated that patient's confidence was also enhanced by the test.

Spontaneous Improvement After Myocardial Infarction

Studies have documented that exercise capacity increases spontaneously after an MI, even in patients not in a formal exercise program. Therefore treadmill test performance can be expected to improve if serial tests are performed.[3,4]

Effect of Q-Wave Location on ST-Segment Shifts

Although ST-segment depression is normally most prevalent in the lateral leads (V_4 to V_6), Q-wave patterns may alter the direction of the ST-segment vector. Particularly after a lateral Q-wave infarct, ST-segment depression may be isolated to the anterior (V_2 and V_3) or inferior (II and aV_F) leads.[5-7]

RESULTS OF EXERCISE TESTING FOR PREDICTING CORONARY ANGIOGRAPHIC FINDINGS

Exercise testing results would be most helpful clinically in deciding whether to perform coronary artery bypass surgery (CABS) if the exercise test could predict which patients have anatomical findings associated with improved survival if CABS was performed (i.e., which patients have left main or triple-vessel disease accompanied by an ejection fraction [EF] of 30% to 50%). Studies in which the results of exercise testing were used to predict the results of coronary angiography after acute MI are summarized in Table 6-1. The average sensitivity of these exercise tests for ST-segment depression indicating severe angiographic disease was 58%, and the average specificity was 82%.[8-21]

What, then, can be our expectations for using exercise tests to identify high-risk patients? The exercise test can be expected to identify patients with much muscle in jeopardy from lesions causing ischemia. However, it cannot be expected to recognize individuals with decreased ventricular function. Such patients are best recognized by a combination of a prior history of MI or congestive heart failure, an abnormal ECG, and physical examination and chest x-ray findings.

PROGNOSTIC STUDIES

Studies of the ability of the exercise test after acute MI to predict another MI and mortality have reached conflicting conclusions. The following, therefore, is an analysis of published reports of longitudinal studies using exercise testing in the early post-MI period with a follow-up for cardiac events. To identify differences that might explain their lack of agreement, the studies have been carefully ana-

TABLE 6-1.

Studies in Which the Results of Exercise Testing Were Used to Predict the Results of Coronary Angiography After Acute MI

Investigator	Year Published	Patients Tested	Exercise Test Characteristics				Angiography Time After MI
			Endpoints for Testing	ECG Leads	Protocol	Time After MI	
Weiner	1978	154	Signs and/or symptoms, systolic blood pressure drop, > 4 mm, serious PVCs	12 lead	Bruce‡	2-36 mo	2-36 mo
Paine	1978	100	90% heart rate at maximal effort, signs and/or symptoms, intraventricular conduction defect, 1 mm	V_4 to V_6	Bruce	4 mo	4 mo
Dillahunt	1979	28	Signs and/or symptoms, 1 mm, >3 PVCs /min, 5 min	CM_5, V_2	Naughton	10-18 days	4-20 wk
Sammel	1980	77	SS, 6 METs	12 lead	Green Lane	1 mo	1 mo
Fuller	1981	40	Heart rate 120, signs and/or symptoms, 1 mm, >5 PVCs	12 lead	Low Bruce§	9-18 days	5-12 wk
Starling	1981	57	Signs and/or symptoms, ventricular tachycardia as an endpoint, systolic blood pressure drop, high blood pressure	12 lead	Naughton	9-21 days	3-12 wk
Boschat	1981	65	85% maximum heart rate, 1 mm	12 lead	Bruce	2-12 mo	2-12 mo
Schwartz	1981	48	Signs and/or symptoms, systolic blood pressure drop, ventricular tachycardia, 2 mm, 75% maximum heart rate	12 lead	Low Bruce	18-22 days	3 wk
De Feyter	1982	179	Signs and/or symptoms, ventricular tachycardia	12 lead	Bruce	6-8 wk	6-8 wk
Akhras	1984	119	Signs and/or symptoms	12 lead	Bruce	2 wk	6 wk
Morris	1984	110	Signs and/or symptoms	12 lead	UPR Bike‖	>6 wk	<3 mo
van der Wall	1985	176	Signs and/or symptoms	12 lead	Bruce/TH¶	6-8 wk	6-8 wk

PR, Prior MI; *SE*, subendocardial, or non-Q-wave, MI; *A*, transmural (Q-wave) anterior wall MI; *IP*, transmural inferior and/or posterior MI; *meds*, medications; *dig*, digoxin; *BB*, beta-blockers; *% MVD*, percentage of population with multivessel disease; *sens*, sensitivity; *spec*, specificity; *mm*, amount of ST-segment shift in millimeters taken as an endpoint; *PVCs*, premature ventricular contractions; *CM₅*, a bipolar lead; *ST & ang*, abnormal ST-segment depression and angina induced by the exercise test as the criteria for an abnormal response.
*Ages of all patients and the percentage of women included in the studies.
†Percentage of patients on digitalis or beta-blockers at the time of treadmill testing and often through the follow-up period.
‡Bruce protocol stopped at 85% of the age-predicted maximum heart rate.
§Low Bruce protocol has 0 and $^1/2$ stages that are 0% and 5% grade at 1.7 miles per hour before stage 1 (10% grade at 1.7 miles per hour).
‖UPR Bike protocol uses an upright bike with radionuclide testing.
¶Bruce/TH protocol is the Bruce protocol with thallium imaging.

| Age/% women* | Exclusions | MI % | | Transmural | | % with Angina | Meds † (dig or BB) | % MVD | ST Depression | | Angina | |
		PR	SE	A	IP				Sens	Spec	Sens	Spec
25-65/12%	<85% Heart rate at maximal effort, bundle branch block	0	27	33	41	45	No dig	59	91	65		
48/7%	Unstable angina pectoris, congestive heart failure	22	4	48	48	59	18% BB, 23% dig	66	41	88		
42-69/21%	>Killip 2, hypertension	?	21	50	29		7% dig	61	23	100	29	100
<60/0%	>60, PR, left bundle branch block	0	27	33	43	30	25%, BB, 12% dig	33	48	89		
54/0%	>65, congestive heart failure	25	23	25	53	25	22% BB 10% dig	50	65	ST & ang		90
56/7%	Unstable angina pectoris, congestive heart failure, hypertension	19	25	37	39		25% dig, 33% BB	72	54	75	68	81
50/2.5%	Congestive heart failure, aneurysm, Unstable angina pectoris	0	0	24	41	50	Stopped	65	60	?		
50/10%	Congestive heart failure, unstable angina pectoris	25	31	54	35	15		71	56	ST % ang		86
28-65/10%	>65, bundle branch block	8	12	35	45	29	Stopped	54	67	ST & ang		67
50/6%	Complications, bundle branch block	?	?	?	?		Stopped	73	94	94		
56/12%	Complications	0	0	53	47	31	Stopped	88	30	84	44	95
54/11%	>70, bundle branch block	0	0	43	57	30	Stopped	44	64	70	20	63
							AVERAGES	59	58	82	40	83

lyzed for their methodology, sample selection, detailed description of sample, and description of statistical methods. These studies are summarized in Table 6-2.[22-49] Because they involve the same populations and usually obtained the same results, the studies from the same institution are grouped together. Thus the results from a total of 28 centers are considered.

Prognostic Indicators from the Exercise Test

The five exercise test variables thought to have prognostic importance are a blunted systolic blood pressure (SBP) response (or exertional hypotension), premature ventricular contractions (PVCs), poor exercise capacity (or excessive heart rate response to a low workload), exercise test–induced angina, and ST-segment depression (and sometimes elevation).

Exercise-Induced Dysrhythmias

Only 5 of 28 centers reported that exercise test–induced PVCs indicated a significant increase in risk. Four centers did not include results regarding PVCs; 9 centers reported null or negative associations of PVCs with mortality.

Exercise-Induced ST-Segment Depression

A total of 9 to 28 centers found ST-Segment depression to be significantly predictive of subsequent death; an additional 6 enters reported a positive but insignificant association. Nine centers reported a null effect, and 4 failed to report data on ST-segment depression.

ST Segment Elevation

DeFeyter et al[15] found that ST-segment depression indicated multivessel disease, whereas ST-segment elevation indicated advanced LV wall motion abnormalities and a low EF. Both shifts indicated that multivessel disease and advanced LV wall motion abnormalities existed. In the study of Waters et al,[32] ST-segment elevation generated the same univariate risk as did depression; therefore they were considered together. However, location of the ST-segment shift was not specified. Saunamaki and Anderson considered ST-segment depression and elevation separately but did not specify its location. In their study, the ST-segment responses had little prognostic value. Handler[48] found ST-segment elevation to generate a significant risk ratio of 10. Combined elevation and depression had a significant risk ratio of 13. ST-segment elevation also predicted heart failure.

Exercise Capacity

A total of 9 of 28 centers reported that a low exercise capacity or an excessive heart rate response to exercise indicated a high-risk group. Five additional centers reported nonsignificant positive associations, and Stanford[30] reported a positive association in only one of three studies. A total of 10 of 28 centers failed to report suffcient data on this variable to assess its effect.

Exercise-Induced Angina

Only 5 of 28 centers reported that exercise test–induced angina indicated a significantly increased risk group. Eight centers failed to report angina data. A total of 7 reported nonsignificant positive associations.

Systolic Blood Pressure Response to Exercise

A total of 9 of 28 centers found that inadequate or abnormal SBP response to exercise significantly identified a high-risk group; 11 of the centers failed to report data, and 4 reported a nonsignificant positive association.

Comparison of Exercise Data to Clinical Data

An important question to be resolved is whether the exercise test gives more predictive information than the standard clinical risk predictors. Clinical attempts to establish risk have included scores based on clinical features of the MI and historical information such as the Norris and Peel indexes. Kentala[23] assessed clinical parameters, including a careful history of prior activity level. The prognostic power of clinical and ECG variables recorded soon after MI and in connection with the exercise test were analyzed by stepwise multiple discriminant analysis. Kentala[23] found that clinical and exercise test variables were important. Patients dying within 2 years had a low exercise SBP. With longer follow-up, though, the exercise SBP was a weaker predictor of risk. For patients who suddenly died after 2 years, T-wave changes after exercise, which possibly indicated subendocardial injury, were common. Patients with a high level of physical activity before their MI were less prone to die suddenly. Saunamaki and Anderson[36] demonstrated that exercise testing variables, including PVCs and a poor hemodynamic response to exercise, still were able to predict risk for those with congestive heart failure (CHF), prior MI, and anterior MI. In predicting risk, the exercise test variables outperformed these important clinical parameters.

Clinical Design Features

The column headings used in Table 6-2 and separately listed in the box are the important features of study design that could affect findings.

Myocardial Infarction Mix.   The different types of MIs marked by Q-wave location have a different prognosis and different normal response to exercise. Exercise predictors may be different in each type.

Inclusion of Non-Q-Wave MIs.   After much controversy about the risk of having a subendocardial MI, studies from the Mayo clinic[50] and Framingham[51] appear to clarify the issue. The 30-day fatality rate was higher among patients with transmural MIs and lower among those with subendocardial MIs. No significant difference was found in the rates of reinfarction, CABS, or mortality over the next 5 years. CHF was more common among patients with transmural MIs, and angina was more common among patients with non-Q-wave MIs. This review and other data support the concept that ST-segment depression in exercise testing effectively predicts high-risk patients after a non-Q-wave MI.

Text continued on p. 148.

TABLE 6-2.

Summary of Prospective Studies Evaluating the Ability of the Exercise Test After Acute MI to Allow Prediction of Reinfarction and Mortality

Investigator	Year	MI Pop. Size	Exercise Tested n	Exercise Tested %	End Points	ECG Leads	Protocol	Weeks After MI	Age/% Women[a]	Exclusions	PR	SE	A	IP	Meds (Dig or BB)[b]
Ericsson	73	184	100	54	Heart rate 140, signs and/or symptoms	PC	Treadmill	3	59/7	>65	25	?	51	43	
Kentala	75	298	158	53	Maximal effort	CH$_1$ to CH$_6$	Bike	6-8	53/0	>65, rehabilitation program	28	13	42	58	35% dig, 1% BB
Granath	77	430	205	48	Heart rate 140, signs and/or symptoms	12-lead	TM/Bike	3&9	59/11	>65	18	?	48	33	66% dig
Smith	79	109	62	57	60% heart rate	12-lead	GXT[f]	3	60/?	?	?	5	?	?	10% BB
Hunt	79	633	56	9	70% heart rate, signs and/or symptoms	7-lead	Bike	6	57/11	No complications	?	0	47	53	?
Srinivasan	81	154				7-lead					?	?	?	?	?
Sami	79	200			Signs and/or symptoms	12-lead	Naughton	3-52	57/10	Congestive heart failure, unstable angina pectoris	8	9	29	62	8% dig
Davidson	80	461	195	42	Heart rate, signs and/or symptoms	12-lead	Stanford[g]	3	53/0	>70, cardiac medications, congestive heart failure	8	10	29	61	None
DeBusk	83	702	338	48	Signs and/or symptoms	12-lead	Naughton	3	54/0	>70, congestive heart failure, unstable angina pectoris	?	?	?	?	3% dig
Theroux	79	326	210	64	5 METs, 70% heart rate	CM$_5$	Naughton	1.6	52/0	>70 congestive heart failure, unstable angina pectoris	34	18	31	50	40% BB, 1% dig
Waters	85	330	225	68					53/16		25	21	43	55	6% dig, 32% BB
Koppes	80	410	108	26	Submaximal effort/maximal effort	12-lead	Bruce	3&8	52/13	Congestive heart failure, cardiac medications, angina	?	24	28	48	None
Starling	80	190	130	68	Heart rate 130, signs and/or symptoms	V$_1$, V$_5$, V$_6$	Naughton	2	53/14	Unstable angina pectoris, congestive heart failure	24	29	34	37	26% dig, 16% BB
Weld	81	325	236	73	4 METs, signs and/or symptoms	V$_5$	Low Bruce[i]	2	54/12	>70	21	?	?	?	12% BB, 41% dig
Saunamaki	81	404	317	78	Signs and/or symptoms	PC	Bike	3	57/20	Age, congestive heart failure, angina	10	?	32	?	20% dig, 2% BB
Velasco	81	958	200	21	30watts, signs and/or symptoms	PC	SupBike	2.5	60/22	>66, subendocardial MI, women	3	0	46	55	11% dig, 9% BB

Column groupings: "Exercise Test Characteristics" spans End Points through Weeks After MI. "Population Characteristics" spans Age/% Women through Meds. "MI %" with "Transmural" (A, IP) and PR, SE subcolumns.

n, Number; *PR*, prior MI; *SE*, subendocardial, or non-Q-wave, MI; *A*, transmural (Q-wave) anterior wall MI; *IP*, transmural inferior and/or posterior MI; *meds*, medications; *dig*, digoxin; *BB*, beta-blockers; % *CABS*, percentage of patients who underwent coronary artery bypass surgery during follow-up; *ET*, exercise testing; *RE*, recurrent; *SPB*, abnormal systolic blood pressure response; *PVCs*, abnormal premature ventricular contractions; *ExCap*, abnormally low exercise capacity tolerance; *ST*, abnormal ST-segment response (usually only depression); *NR*, not reported; +, positive nonsignificant association of unusual high risk with death; nx, *n* times increased risk of death with usual high-risk level; ?, insignificant data to test significance; *1*, null effect; −, a negative nonsignificant association of usual high-risk level with death.
[a] Mean age of all patients and percentage of women included in the study.
[b] Percentage of patients on digitalis or beta-blockers at the time of treadmill testing and often through the follow-up period.
[c] Mortality rate in patients who underwent exercise testing (yes) and who were excluded from exercise testing for clinical reasons (no).
[d] Percentage of patients who had another MI if they underwent exercise testing (yes) and if they were excluded from exercise testing (no).
[e] These are responses to exercise testing that have been most commonly reported as having prognostic value. If the risk ratio is statistically significant, it is underlined. Nonsignificant risk ratios permit trends across studies to be detected. The risk ratio means that if the cutoff point for this abnormality was reached, patients with that abnormality have a risk of death at certain times (×) greater than those without the abnormality. Only the hard endpoints of death (and in some studies reinfarction) are considered.
[f] GXT protocol is the Bruce protocol stopped at 85% of the age-predicted maximum heart rate.
[g] The Stanford protocol is another version of the Naughton test.
[h] Proportional hazards regression model for survival analysis.
[i] The low Bruce protocol has 0 and 1/2 stages that are 0% and 5% grade at 1.7 miles per hour before stage 1 (10% grade at 1.7 miles per hour).
[j] Detailed specific alogorithm displayed for clinical use.
[k] This study used a 2.5-mile-per-hour treadmill protocol with increasing grades.

| Follow-up Period | | | | | Exercise Test Risk Markers[e] | | | | | |
Mean or Median	Range	% CABS	Mortality If ET Performed: Yes/No[c]	RE MI If ET Performed: Yes/No[d]	SBP	PVC	ExCap	Angina	ST	Statistical Method
3 mo	3 mo-?	?	5%/		NR[f]	4×	?	?	NR	Descriptive
6 yr	?	0%	32%/	?	+	+	NR	NR	+[a]	Univariate, some discriminant function analysis
2-5 yr	2-5 yr	?	25%/		NR	2×[a]	2×	2×	NR	Univariate
1.5 yr	?	?	10%/17%	?	NR	—	NR	NR	6×[a]	Univariate
1 yr	?	?	14%/18%	?	NR	1	NR	4×[a]	3×[a]	Descriptive, univariate
1.25 yr	1-2 yr	?	8%	?	NR	?	NR	3×[a]	7×[a]	Not cited (univariate)
19 mo	2-51 mo	10%	2%/	5%/	NR	—	1	NR	3×[a]	Univariate
26 mo	1-60 mo	10%	1.5%/	6%/	?	?	+[a]	1	+[a]	Multivariate—logistic regression, clinical life-table, Kaplan-Meier estimates
34 mo	?	6%	2.1%/5.5%	2%/	NR	NR	NR	NR	8×[a]	Univariate; Cox[h] to select some variables
1 yr	1 yr	5.7%	9.5%/	6%/	NR	2×	NR	—	13×[a]	Univariate
2 yr	5-7 yr	16%	11%-3%		+[a]	+	+	NR	8×[a]	Univariate (Cox[h]), multivariate-Cox/conditional with regard to time
2 yr	?		2%/		?	?	?	?	?	Univariate
11 mo	6-20 mo	?	8%/	9%/	5×	2×	NR	4×	4×	Univariate
1 yr	?	?	9%/		5×[a]	2×[a]	19×[a]	2×	2×	Multivariate—logistic regression, univariate estimate
5.7 yr	5-6 yr	?	35.6%/	?	3×[a]	2×[a]	NR	NR	1	Clinical life tables within clinical subsets
3 yr	3 mo-6 yr	?	11%/	3%/	3×	2×	NR	3×[a]	4×[a]	Univariate
28 mo	13-40 mo	13%	6%/	7%/	NR	3×	+	2×	1	Univariate
2.3 yr	10d-62 mo	?	7%/	19%/	—	NR	+	2×[a]	1	Univariate

Continued.

TABLE 6-2—cont'd.

Summary of Prospective Studies Evaluating the Ability of the Exercise Test After Acute MI to Allow Prediction of Reinfarction and Mortality

Investigator	Year	MI Pop. Size	Exercise Tested n	%	End Points	ECG Leads	Protocol	Weeks After MI	Age/% of Women[a]	Exclusions	MI % Transmural PR	SE	A	IP	Meds (Dig or BB)[b]
De Feyter	82	222	179	81	Signs and/or symptoms	12-lead	Bruce	6-8	52/0	>65, referrals	8	12	35	45	Stopped
Jelinek	82		188		Symptoms	V_4, V_5, V_6	Bike	1.5	52/10	Angina, congestive heart failure	18	28	29	42	?
Madsen	83	886	456	52	Signs and/or symptoms	9-lead	Bike	2.6	51/?	>75, unstable angina pectoris, congestive heart failure	31	6	35	?	12% dig, 2% BB
Gibson	83	229	140	61	Heart rate 120, signs and/or symptoms	3-lead	Naughton	1.6	63/13	>65, congestive heart failure	19	26	35	53	2% dig, 61% BB
Norris	84	395	315	80	Signs and/or symptoms	?	2.5 mph[k]	4	51/13	>60	0	27	29	42	30% BB
Williams	84	226	205	91	6 METs	3-lead	Bruce	1.7	50/0	>70	23	22	33	46	16% dig, 19% BB
Jennings	84	503	103	20	5 METs, signs and/or symptoms	V_5	2 mph	1.7	56/18		?	?	51	49	4% dig, 10% BB
Fioretti	84	293	214	72	Symptoms	XYZ	Bike	2	54/13	>66, congestive heart failure, angina		?			40% BB
	85	405	300	74					54/16	Congestive heart failure, angina	27		36	?	18% dig, 52% BB
Krone	85	1417	667	47	5 METs	3-lead	Low Bruce	2	?/20	>70	22	22	31	42	28% dig, 31% BB
Dwyer	85								60% <60						
Handler	85	296	222	75	5 METs, 70% heart rate	3-lead	Naughton	1.4	54/16	>65, coronary artery bypass surgery, bundle branch block	?	21	42	37	1% dig, 17% BB
SCOR	85	1469	295	20	75% heart rate, signs and/or symptoms	12-lead	Mixed treadmill	1.7	58/18	Physician judgment	21	18	38	44	26% dig, 53% BB
Jespersen	85		126		Maximal effort, signs and/or symptoms	II, V_4 and V_6	Bike	3.4	57/14	> 71, unstable angina pectoris, congestive heart failure	0	36	31	33	13% dig, 20% BB
Paolila	85	362	263	73	Maximal effort	12-lead	Bike	7	50/0	>65, unstable angina pectoris, congestive heart failure, women	3	11	32	57	2% dig, 2% BB
Murray	86	350	300	86	Submaximal effort		Treadmill	2	53/17	>66, congestive heart failure	?	?	?	?	20% BB
Cleempoel	86	202	198	98	Submaximal effort	4-lead	Treadmill	1.6	58/0	>70, women, congestive heart failure	?	?	?	?	10% dig, 50% BB
Stone	86	719	473	66	Maximal effort	12-lead	Treadmill	24	54/21	> 75, unstable angina pectoris, congestive heart failure, PVCs	22	28	?	?	26% dig, 39% BB
TOTAL			7029												

Follow-up Period					Exercise Test Risk Markers[e]					
Mean or Median	Range	% CABS	Mortality If ET Performed: Yes/No[c]	RE MI If ET Performed: Yes/No[d]	SBP	PVC	ExCap	Angina	ST	Statistical Method
28 mo	13-40 mo	13%	6%/	7%/	NR	3×	+	2×	1	Univariate
2.3 yr	10d-62 mo	?	7%/	19%/	—	NR	+	2×[a]	1	Univariate
1 yr		0%	6.6%/28%	4%/12%	+[a]	+[a]	+[a]	?	1	Multivariate—discriminant function analysis; Cox;algorithm[j]
1.3 yr	1-3 yr	14%	5%/	6%/	NR	NR	NR	+	+	Univariate
3.5 yr	1-6 yr	24%	13%/33%	12%/	NR	NR	?	?	1	Univariate—logistic regression; Cox cited
1 yr	1 yr	12%	6%/31%	6.8%/	2×	—	2×[a]	2×	1	Multivariate—discriminant function analysis; univariate estimates
1 yr	?	5%	9%/21%	3%/	8×[a]	1	8×[a]	?	1	Univariate
1.2 yr		8%	9%/23%		+[a]	2×	+	1	2×	Univariate
1 yr	1 yr	8%	7%/28%	4%/	+[a]	+	+[a]	1	—	Multivariate—discriminant function analysis; algorithm
1 yr	1 yr	12%	5%/14%		8×[a]	2×	3×[a]	3×[a]	1	Univariate; multivariate—logistic regression
				5%/10%	NR	?	?	?	?	Univariate multivariate—logistic regression
1.2 yr	6-36 mo	9%	7%/	4%/	5×[a]	1	8×[a]	1	2×	Univariate
1 yr	?	?	7%/15%		1	2×	9×[a]	2×	3×	Univariate, multivariate—discriminant function analysis
1 yr	1 yr	<1%	7%	2%	1	1	1	1	3×[a]	Univariate, Kapplan-Meier
2.6 yr	3-57 mo	6%	4.1%/	8.3%/	1	1	1	1	4×	Univariate
13 mo	6 mo-?	?	18%/	30%/	NR	NR	NR	+	+	Univariate
0.16 yr	2 mo	?	5%/	?	NR	NR	+	NR	1	Univariate, multivariate—discriminant function analysis
1 yr	?	2	3%/16%	5%/	5×	6×	6×	1	1	Univariate, multivariate, logistic regression

	SBP RR	PVC RR	ExCap RR	Ang RR	ST RR
Number of studies demonstrating significant risk predictor	9	5	9	5	9
Number with positive risk	13	14	14	12	15
Number with reported effect	18	23	18	20	24

METHODOLOGICAL CHARACTERISTICS
THAT DIFFER BETWEEN STUDIES

Infarct mix (i.e., non-Q-wave, inferior/anterior/lateral Q-wave)
Endpoints of test
Leads monitored and ways that ST-segment elevation is considered
Exercise protocol
Time after MI when test was performed
Age range, gender
Entrance criteria
Patients excluded
History of CHF and angina
Patients with prior MI and those with or without complications
MI size
Follow-up thoroughness and length
Percentage of patients undergoing CABS or PTCA during follow-up study and
   whether they are censored
Prior CABS
Cardiac events (CABS should not be used as an endpoint.)
Mortality rate during follow-up (Are they a high-risk or a low-risk group?)
Reinfarction rate
Test responses considered and their cutoff points (SBP, PVCs, exercise
   capacity, angina, ST)
Statistical methods (multivariate survival analysis techniques are required; if
   univariate techniques are used, they should include Kaplan-Meier survival
   curves)

Klein, Froelicher, and Detrano[52] found exercise-induced ST-segment depression to be associated with cardiovascular death in patients with non-Q-wave MIs and not in those with Q-wave MIs. Abnormal ST-segment depression was associated with twice the risk for death, and the risk increased to 11 times in patients without diagnostic Q waves, similar to the results by Krone, Dwyer, and Greenberg[53] in patients with an initial non-Q-wave MI. These results suggest that the differences among studies in the prognostic value of the post MI exercise ECG is due to variations in the prevalence of the patterns of the rest ECG among study populations. Angiographic studies, however, have demonstrated that exercise-induced ST-segment depression is associated with severe coronary artery disease whether Q waves are present. The conflicting results from follow-up and angiographic studies are probably due to the fact that early mortality is strongly associated with LV damage, whereas later mortality is associated with ischemia and severe coronary artery disease.

Endpoints of Exercise Test. If the exercise test was stopped at a certain amount of ST-segment shift, MET level, or heart rate, the test response could not be considered as a continuous variable nor could a higher value, which might be more discriminating, be reached.

Exercise Protocol.   Whether the test was maximal or submaximal has an impact on the responses.

Time After Myocardial Infarction When Exercise Test Was Performed.   The studies that performed exercise testing at multiple times found the same responses to have different predictive values at the specific times the tests were performed. "Stunned" myocardium and deconditioning affect predischarge testing more than they affect later hemodynamic responses. ST-segment responses appear more labile soon after MI. The responses differ at various times after MI as well, with a spontaneous improvement in hemodynamics occuring by 2 months. A spontaneous improvement during the first year after MI in the blunted blood pressure response to exercise particularly occurs in patients with large anterior MIs.

Age Range and Gender.   Women are thought to have a higher MI mortality and certainly are known to respond differently than men to exercise testing. Because of this, they should be considered separately, but the studies do not contain a sufficent number for valid analysis. Death rates are directly related to age.

Exclusion Criteria.   To identify the highest risk group, patients are excluded from exercise testing on the basis of clinical judgments about illness, age, cardiac dysfunction, and ischemia in the post-MI population. Alternate testing methods that have been compared favorably with exercise testing have included right atrial pacing and electrophysiological stimulation studies.

Inclusion of Patients with Prior MI.   Prior MI is an important predictive variable that depends on the severity of the prior MI or MIs. Patients with prior large MIs are more likely to be admitted with non-Q-wave MIs, since another transmural MI increases their likelihood of dying before hospitalization. Few studies have tried to account for the number or severity of prior MIs.

Medications Taken After Discharge from Hospital and at the Time of the Test.   Digoxin causes ST-segment depression but is usually taken for CHF, thus implicating an ischemic etiology for a potential death from dysfunction. Beta-blockers affect blood pressure and heart rate response and improve survival.

Percentage of Patients Undergoing CABS or PTCA During Follow-Up.   CABS or PTCA could alter mortality and affect outcome prediction. Also, patients with ischemic predictors would be selected to have this procedure more frequently. These patients should be censored at the time of intervention, but such censoring is not random.

Cardiac Events Considered Endpoints.   The only hard endpoints that should be considered are death and reinfarction. However, distinguishing sudden death as an endpoint makes little sense and may confuse the analysis, particularly if those with sudden death are compared with all others (including those with non-sudden cardiac death). Nonsudden cardiac deaths are often difficult to distinguish, lead to biased results, and may play a confusing role, particularly in older populations. CABS is not a valid endpoint and should be censored.

Metaanalysis Considerations

Metaanalysis is a statistical approach used to develop a consensus from an existing body of research. It is a quantitative approach to reviewing research by using a variety of statistical techniques for sorting, classifying, and summarizing information from the findings of many studies. It is also the application of research methodology to the characteristics and findings of studies, including problem selection, hypothesis formulation, the definition and measurement of constructs and variables, sampling, and data analysis.

Metaanalysis is applied to a body of research in three stages. First, a complete literature search is conducted (analogous to the collection of data in an experimental study). Second, the important characteristics and findings of relevant studies are classified. Third, statistical techniques are applied to the compiled data. This last stage can involve descriptive, correlational, and inferential statistical analysis. The statistical techniques applied here are sign testing, correlation analysis, and weighted regression analysis.

Sign testing is a statistical test that evaluates the proportions of findings and determines if they are related by more than chance. As a part of metaanalysis, it was applied to the findings in Table 6-2. Because it is not possible to ascertain the directions of the nonsignificant associations listed as *?* in Table 6-2, metaanalysis conclusions must be tentative. Some researchers probably did not evaluate markers that are not reported *(NR)*, but others are likely to have failed to report null or negative findings. The most generous approach would be to omit studies that did not report results for a particular marker; the most conservative approach would be to include these studies and to assume that any unreported results were not positive associations. Results are presented for both approaches, with upper and lower bounds for the overall published results evaluating exercise test markers as predictors of death.

If there were not a true underlying association of a risk marker with death, we would expect that 50% of studies would report positive associations based on chance. *Statistical significance* is not considered here; only the directions of the *observed* associations. Using only studies with any reported effect as the denominator, the generous estimates of the percentages of positive associations reported for SBP (12 centers reporting positive associations/18 centers presenting any results for SBP), PVCs (14/23), exercise capacity (14/18), angina (12/20), and ST-segment changes (15/19) are 72%, 61%, 78%, 60%, and 63%. Only the *SBP* and *exercise capacity* proportions are significantly different by a sign test from those by chance. The conservative estimates using all 28 studies as the denominator are 46%, 50%, 50%, 43%, and 54%. None of these are different from those based on chance. Considering probable bias against publishing negative findings, the true situations are likely to be closer to the conservative computations than to the generous ones.

Subgrouping by predischarge testing (arbitrarily set at less than 3 weeks after

MI) and postdischarge testing (3 weeks or greater) yielded the findings in Table 6-3. Note that all of the predictors except for ST-segment shifts were reported positively more than 50% of the time during predischarge testing and not during postdischarge testing. To see whether these differences were due to maximal or submaximal endpoints for exercise testing, Table 6-4 was constructed. Although during submaximal testing the exercise predictors were more likely to be associated with positivity than during maximal testing, the finding was not as strong.

TABLE 6-3.

Results of Studies Grouped by Whether Testing Was Done Before 3 Weeks After MI or at 3 Weeks or Later

		Exercise Test Risk Markers				
Investigator	Endpoint	SBP	PVCs	ExCap	Angina	ST
Early or predischarge (13 institutional studies)						
MHI	Submaximal	+*	+	+	NR	8×*
Starling	Submaximal	5×	2×	NR	4×	4×
Weld	Submaximal	5×*	2×*	19×*	2×	2×
Velasco	Submaximal	3×	2×	NR	3×	4×*
Jelinek	Maximal	−	NR	+	2×*	1
Madsen	Maximal	+*	+*	+*	?	1
Gibson	Submaximal	NR	NR	NR	+	+
Williams	Submaximal	2×	−	2×*	2×	1
Jennings	Submaximal	8×*	1	8×*	?	1
Fioretti	Maximal	+*	+	+*	1	−
MCPMIgrp	Submaximal	8×*	2×	3×*	3×*	1
Handler	Submaximal	5×*	1	8×*	1	2×
SCOR	Submaximal	1	2×	9×*	2×	3×
No. significant out of 13		7	2	8	3	2
No. reporting positively		10	8	10	7	7
No. reporting analysis		12	11	10	12	13
Late or postdischarge (11 institutional studies)						
Ericsson	Submaximal	NR	4×	?	?	NR
Kentala	Maximal	+	+	NR	NR	+*
Granath	Submaximal	NR	2×*	2×	2×	NR
Smith	Submaximal	NR	−	NR	NR	6×*
Hunt	Submaximal	NR	1	NR	4×*	3×*
Stanford	Maximal	NR	NR	+*	1	8×*
Koppes	Maximal	?	?	?	?	?
Saunamaki	Maximal	3×*	2×*	NR	NR	1
De Feyter	Maximal	NR	3×	+	2×	1
Norris	Maximal	NR	NR	?	?	1
Jespersen	Maximal	1	1	1	1	3×*
No. significant out of 11		1	2	1	1	5
No. reporting positively		2	5	3	3	5
No. reporting analysis		4	9	7	8	9

ExCap, Abnormally low exercise capacity tolerance; *ST*, abnormal ST-segment response (usually only depression); +, positive nonsignificant association of unusual high risk with death; *NR*, not reported; n×, *n* times increased risk of death with usual high-risk level; −, a negative nonsignificant association of usual high-risk level with death; *1*, null effect; *?*, insignificant data to test significance.
*Statistically significant.

TABLE 6-4.

Results of Studies Grouped by Whether the Endpoint Was Maximal or Submaximal

Investigators	Exercise Test Risk Markers				
	SBP	PVCs	ExCap	Angina	ST
Submaximal testing (14 institutional studies)					
Ericcson	NR	4×	?	?	NR
Granath	NR	2×*	2×	2×	NR
Smith	NR	−	NR	NR	6×*
Hunt	NR	1	NR	4×*	3×*
MHI	+*	+	+	NR	8×*
Starling	5×	2×	NR	4×	4×
Weld	5×*	2×*	19×*	2×	2×
Velasco	3×	2×	NR	3×*	4×*
Gibson	NR	NR	NR	+	+
Williams	2×	−	2×*	2×	1
Jennings	8×*	1	8×*	?	1
MCPMIgrp	8×*	2×	3×*	3×*	1
Handler	5×*	1	8×*	1	2×
SCOR	1	2×	9×*	2×	3×
No. significant out of 14	5	2	6	3	4
No. reporting postively	8	8	8	9	9
No. reporting analysis	9	13	9	12	12
Maximal testing (10 institutional studies)					
Kentala	+	+	NR	NR	+*
Stanford	NR	NR	+*	1	8×*
Koppes	?	?	?	?	?
Saunamaki	3×*	2×*	NR	NR	1
De Feyter	NR	3×	+	2×	1
Jelinek	−	NR	+	2×*	1
Madsen	+*	+*	+*	?	1
Norris	NR	NR	?	?	1
Fioretti	+*	+	+*	1	−
Jespersen	1	1	1	1	3×*
No. significant out of 10	3	2	3	1	3
No. reporting positively	4	5	5	2	3
No. reporting analysis	7	7	8	8	10

*Statistically significant.
ExCap, Abnormally low exercise capacity tolerance; *ST*, abnormal ST-segment response (usually only depression); +, positive nonsignificant association of unusual high risk with death; *NR*, not reported; n×, *n* times increased risk of death with usual high-risk level; −, a negative nonsignificant association of usual high-risk level with death; *1*, null effect; ?, insignificant data to test significance.

Subgrouping the studies by whether they were performed before or after discharge, as was done in Table 6-3, shows that the highest rate of positive predictors and the highest risk ratios occur with predischarge testing. Using only studies of predischarge exercise testing with any reported effect as the denominator, the generous estimates of the percentages of positive associations reported for SBP (10 centers reporting positive associations/12 centers presenting any results for SBP), PVCs (8/12), exercise capacity (10/10), angina (7/12), and ST-segment changes (7/13) are 83%, 67%, 100%, 58%, and 54%. Only the responses for SBP and exercise capacity were significant, but none of the exercise test responses were significant for testing done after discharge (50%, 56%, 43%, 38%, and 56%). In Table 6-4, the studies are divided into those that used maximal and those that used submaximal endpoints for exercise testing. Using only studies of submaximal exercise testing with any reported effect as the denominator, the generous estimates of the percentages of positive associations reported for SBP (8 centers reporting positive associations/9 centers presenting any results for SBP), PVCs (8/13), exercise capacity (8/9), angina (8/10), and ST-segment changes (9/12) are 89%, 63%, 89%, 80%, and 75%. All exercise responses except for PVCs were significantly associated with a poor outcome with submaximal testing, and none of the exercise test responses with maximal testing were significant (57%, 71%, 63%, 25%, and 30%).

PATIENTS WHO SHOULD UNDERGO CORONARY ANGIOGRAPHY AFTER MI FOR CONSIDERATION OF CABS TO IMPROVE SURVIVAL

By working backward through known associations and relationships, the clinical description of the high-risk patient who could potentially have improved survival with CABS can be derived. The randomized trials of CABS have demonstrated that patients with triple-vessel or left main disease with an EF of 30% to 50% have improved survival with surgery as compared with medical therapy. Although coronary heart disease can cause myocardial fibrosis and decreased ventricular function without overt MIs by signs or symptoms, this occurrence is unusual. Studies have shown 15% to 25% of MIs are silent, but in these cases the diagnosis was made by the ECG. The clinical picture, either by history or by ECG, that would result in an EF from 30% to 50% would include patients with large anterior MIs, a history or ECG pattern of multiple MIs, transmural MIs followed by subendocardial MIs, or a history of transient CHF with an MI. In addition, physical findings of ventricular dyskinesia or cardiomegaly on palpation would support this picture. Thus clinical and ECG features predict those with decreased ventricular function. Noninvasive testing (e.g., radionuclide ventriculography and echocardiography) could also be used. Although its sensitivity is decreased in single- or double-vessel disease, the exercise ECG is approximately 90% sensitive for triple-vessel or left main disease. Angina is also very common in this group of patients. Therefore the following profile identifies the high-risk patient after an MI who should undergo coronary angiography: the patient with a history or ECG findings of a large anterior MI, multiple MIs, abnormal precordial movements, a history of transient CHF, or signs and symptoms of severe myocardial ischemia on the exercise test. Severe ischemia is characterized by the occurrence of ST-segment depression or angina at a double product less than 20,000 and less than 5 METs exercise capacity. If there are no contraindications to CABS in these patients, they should be considered for coronary angiography. Post-MI patients who should be considered for reasons other than improved survival are those whose angina is not controlled satisfactorily with medications and those in whom the diagnosis of

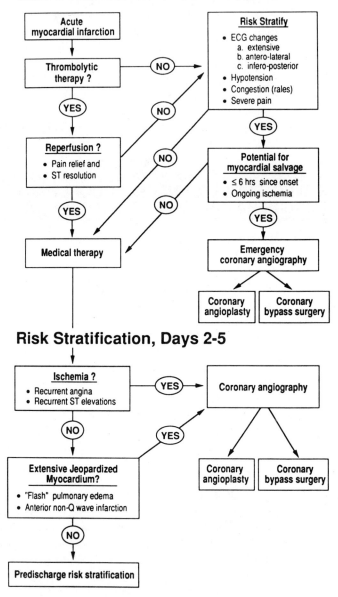

Risk Stratification: Initial Presentation

Risk Stratification, Days 2-5

FIG 6-1.
Krone's scheme for initial treatment of a patient with an acute MI. (From Krone RJ: *Ann Intern Med* 116:223-237, 1992.)

Risk Stratification: Predischarge

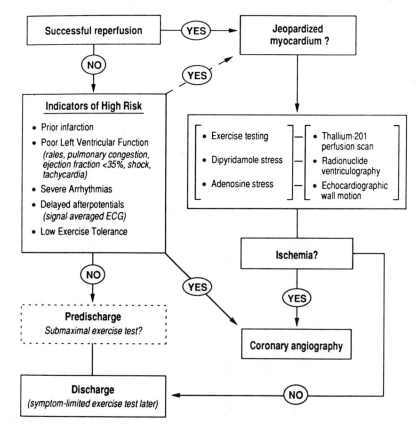

FIG 6-2.
The risk stratification plan synthesized by Krone for predischarge after MI. (From Krone RJ: *Ann Intern Med* 116:223-237, 1992.)

MI or the etiology of chest pain after MI is uncertain. This logical algorithm still requires validation.

Although exercise-induced ST-segment depression is associated with cardiovascular death in non-Q-wave MIs and not in Q-wave MIs, angiographic studies have demonstrated that exercise-induced ST-segment depression is associated with severe coronary artery disease whether Q waves are present. The conflicting results from follow-up and angiographic studies probably relate to the fact that early mortality is strongly associated with LV damage and later mortality is associated with ischemia and severe coronary artery disease.

Krone has nicely summarized recommendations for the use of noninvasive testing in risk stratification after MI.[54] Figs 6-1 and 6-2 illustrate these recommendations, which are pertinent to clinical practice.

SUMMARY

The many practical clinical purposes of the post-MI exercise test have been described. The test can demonstrate to the patient, relatives, or employer the effect of the MI on the capacity for physical performance. Psychologically, it can cause an improvement in the patient's self-confidence by making the patient less anxious about daily physical activities. The test has been helpful in reassuring spouses of post-MI patients of their physical capabilities. The psychological impact of performing well on the exercise test is impressive. Many patients increase their activity and actually rehabilitate themselves after being encouraged and reassured by their response to this test.

The angiographic studies correlating results with post-MI exercise testing involved populations that were very selected, in particular containing a higher prevalence of patients with angina because they are more likely to undergo angiography. In some studies, an abnormal test result was considered to indicate angina or ST-segment depression, and the results for each response could not be distinguished. Few of these studies considered the other exercise test responses that have been associated with a poor prognosis. Review of the studies demonstrated a limited sensitivity and specificity for identification of patients with multivessel disease. Certainly the sensitivity for detecting those with left main and triple-vessel disease is higher. The poor specificity could lead to more angiography than is necessary and, in turn, to unnecessary interventions, since there is always the tendency to "do something," despite the absence of data that survival is improved.

One consistent finding in the review of post-MI exercise test studies that included a follow-up for cardiac endpoints is that patients who met whatever criteria were set forth for exercise testing were at lower risk than patients not tested. This finding supports the clinical judgment of the skilled clinician. In the complete set of data from the review, only an abnormal SBP response or a low exercise capacity were significantly associated with a poor outcome. These responses are so powerful because they can be associated with ischemic or CHF cardiovascular deaths. When the studies were subgrouped by whether testing was done before or after discharge, a high proportion of predischarge test results indicated a poor outcome. This may mean that the risk predictors from exercise testing can only identify the patients that die early after an MI, before later testing can be done. Submaximal testing resulted in the highest proportion of positive associations and the highest risk ratios, which may mean that abnormal responses at higher workloads are not as predictive as those at lower workloads.

REFERENCES

1. Taylor CB et al: Exercise testing to enhance wives' confidence in their husband's cardiac capability soon after clinically uncomplicated acute myocardial infarction, *Am J Cardiol* 55:635-638, 1985.
2. Ewart CK et al: Effects of early postmyocardial infarction exercise testing on self-perception and subsequent physical activity, *Am J Cardiol* 51:1076-1080, 1983.

3. Wohl AJ et al: Cardiovascular function during early recovery from acute myocardial infarction, *Circulation* 56:931-937, 1977.

4. Haskell WL et al: Factors influencing estimated oxygen uptake during exercise testing soon after myocardial infarction, *Am J Cardiol* 50:299-304, 1982.

5. Castellanet MJ, Greenberg PS, Ellestad MH: Comparison of ST-segment changes on exercise testing with angiographic findings in patients with prior myocardial infarction, *Am J Cardiol* 42:29-35, 1978.

6. Ahnve S et al: Can ischemia be recognized when Q waves are present on the resting electrocardiogram? *Am Heart J* 110:1016-1020, 1986.

7. Miranda C et al: Post MI exercise testing: non Q wave vs Q wave, *Circulation* 84:2357-2365, 1991.

8. Paine TD et al: Relation of graded exercise test findings after myocardial infarction to extent of coronary artery disease and left ventricular dysfunction, *Am J Cardiol* 42:716-723, 1978.

9. Dillahunt PH, Miller AB: Early treadmill testing after myocardial infarction, *Chest* 76:150-155, 1979.

10. Sammel NL et al: Angiocardiography and exercise testing at one month after a first myocardial infarction, *Aust NZ J Med* 10:182-187, 1980.

11. Fuller CM et al: Early post-myocardial infarction treadmill stress testing: an accurate predictor of multivessel coronary disease and subsequent cardiac events, *Ann Intern Med* 94:734-739, 1981.

12. Boschat J et al: Treadmill exercise testing and coronary cineangiography following first myocardial infarction, *J Cardiac Rehab* 1:206-211, 1981.

13. Schwartz KM et al: Limited exercise testing soon after myocardial infarction: correlation with early coronary and left ventricular angiography, *Ann Intern Med* 94:727-734, 1981.

14. Starling MR et al: Predictive value of early postmyocardial infarction modified treadmill exercise testing in multivessel coronary artery disease detection, *Am Heart J* 102:169-175, 1981.

15. De Feyter PJ et al: Early angiography after myocardial infarction: what have we learned? *Am Heart J* 109:194-199, 1985.

16. Akhras F et al: Early exercise testing and elective coronary artery bypass surgery after uncomplicated myocardial infarction: effect on morbidity and mortality, *Br Heart J* 52:413-417, 1984.

17. Morris DD et al: Noninvasive prediction of the angiographic extent of coronary artery disease after myocardial infarction: comparison of clinical bicycle exercise, electrocardiographic and ventriculographic parameters, *Circulation* 70:192-201, 1984.

18. van der Wall EE et al: Thallium-201 exercise testing in patients 6-8 weeks after myocardial infarction: limited value for the detection of multivessel disease, *Euro Heart J* 6:29-36, 1985.

19. Veenbrink WG et al: Is there an indication for coronary angiography in patients under 60 years of age with no or minimal angina pectoris after a first myocardial infarction? *Br Heart J* 53:30-35, 1985.

20. Sia STB et al: Usefulness of early exercise testing after non-Q-wave myocardial infarction in predicting prognosis, *Am J Cardiol* 57:738-744, 1986.

21. Laupacis A et al: The cost-effectiveness of routine post myocardial infarction exercise stress testing, *Can J Cardiol* 6:157-163, 1990.

22. Ericsson M et al: Arrhythmias and symptoms during treadmill testing three weeks after myocardial infarction in 100 patients, *Br Heart J* 35:787-790, 1973.

23. Kentala E: Physical fitness and feasibility of physical rehabilitation after myocardial infarction in men of working age, *Ann Clin Res* 4(suppl 9):1-77, 1975.

24. Granath A et al: Early work load tests for evaluation of long-term prognosis of acute myocardial infarction, *Br Heart J* 39:758-763, 1977.

25. Smith JW et al: Exercise testing three weeks after myocardial infarction, *Chest* 75:12-16, 1979.

26. Hunt D et al: Predictors of reinfarction and sudden death in a high-risk group of acute myocardial infarction survivors, *Lancet* 1:233-236, 1979.

27. Srinivasan M et al: The value of postcardiac infarction exercise stress testing: identification of a group at high risk, *Med J Aust* 2:466-467, 1981.

28. Sami M, Kraemer H, DeBusk RF: The prognostic significance of serial exercise testing after myocardial infarction, *Circulation* 60:1238-1246, 1979.

29. Davidson DM, DeBusk RF: Prognostic value of a single exercise test 3 weeks after uncomplicated myocardial infarction, *Circulation* 61:236-241, 1980.

30. DeBusk RF, Dennis CA: "Submaximal" predischarge exercise testing after acute myocardial infarction: who needs it? *Am J Cardiol* 55:499-500, 1985.

31. Theroux P, Marpole DGF, Bourassa MG: Exercise stress testing in the post-myocardial infarction patient, *Am J Cardiol* 52:664-667, 1983.

32. Waters DA et al: Comparison of clinical variables and variables derived from a limited predischarge exercise test as predictors of early and late mortality after myocardial infarction, *J Am Coll Cardiol* 5:1-8, 1985.

33. Koppes GM et al: Response to exercise early after uncomplicated acute myocardial infarction in patients receiving no medication: long-term follow-up, *Am J Cardiol* 46:764-769, 1980.

34. Starling MR et al: Comparative predictive value of ST-segment depression or angina during early and repeat postinfarction exercise tests, *Chest* 86:845-849, 1984.

35. Saunamaki KI, Anderson JD: Early exercise test in the assessment of long-term prognosis after acute myocardial infarction, *Acta Med Scand* 209:185-191, 1981.

36. Saunamaki KI, Anderson JD: Early exercise test vs clinical variables in the long-term prognostic management after myocardial infarction, *Acta Med Scand* 212:47-52, 1982.

37. Velasco J. et al: Early exercise test for evaluation of long-term prognosis after uncomplicated myocardial infarction, *Euro Heart J* 2:401-407, 1981.

38. Weld FM: Exercise testing after myocardial infarction, *J Cardiac Rehab* 5:20-27, 1985.

39. Jelinek VM et al: Early exercise testing and mobilization after myocardial infarction, *Med J Aust* 2:589-593, 1977.

40. Madsen EB, Gilpin E: Prognostic value of exercise test variables after myocardial infarction, *J Cardiac Rehab* 3:481-488, 1983.

41. Gibson RS et al: Prediction of cardiac events after uncomplicated myocardial infarction: a prospective study comparing predischarge exercise thallium-201 scintigraphy and coronary angiography, *Circulation* 68:321-336, 1983.

42. Norris RM et al: Prognosis after recovery from first acute myocardial infarction: determinants of reinfarction and sudden death, *Am J Cardiol* 53:408-413, 1984.

43. Williams WL et al: Comparison of clinical and treadmill variables for the prediction of outcome after myocardial infarction, *J Am Coll Cardiol* 4:477-486, 1984.

44. Jennings K et al: Role of exercise testing early after myocardial infarction in identifying candidates for coronary surgery, *Br Med J* 288:185-187, 1984.

45. Fioretti P et al: Predischarge stress test after myocardial infarction: results and prognostic value, *Euro Heart J* 5:101-104, 1984.

46. Krone RJ et al: Low-level exercise testing after myocardial infarction: usefulness in enhancing clinical risk stratification, *Circulation* 71:80-89, 1985.

47. Dwyer EM, McMaster P, Greenberg H: Nonfatal cardiac events and recurrent infarction in the year after acute myocardial infarction, *J Am Coll Cardiol* 4:695-702, 1984.

48. Handler CE: Exercise testing to identify high risk patients after myocardial infarction, *J R Coll Physicians Lond* 18:124-127, 1984.

49. Jespersen CM et al: The prognostic value of maximal exercise testing soon after first MI, *Euro Heart J* 6:769-772, 1985.

50. Connolly DC, Elveback LR: Coronary heart disease in residents of Rochester, Minnesota. VI. Hospital and posthospital course of patients with transmural and subendocardial myocardial infarction, *Mayo Clin Proc* 60:375-381, 1985.

51. Berger C et al: Prognosis after first MI: comparison of Q wave and non-Q wave MI in the Framingham Heart Study, *JAMA* 268:1545-1551, 1992.

52. Klein J, Froelicher V, Detrano R: Does the rest ECG after MI determine the predictive value of exercise-induced ST depression? *J Am Coll Cardiol* 14:305-311, 1989.

53. Krone R, Dwyer E, Greenberg H: Risk stratification in patients with first non-Q wave MI: the Multicenter Post-MI Research Group, *J Am Coll Cardiol* 14:31-37, 1989.

54. Krone RJ: The role of risk stratification in the early management of a myocardial infarction, *Ann Intern Med* 116:223-237, 1992.

CHAPTER 7

Special Applications: Screening Apparently Healthy Individuals

DEFINITION

Screening can be defined as the presumptive diagnosis of previously unrecognized disease by using procedures that can be applied rapidly. By identifying individuals who have asymptomatic or latent coronary heart disease (CHD), secondary preventive action can be taken. Limited data suggest that angiographically documented asymptomatic coronary disease has a relatively good prognosis compared with symptomatic disease and rarely should lead to coronary artery bypass surgery. Therefore asymptomatic individuals diagnosed by screening should be treated through behavior modification to the usual course of this disease. Because of the high probability of restenosis (and of making asymptomatic disease symptomatic), percutaneous transluminal coronary angioplasty (PTCA) should rarely be used to treat these individuals.

CRITERIA

Eight criteria have been proposed for the selection of a screening procedure:

1. The procedure is acceptable and appropriate.
2. The quantity or quality of life can be favorably altered.
3. The results of intervention outweigh any adverse effects.
4. The target disease has an asymptomatic period during which its outcome can be altered.
5. Acceptable treatments are available.
6. The prevalence and seriousness of the disease justify the costs of intervention.
7. The procedure is relatively easy and inexpensive.
8. Sufficient resources are available.

In addition, seven guidelines have been recommended for deciding whether a community screening program does more harm than good:

1. Has the program's effectiveness been demonstrated in a randomized trial?
2. If so, are efficacious treatments available?
3. Does the current burden of suffering warrant screening?
4. Is there a good screening test?
5. Does the program reach those who could benefit from it?
6. Can the health care system cope with the screening program?
7. Will those who had a positive screening comply with subsequent advice and interventions?

Screening has also been recommended for evaluating asymptomatic individuals in whom sudden incapacitation could compromise public safety. Such individuals include pilots, firefighters, and police officers. Others who might be screened are railroad engineers, air traffic controllers, and drivers of large commercial vehicles. Because a high-level exercise program designed to develop athletic performance does present a risk to sedentary, coronary-prone middle-aged men, it may be prudent to evaluate such individuals with screening before beginning such an exercise program.

SENSITIVITY AND SPECIFICITY

To evaluate the value of any screening test, its sensitivity, specificity, predictive value, and relative risk must be demonstrated. Sensitivity is the percentage of times a test gives an abnormal response when those with disease are tested. Specificity is the percentage of times a test gives a normal response when those without disease are tested—a definition quite different from that implied by the conventional use of the word *specific*. These two values are inversely related and are determined by the discriminant values, or cutoff points, chosen for the test to distinguish abnormal from normal results. The predictive value of an abnormal test response is the percentage of individuals with an abnormal test response who have disease. The relative risk of an abnormal test response is the relative chance of having disease if the test result is abnormal compared with the chance of having disease if the test result is normal. The values for these last two terms depend on the prevalance of disease in the population being tested.

A basic step in applying any testing procedure to distinguish normal subjects from patients with a disease is to determine a test value that best separates the two groups. One problem is that there is usually a considerable overlap of measurement values of a test in the groups with and without disease. Consider two bell-shaped normal distribution curves, one representing a normal population and the other representing a population with disease, with a certain amount of overlap of the two curves (see Fig 4-1). Along the vertical axis is the number of patients, and along the horizontal axis could be the value for measurements such as Q-wave size, exercise-induced ST-segment depression, or creatine kinase level. The optimal test would be able to achieve the most marked separation of these two bell-shaped curves and minimize the overlap. Unfortunately, most tests have a considerable overlap of the range of measurements for the normal population and for those with heart disease. Therefore problems arise when a certain value is used to distinguish these two groups (e.g., Q-wave amplitude or width, 0.1 mV of ST-segment depression, a 10 mm Hg drop in systolic blood pressure, less than 5 metabolic equivalents [METs] exercise capacity, or 3 ventricular beats). If the value is set far to the right (e.g., 0.2 mV of ST-segment depression) to identify nearly all the normal subjects as being free of disease, the test will have a high specificity. However, a substantial number of those with disease will be called *normal*. If a value is chosen far to the left (e.g., 0.05 mV ST-segment depression) to identify nearly all those with disease as being abnormal and giving the test a high sensitivity, then many of those without disease will be identified as abnormal. If a cutoff point is chosen that equally mislabels those without disease and those with disease, the test will have its highest predictive accuracy. However, there may be reasons for wanting to adjust a test to have a relatively higher sensitivity or relatively higher specificity than possible when predictive accuracy is optimal. For instance, sensitivity should be highest in the emergency room and specificity highest when doing insurance examinations. Remember that sensitivity and specificity are inversely related. That is, when sensitivity is the highest, specificity is the lowest and vice versa. Any test has a range of inversely related sensitivities and specificities that can be chosen by selecting a certain discriminant, or diagnostic, value. Attempts have been made to use a series of tests to improve diagnostic power, but test interaction is complex. Usually the highest sensitivity and the lowest specificity of the tests represent their combined performance.

The resting electrocardiogram (ECG) as a screening technique has limited predictive accuracy, resulting in much misclassification in a population with a low prevalence of coronary artery disease (CAD).[1-7] For example, cardiac catheterization was used to evaluate 298 asymptomatic, apparently healthy aircrewmen with ECG abnormalities, including bundle branch block.[8] The predictive value of any abnormality was very low because of the low prevalence of CAD in such a population.

FOLLOW-UP STUDIES THAT HAVE USED EXERCISE TESTING

There has been controversy over whether in the absence of conventional risk factors, exercise testing provides additional prognostic information in normal men. Another concern is whether the knowledge of having an abnormal exercise test makes an individual more likely to report angina. The following discussion of follow-up studies using exercise testing in apparently healthy individuals will examine these concerns.

The follow-up studies that used maximal or near-maximal exercise testing to screen asymptomatic individuals for latent CHD tested and followed their populations for the CHD endpoints of angina, acute myocardial infarction (MI), and sudden death. For this discussion, distinction will be made between the results of these studies by dividing them into two groups according to the endpoints used:

angina included as an endpoint (Table 7-1) and hard endpoints (Table 7-2). Table 7-3 lists the endpoints in all of the studies for comparison.

Bruce and McDonough[9] studied 221 clinically normal men in Seattle who were 35 to 82 years of age. Aronow and Cassidy[10] tested 100 normal men in Los Angeles, ages 38 to 64 years, and followed them for 5 years. Cumming et al[11] reported their 3-year follow-up for CHD endpoints in 510 asymptomatic men 40 to 65 years of age.[12] Allen et al[13] reported a 5-year follow-up of 888 asymptomatic men and women without known CHD who had initially undergone maximal treadmill testing. In Italy, Manca et al[14] studied 947 men and 508 women who were referred for exercise testing because of atypical chest pain. Bruce, Fisher, and Hossack[15] later reported a 6-year follow-up of 2365 clinically healthy men (mean age 45 years) who were exercise tested as part of the Seattle Heart Watch. MacIntyre et al[16] performed maximal exercise tests on 548 fit, healthy middle-aged former aviators at the Naval Aerospace Medical Laboratory. McHenry et al[17] reported the results of an 8- to 15-year follow-up of 916 apparently healthy men between the ages of 27 and 55 who underwent serial medical and exercise test evaluations.

TABLE 7-1.

Screening Studies That Included Angina as an Endpoint

	Number	Years Followed	Incidence of CHD (%)	Sens (%)	Spec (%)	Predictive Value + %	Risk Ratio
Bruce	221	5	2.3	60	91	14	14×
Aronow	100	5	9.0	67	92	46	14×
Cumming	510	3	4.7	58	90	25	10×
Froelicher	1390	6	3.3	61	92	20	14×
Allen	356	5	9.6	41	79	17	2.4×
Manca	947	5	5.0	67	84	18	10×
	508(w)	5	1.6	88	73	5	15×
MacIntyre	578	8	6.9	16	97	26	4×
McHenry	916	13	7.1	14	98	39	6×
			AVERAGES*	48	90	26	9×

Sens, Sensitivity; *Spec*, specificity; *w*, women.
*Averages do not include women.

TABLE 7-2.

Four Screening Studies with Hard Endpoints (Not Angina)

	Number	Years Followed	Incidence of CHD (%)	Sens (%)	Spec (%)	Predictive Value + %	Risk Value
Seattle Heart Watch	2365	6	2.0	30	91	5	3.5×
MRFIT (SI)	6217	6-8	1.7	17	88	2.2	1.4×
(UC)	6205		1.9	34	88	5.2	3.7×
LRC (Gordon)	3630	8	2.2	28	96	12	6×
(Ekelund)	3806	7	1.8	29	95	7	5×
			AVERAGES	27	91	6	4×

Sens, Sensitivity; *Spec*, specificity; *UC*, usual care group.

TABLE 7-3.

Events Used as Endpoints for Follow-Up Studies

	Number	Events	Total Deaths	Cardiovascular Deaths	MI	CABS	AP
Aronow	100	9	3	3	4	1	1
Bruce	221	5	NR	1	1		3
Cumming	510	26	5	3	8		13
McHenry	916	65	8	8	26		30
MacIntyre	548	38	NR	10	16	6	6
Allen	888	48	NR	?	?	NR	?
Froelicher	1390	65	47	25	82	35	11
Seattle Heart Watch	2365	65	47	25	82	35	11
MRFIT (SI)	6427	265	115	NR	NR	NR	NR
(UC)	6438	260	124	NR	NR	NR	NR
LRC	3630	NR	151	75	NR	NR	NR

CABS, Coronary bypass surgery; *AP*, angina pectoris; *NR*, not reported; *?*, used as endpoint; *UC*, usual care group.

The Multiple Risk Factor Intervention Trial (MRFIT), a coronary heart disease primary prevention trial, examined the effect of a special intervention (SI)[18] program to reduce cholesterol, high blood pressure, and cigarette smoking in men 35 to 57 years old. This study certainly is the largest and probably the most reliable for demonstrating the predictive accuracy of exercise testing in an asymptomatic population, since only cardiac death was considered the endpoint as opposed to angina in most of the other studies. Rautaharju et al[19] presented the prognostic value of the exercise ECG in the 6438 men of MRFIT receiving usual care in relation to fatal and nonfatal CHD events, rest ECG abnormalities, and CHD risk factors. Gordon et al[20,21] presented an analysis of the exercise test results from the Lipid Research Clinics (LRC) Mortality Follow-Up Study. Ekelund et al[22] attempted to predict CHD morbidity and mortality in hypercholesterolemic men from an exercise test performed as part of the LRC Coronary Primary Prevention Trial. To study whether the test was more predictive for hypercholesterolemic men (thus increasing the pretest probability for disease), data from 3806 asymptomatic hypercholesterolemic men was analyzed. Josephson et al[23] analyzed the results of serial exercise tests performed at two to four intervals in 726 male and female volunteers, ages 22 to 84 (mean of 55), from the Baltimore Longitudinal Study of Aging.

Relevance to Silent Ischemia Issue

The use of the exercise ECG for predicting prognosis in asymptomatic individuals has again become of interest because of the poor predictive power of the ST-segment response being reported and referral to these studies in regard to silent ischemia. The Seattle Heart Watch study[15] was the first study that reported quite different results from previous studies. The explanation became apparent from considering the endpoints used. The earlier studies all considered angina pectoris as one of the cardiac events or endpoints. In the Seattle Heart Watch study, the

TABLE 7-4.

Results of Screening in Asymptomatic and Symptomatic Populations

History of CHD*	ST Depression on Holter	Number	MI†/Deaths	Risk Ratio
Yes	No	34	2(5.9%)	2.6×
	Yes	19	7(39%)	16×
No	No	262	6(2.3%)	1×
	Yes	79	8(10.8%)	4.4×

Data from Hedblad B: *Euro Heart J* 10:149-158, 1989.
*Positive Rose questionnaire result.
†Previous MI.

angina endpoint had to be associated with a hospital admission diagnosis of angina, making it a more definite cardiac endpoint. The other more recent studies considered only hard endpoints, such as death or MI, and not angina.

When the studies are separated, those that used angina as an endpoint (Table 7-1) had an average sensitivity of 48%, predictive value of 26%, and risk ratio of 9 times. In other words, 26%, or 1 out of 4, with ST-segment depression would have a cardiac event including angina during approximately 5 years of follow-up. However, when the studies that used only hard endpoints were considered (Table 7-2), much poorer results were obtained. The sensitivity was 27%, and the predictive value was 6%. Only 6%, or 1 out of 17, with ST-segment depression would have a hard endpoint during follow-up. Rather than 1 cardiac event out of 4 for those with ST-segment depression, it turned out to be 1 out of 17. This means that 16 out of 17 abnormal responses were false positives. This misclassification must be considered because these studies are being cited as showing the dangers of silent ischemia. Silent ischemia induced by exercise testing in apparently healthy men is not as predictive of a poor outcome as once thought. Also, the use of the exercise test for screening asymptomatic individuals is even more misleading than previously appreciated because of the higher false-positive rate. The earlier better results can be explained by the cardiac concerns caused by an abnormal exercise test. Individuals with abnormal tests would be more likely to report chest pain, and doctors would be more likely to diagnose it as angina given the exercise test results. In the only study of its kind (summarized in Table 7-4), Hedblad[24] obtained misleading results similar to those from exercise test studies when using ambulatory Holter monitoring.

The nonselective use of exercise testing for screening apparently healthy individuals should be discouraged because of the poor predictive value of only 1 mm of ST-segment depression. Unfortunately, this "abnormal" response can lead to psychological and vocational disability as well as unnecessary medical expenses and risks. When this response is no longer equated with disease, then perhaps the test could be used in such individuals for setting exercise prescriptions and for motivational purposes. Only combinations of other abnormal responses and 2 mm of ST-segment depression should be considered as predictive of increased risk for exercise-related cardiovascular events.

Exercise Testing and Coronary Angiography in Asymptomatic Populations

Froelicher et al[12] used cardiac catheterization to evaluate 111 asymptomatic men with an abnormal ST-segment depression in response to a treadmill test. Only a third of the subjects had at least one lesion equal to or greater than a 50% luminal narrowing of a major coronary artery. However, resting mild ST-segment depression that appears on serial ECGs and persists increases the predictive value of an abnormal exercise test. Borer et al[25] reported angiographic findings in 11 asymptomatic individuals with hyperlipidemia and an abnormal exercise test. Only 37% had coronary artery occlusions.

Barnard et al[26] used near-maximal treadmill testing to screen randomly selected Los Angeles firefighters. Despite few risk factors for coronary disease, 10% had abnormal exercise-induced ST-segment depression. Six men with an abnormal exercise test elected to undergo cardiac catheterization. One had severe triple-vessel disease, and another had a 50% obstruction of the left circumflex coronary artery. The other four men had normal studies.

Uhl et al[27] have reported their findings in 255 asymptomatic men who underwent coronary angiography for an abnormal ST-segment response to exercise testing over a 7-year period at the United States Air Force School of Aerospace Medicine (USAFSAM). None of the clinical or ECG variables were able to detect those with significant diseases. The three exercise test responses with a high likelihood ratio were (1) at least 0.3 mV depression, (2) persistence of ST-segment depression 6 minutes after exercise, and (3) an estimated oxygen uptake of less than 9 METs. However, because of their low sensitivity and predictive value, it was necessary to combine these responses with risk factors. A combination of any risk factor and two exercise responses was highly predictive (89%) but insensitive (39%) for presence of coronary disease. However, this combination had a sensitivity of 55% and a predictive value of 84% for double- or triple-vessel diseases.

Erikssen et al[28] reported angiographic findings in 105 men ages 40 to 59 of a working population with one or more of the following criteria: (1) a questionnaire for angina pectoris positive on interview, (2) typical angina, or (3) ST-segment depression as a response to a near-maximal bicycle test. The exercise test had a predictive value of 84% if a slowly ascending ST segment was included. The higher predictive value in this study may result from the older age of its population and its inclusion of men with angina. Of the 36 who had normal coronary arteries, a 7-year follow-up revealed that 3 died of sudden death, 4 received a diagnosis of cardiomyopathy, and 1 developed aortic valve disease.[29] They had a relative decline in their physical performance over the follow-up period. Thallium studies were normal, but the radionuclide ventriculogram revealed a subnormal increase in EF during exercise in half of them.

Kemp et al[30] evaluated 7-year survival in patients having normal or near-normal coronary arteriograms using data from the Coronary Artery Surgery Study (CASS) registry of 21,487 consecutive coronary arteriograms taken in 15 clinical sites. Of these, 4051 arteriograms were normal or near normal, and the patients had normal left ventricular function as judged by absence of a history of congestive heart failure, no reported segmental wall motion abnormality, and an EF of at least 50%; 3136 arteriograms were entirely normal, and the remaining 915 revealed mild disease with less than 50% stenosis in one or more segments. Of the total number, 843 patients had exercise tests, and of these, 195 had abnormal ST-segment depression. The 7-year survival rate was 96% for the patients with a normal arteriogram and 92% for those whose study revealed mild disease. The ECG response to exercise was a nonpredictive variable. In contrast, the 7-year follow-up study of only 36 apparently healthy middle-aged men with positive exercise tests and normal coronary arteriograms reported by Erikssen et al[29] concluded that patients with abnormal exercise tests could not be ensured good prognoses on the basis of normal coronary arteriograms. The CASS data, however, do not support this conclusion. There were 195 subjects with abnormal ST-segment depression, and Kemp et al[30] were unable to show any predictive value of even marked amounts of depression. If exercise-induced ST-segment depression is due to ischemia in patients with normal coronaries, it is not related to a disease process that has an impact on mortality over 7 years of follow-up. In general, these angiographic studies confirm the low predictive value of an abnormal exercise test response also found in the epidemiological studies of populations with a low prevalence of coronary disease.

Labile ST-Segment Shifts

McHenry[31] performed serial exercise tests on 900 presumably healthy men and identified 14 men with labile ST-T changes on standing or hyperventilation and abnormal ST-segment depression at exercise. At 7-year follow-up, none had manifested a coronary event. In contrast, of 24 men with exercise-induced ST-segment changes but no labile ST-T wave phenomena before the exercise test, 10 (42%) had a coronary event.[32]

Exercise-Induced Dysrhythmias

Few studies in asymptomatic subjects have evaluated exercise-induced ventricular premature beats for detecting coronary disease. In the USAFSAM study[27] of 1390 men, only 39 men (2.1%) of the population developed "ominous" dysrhythmias. The risk ratio of developing coronary disease over 6 years of follow-up with these dysrhythmias was 3:1, however, the predictive value was only 10%, and sensitivity only 6.7%. Thus dysrhythmias induced by exercise testing have not been helpful in detecting latent coronary disease in apparently healthy men.

Busby, Shefrin, and Fleg[33] studied 1160 subjects ages 21 to 96 who underwent maximal exercise treadmill testing an average of 2.4 times. A total of 80 (6.9%) developed frequent (≥10% of beats in any 1 minute) or repetitive (≥3 beats in a row) ventricular ectopic beats on at least one test. These 80 individuals were older than the group without such dysrhythmia. A striking age-related increase in the prevalence of frequent or repetitive exercise-induced ventricular ectopic beats was seen in men but not in women. There were no differences in the prevalence of ECG abnormalities at rest, exercise-induced ST-segment depression and thallium perfusion defects, duration of treadmill exercise, maximum heart rate, systolic blood pressure, and rate-pressure product between these 80 study subjects with frequent exercise-induced ventricular ectopic beats and a control group matched for age and gender. Furthermore, the study and control groups had similar percentages (10% versus 12.5%) for the incidence of cardiac events (angina pectoris, nonfatal MI, cardiac syncope, or cardiac death), as well as for noncardiac mortality (each 7.5%) over a mean follow-up of 5.6 years. No study subjects required antidysrhythmic drugs during this time. Thus frequent or repetitive exercise-induced ventricular ectopic beats in these predominantly older, asymptomatic individuals without apparent heart disease do not predict increased cardiac morbidity or mortality and therefore do not require specific therapy.

Techniques to Improve Screening

Numerous techniques have been recommended to improve the sensitivity and specificity of exercise testing. Various computerized criteria for ischemia as well as new standard visual ST criteria have been proposed. In addition, ancillary techniques could improve the discriminating power of the exercise test. These methods are listed in the box.

ECG Criteria

Numerous computerized treadmill scores and measurements have been proposed, but none have been validated.[34,35]

Thallium Exercise Testing

Numerous studies have demonstrated that thallium exercise testing is the usual next best test in clarifying an abnormal ST-segment response in asymptomatic individuals with abnormal ST-segment responses to exercise testing.[36-38] To examine whether thallium scintigraphy improved the predictive value of exercise-induced ST-segment depression, Fleg et al[39] performed maximal treadmill tests

---

ANCILLARY TECHNIQUES USED TO SCREEN FOR ASYMPTOMATIC CHD

Thallium perfusion imaging
Radionuclide ventriculography during bicycle exercise and after treadmill exercise
Cardiac fluoroscopy for coronary artery calcification (enhanced with digital subtraction angiography)
Cardiokymography
Total cholesterol/high-density lipoprotein ratio, conventional risk factors
ECG-gated chest x-ray film before and after exercise
Computerized multifactorial risk prediction using Bayesian statistics
Systolic time intervals during and after exercise
Digital subtraction angiography with intravenous injection of contrast to visualize coronary arteries
Echocardiography (or Doppler) during and after exercise (even after treadmill)

and thallium scans on 407 asymptomatic volunteers, 40 to 96 years of age (mean of 60), from the Baltimore Longitudinal Study on Aging. The prevalence of exercise-induced silent ischemia, defined by concordant ST-segment depression and a thallium perfusion defect, increased more than 7-fold from 2% in the fifth and sixth decades to 15% in the ninth decade. Over a mean follow-up of 4.6 years, cardiac events developed in 9.8% of subjects and consisted of 20 cases of new angina pectoris, 13 MI, and 7 deaths. Events occurred in 7% of individuals with negative thallium scans and ECGs, 8% of those with positive results for either test, and 48% of those with positive results for both tests ($p < 0.001$). According to proportional hazards analysis of the results, age, hypertension, exercise duration, and a concordant positive ECG and thallium scan result were independent predictors of coronary events. Furthermore, those with positive ECG and thallium scan results had a 3.6-fold relative risk for subsequent coronary events, independent of conventional risk factors.

Radionuclide Ventriculography

Radionuclide left ventricular angiography during exercise has not been reported in any substantial number of asymptomatic subjects, but its low specificity makes its use impractical.

Coronary Artery Calcification on Fluoroscopic Examination

Langou et al[40] reported the use of cardiac fluoroscopy as a prescreening tool in asymptomatic men before exercise tests. To evaluate the reported accuracy of fluoroscopically detected coronary calcific deposits for predicting angiographic disease, Gianrossi et al[41] applied metanalysis to 13 consecutively published reports comparing the results of cardiac fluoroscopy with coronary angiography. Population characteristics and technical and methodological factors were analyzed. Sensitivity and specificity for predicting serious coronary disease compared quite well with those from the literature on the exercise ECG and the thallium scintigram. For any presence of disease, sensitivity averaged 58% and specificity 82%, and for severe disease, sensitivity averaged 87% and specificity 59%. Sensitivity increases and specificity decreases more significantly with patient age. In addition, sensitivity is paradoxically lower in laboratories testing patients with more severe disease, as well as when a 70% rather than a 50% diameter narrowing is used to define angiographic disease. Workup and test review bias were also significantly related to reported accuracy.[42]

Lipid Screening

Total cholesterol to high-density lipoprotein cholesterol ratios are directly correlated with CHD risk.[43]

Computer Probability Estimates

Diamond and Forrester[44] have reviewed the literature to estimate pretest likelihood of disease by age, gender, symptoms, and the Framingham risk equation (based on blood pressure, smoking, glucose intolerance, resting ECG, and cholesterol).

Prognosis in Asymptomatic Patients with Angiographic CAD

Hammermeister, De Rouer, and Dodge[45] reported the effects of coronary artery bypass surgery on asymptomatic or mildly symptomatic angina patients who were studied as part of the Seattle Heart Watch program. Hickman et al[46] at USAFSAM followed for 5 years 90 men aged from 45 to 54, with asymptomatic angiographic coronary disease without previous MI. Kent et al[47] reported on 147 asymptomatic or mildly symptomatic patients with CHD who were followed prospectively for an average of 2 years.

Secondary Prevention and Testing

If a method of secondary prevention were proven and available today, the following three-step approach to screening for asymptomatic CHD in men over 35 years old would appear reasonable. First, a chest pain history, a risk factor analysis, and a resting ECG should be obtained. If any of this data placed the individual at risk, the second step should be a maximal exercise test. If the test results were interpreted as abnormal, based on ST-segment shifts and perhaps other abnormal responses, the third step should be use of thallium exercise scintigraphy. Good clinical judgment must be exercised to avoid producing "cardiac cripples" by mislabeling healthy people. The severity of the abnormal response must be considered. Most often it is appropriate to follow an asymptomatic individual with only abnormal ST-segment depression at maximal exercise, particularly if the exercise capacity is good.

Exercise Testing for Exercise Programs

There are multiple reasons for doing an exercise test before initiating an exercise program. The optimal exercise prescription, based on a percentage of an individual's maximum heart rate or oxygen consumption (50% to 80%) to exceed the gas exchange anaerobic threshold, can only be written after performing an exercise test. The best way to assess the risk of an adverse reaction during exercise is to observe the individual during exercise. The level of exercise training then can be set at a level below that at which adverse responses or symptoms occur. Some individuals motivated by popular misconceptions about the benefits of exercise may disregard their natural warning systems and push themselves into dangerous levels of ischemia.

An individual with a good exercise capacity and only 0.1 mV of ST-segment depression at maximal exercise has a relatively low risk of cardiovascular events in the next several years compared with an individual with marked ST-segment depression at a low heart rate or systolic blood pressure. Most individuals with an abnormal test can be put safely into an exercise program if the level of intensity of the exercise at which the response occurs is considered. Such patients can be treated by risk factor modification rather than by being excluded from exercise or their livelihood.

Siscovick et al[48] determined whether the exercise ECG predicted acute cardiac events during moderate or strenuous physical activity among 3617 asymptomatic, hypercholesterolemic men (ages 35 to 59) who were followed up in the Coronary

Primary Prevention Trial. Submaximal exercise test results were obtained at entry and at annual follow-up visits in years 2 through 7. ST-segment depression or elevation (≥ 1 mm or 10 μV-sec) was considered to be an abnormal result. The circumstances that surrounded each nonfatal MI and CHD death were determined through a record review. The cumulative incidence of activity-related acute cardiac events was 2% during a mean follow-up of 7.4 years. The risk was increased 2.6-fold in the presence of clinically silent, exercise-induced ST-segment changes at entry after adjustment for 11 other potential risk factors. Of 62 men who experienced an activity-related event, 11 had abnormal test results at entry (sensitivity of 18%). The specificity of the entry exercise test was 92%. The sensitivity and specificity were similar when the length of follow-up was restricted to 1 year after testing. For a newly abnormal test result on a follow-up visit, the sensitivity was 24%, and the specificity was 85%; for any abnormal test result during the study (mean number of tests per subject was 6.2), the sensitivity was 37%, and the specificity was 79%. These findings suggested that the presence of clinically silent, exercise-induced, ischemic ST-segment changes on a submaximal test was associated with an increased risk of activity-related acute cardiac events. However, the test was not sensitive when used to predict the occurrence of activity-related events among asymptomatic, hypercholesterolemic men. For this reason, the use of the exercise test to assess the safety of physical activity among asymptomatic men at risk of CHD is limited.

Exercise testing is recommended, however, before entering an exercise program for individuals with a strong family history of coronary disease (i.e., family members aged less than 60 with a coronary event), with the presence of increased risk factors (particularly serum cholesterol), or with any symptoms suggestive of myocardial ischemia currently or in the past. In addition, there are clearly a group of patients who select themselves for exercise testing. They may request the test even though they deny having any symptoms.

Further Testing

A major problem with performing an exercise test in apparently healthy people is the difficulty associated with a "positive" response. The thallium test appears to have relatively high sensitivity (80%) and specificity (90%), but it requires experienced readers and a good laboratory.[49] It is, however, superior to radionuclide ventriculography, which in some studies has had a specificity as low as 60%. In some patients, a clearly abnormal secondary study may ultimately require coronary arteriography to assess coronary structures. However, it is necessary to see if there is an overlap in calling both tests false positives; for example, both the exercise ECG and the thallium test could be abnormal in women because of attenuation by breast tissue causing cold spots and because of the microcirculatory abnormalities causing ST-segment depression.[50] Also, for unknown reasons, the thallium test, like the exercise ECG, may be falsely positive for mitral valve prolapse. It must be remembered that a low specificity must be avoided during screening.

Exercise Testing For Special Screening Purposes

Pilots

Unfortunately, politics and economic factors are two of the strongest factors influencing the use of exercise testing in subjects with flying responsibilities.[51] The pool of available pilots is obviously an important national resource. If there are many pilots available, society is more likely to be more strict with regulations regarding flying standards. Clearly, physicians must be concerned with public safety. Allowing an individual with an increased health risk to take responsibility for many other peoples' lives could result in a tragedy. The presence of a backup pilot and the impact of modern technology on flying do not lessen the stresses of this occupation. There are numerous situations of very high stress, such as take-offs and landings, in which it might not be possible for other cockpit personnel to take control of the aircraft and avert disaster if the key pilot was to have a cardiac event. In general, pilots are a highly motivated, intelligent group of people who feel a high level of reponsibility for the performance of their work. Flying is their livelihood, however, and most of them love it so dearly that they may conceal medical information that could endanger their flying status. In addition, the stress of work often leaves them unable to maintain a healthy lifestyle. The stress of altering the circadian cycle and trying to navigate in and out of today's busy airports leaves many of them overweight, deconditioned, and smoking heavily. When possible, health professionals should recommend that these men and women have the full benefits of modern preventive medicine, including the periodic assessment of physical work capacity, response to stress, and probability of coronary atherosclerosis.

SUMMARY

Recent studies have markedly changed our understanding of the application of exercise testing as a screening tool. These studies were additional follow-up studies and one angiographic study from the CASS population in which 195 individuals with abnormal exercise-induced ST-segment depression and normal coronary angiograms were followed for 7 years. No increased incidence of cardiac events was found, so the concerns raised by Erikssen's findings[29] in 36 subjects that they were still at increased risk have not been substantiated. These new follow-up studies (MRFIT,[18] Seattle Heart Watch,[15] and LRC[20,21]) have shown quite different results compared with those of prior studies, mainly because hard cardiac endpoints and not angina were required. The first eight prospective studies[9-17] of exercise testing in asymptomatic individuals included angina as a cardiac disease endpoint, and they showed a higher predictive value for exercise testing. However, this higher correspondence between abnormal responses and angina was probably caused by individuals with abnormal test results being more likely to subsequently report angina or to be diagnosed as having angina. When only hard endpoints (death or MI) were used, as in the MRFIT, LRC, or the Seattle Heart Watch studies, the results indicated that the exercise test was not an effective predictor. The test could only identify one third of patients with hard endpoints, and

95% of abnormal responders were false positives; that is, patients did not die or have an MI. The predictive value of the abnormal maximal exercise ECG ranged from 5% to 46% in the studies reviewed. However, in the studies using appropriate endpoints (i.e., not angina pectoris), only 5% of the abnormal responders developed CHD over the follow-up period. Thus more than 90% of the abnormal responders were false-positives. Some of these individuals have coronary disease that has yet to manifest itself, but angiographic studies have supported this high false-positive rate when using the exercise test in asymptomatic populations. Moreover, the CASS study[30] indicates that such individuals have a good prognosis. In a second LRC study,[21] only patients with elevated cholesterol levels were considered, and yet only a 6% positive prediction value was found. These results in a population first screened for a risk factor to increase the pretest prevalence of disease argue strongly against the routine use of exercise testing as a screening tool. The iatrogenic problems resulting from screening must be considered.

Some individuals who eventually develop coronary disease will change on retesting from a normal to an abnormal response. However, McHenry et al[17] and Fleg et al[39] have reported that a change from a negative to a positive test is no more predictive than is an initially abnormal test. One individual has even been reported who changed from a normal to an abnormal test but was free of angiographically significant disease.[52] Fleg et al[39] has also demonstrated that thallium scintigraphy should be the first choice in evaluating asymptomatic individuals with an abnormal exercise ECG.

Exercise testing may prove to have value in asymptomatic populations other than for screening. Bruce, De Rouen, and Hossack[53] examined the motivational effects of maximal exercise testing for modifying risk factors and health habits. A questionnaire was sent to nearly 3000 men, ages 35 to 65, who had undergone symptom-limited treadmill testing at least 1 year earlier. Individuals were asked whether the treadmill test motivated them to stop smoking (if already a smoker), increase daily exercise, purposely lose weight, reduce the amount of dietary fat, or take medication for hypertension. There was a 69% response to this questionnaire, and 63% of the responders indicated that they had modified one or more risk factors and health habits and that they attributed this change to the exercise test. In fact, a greater percentage of patients with decreased exercise capacity than subjects with normal results reported a modification of risk factors or health habits.

Given the current approaches competing for health care resources, it is best to screen only those who request it, those with multiple abnormal risk factors, those with worrisome medical histories, or those with a family history of premature cardiovascular disease. It is difficult to choose a chronological age after which exercise testing is necessary as a screening technique before beginning an exercise program, since physiological age is important. In general, if the exercise is more strenuous than vigorous walking, most individuals over the age of 50 will benefit from such screening. The potential problems resulting from screening must be considered, and the results of testing must be applied using the predictive model and bayesian statistics. Test results must be thought of as probability statements and not as absolutes. The recent data from treadmill screening studies convincingly demonstrate the inappropriateness of including exercise testing as part of routine health maintenance in apparently healthy individuals. If it is used to decide whether asymptomatic individuals have CAD, it is very ineffective and causes more psychological and economic harm through, for example, work and insurance status and costs for more tests than good by misclassifying approximately 10% of those without CAD as having disease.

REFERENCES

1. Oster E et al: Electrocardiographic findings and their association with mortality in the Copenhagen City Heart Study, *Euro Heart J* 2:317-328, 1981.
2. Rose G et al: Prevalence and prognosis of electrocardiogram findings in middle-aged men, *Br Heart J* 15:636-643, 1978.
3. Cullen K et al: Electrocardiograms and 13 year cardiovascular mortality in Busselton study, *Br Heart J* 47:209-212, 1982.
4. Rabkin SW, Mathewson FAL, Tate RB: The electrocardiogram in apparently healthy men and the risk of sudden death, *Br Heart J* 47:546-552, 1982.
5. Dawber TR et al: The Framingham Study, *Circulation* 5:559-566, 1952.
6. Levine HD, Phillips E: The electrocardiogram and MI, *New Engl J Med* 245:833-842, 1951.
7. Liao Y et al: Major and minor electrocardiographic abnormalities and risk of death from coronary heart disease, cardiovascular diseases and all causes in men and women, *J Am Coll Cardiol* 12:1494-1500, 1988.
8. Froelicher VF et al: Angiographic findings in asymptomatic aircrewmen with electrocardiographic abnormalities, *Am J Cardiol* 39:32-39, 1977.
9. Bruce RA, McDonough JR: Stress testing in screening for cardiovascular disease, *Bull NY Acad Med* 45:1288-1295, 1969.
10. Aronow WS, Cassidy J: Five year follow-up of double Master's test, maximal treadmill stress test, and resting and postexercise apexcardiogram in asymptomatic persons, *Circulation* 52:616-622, 1975.
11. Cumming GR et al: Electrocardiographic changes during exercise in asymptomatic men: 3-year follow-up, *Can Med Assoc J* 112:578-585, 1975.
12. Froelicher VF et al: An epidemiological study of asymptomatic men screened with exercise testing for latent coronary heart disease, *Am J Cardiol* 34:770-779, 1975.
13. Allen WH et al: Five-year follow-up of maximal treadmill stress test in asymptomatic men and women, *Circulation* 62:522-531, 1980.
14. Manca C et al: Multivariate analysis of exercise ST depression and coronary risk factors in asymptomatic men, *Euro Heart J* 3:2-8, 1982.
15. Bruce RA, Fisher LD, Hossack KF: Validation of exercise-enhanced risk assessment of coronary heart disease events: longitudinal changes in incidence in Seattle community practice, *J Am Coll Cardiol* 5:875-881, 1985.
16. MacIntyre NR et al: Eight-year follow-up of exercise electrocardiograms in healthy, middle-aged aviators, *Aviat Space Environ Med* 52:256-259, 1981.
17. McHenry PL et al: The abnormal exercise electrocardiogram in apparently healthy men: a predictor of angina pectoris as an initial coronary event during long-term follow-up, *Circulation* 70:547-551, 1984.
18. Multiple Risk Factor Intervention Research Group: Exercise electrocardiogram and

coronary heart disease mortality in the Multiple Risk Factor Intervention Trial, *Am J Cardiol* 55:16-24, 1985.

19. Rautaharju PM et al: Prognostic value of exercise electrocardiogram in men at high risk of future coronary heart disease: multiple risk factor intervention trial experience, *J Am Coll Cardiol* 8:1-10, 1986.

20. Gordon DL et al: Predictive value of the exercise tolerance test for mortality in North American men: the Lipid Research Clinics Mortality Follow-Up Study, *Circulation* 74:252-261, 1986.

21. Gordon DL et al: Smoking, physical activity, and other predictors of endurance and heart rate response to exercise in asymptomatic hypercholesterolemic men, *Am J Epidemiol* 125:587-600, 1987.

22. Ekelund LG et al: Coronary heart disease morbidity and mortality in hypercholesterolemic men predicted from an exercise test: the Lipid Research Clinics Coronary Primary Prevention Trial, *J Am Coll Cardiol* 14:556-563, 1989.

23. Josephson RA et al: Can serial exercise testing improve the prediction of coronary events in asymptomatic individuals? *Circulation* 81:20-24, 1990.

24. Hedblad B: Screening for silent ischemia using ambulatory monitoring, *Euro Heart J* 10:149-158, 1989.

25. Borer JS et al: Limitations of the electrocardiographic response to exercise in predicting coronary artery disease, *New Engl J Med* 193:367-375, 1975.

26. Barnard RJ et al: Near-maximal ECG stress testing and coronary artery disease risk factor analysis in Los Angeles City fire fighters, *J Occup Med* 18:818-827, 1975.

27. Uhl GS et al: Predictive implications of clinical and exercise variables in detecting significant coronary artery disease in asymptomatic men, *J Cardiac Rehab* 4:245-252, 1984.

28. Erikssen J et al: False positive diagnostic tests and coronary angiographic findings in 105 presumably healthy males, *Circulation* 54:371-376, 1976.

29. Erikssen J et al: False suspicion of coronary heart disease: a 7 year follow-up study of 36 apparently healthy middle-aged men, *Circulation* 68:490-497, 1983.

30. Kemp HG et al: Seven year survival of patients with normal and near normal coronary arteriograms: a CASS registy study, *J Am Coll Cardiol* 7:479-483, 1986.

31. McHenry PL. *Exercise-induced ventricular arrhythmias: prevalence, mechanisms, and prognostic implications,* New York. 1992, Lippincott.

32. McHenry P, Morris S, Karalier M: Comparative study of exercise induced PVCs in normals and CAD patients, *Am J Cardiol* 37:609-616, 1976.

33. Busby MJ, Shefrin EA, Fleg JL: Prevalence and long-term significance of exercise-induced frequent or repetitive ventricular ectopic beats in apparently healthy volunteers, *J Am Coll Cardiol* 14:1659-1665, 1989.

34. Hollenberg M et al: Comparison of a quantitative treadmill exercise score with standard electrocardiographic criteria in screening asymptomatic young men for coronary artery disease, *New Engl J Med* 313 (10):600-606, 1985.

35. Okin PM et al: Heart rate adjustment of exercise-induced ST segment depression: improved risk stratification in the Framingham Offspring Study, *Circulation* 83:866-874, 1991.

36. Caralis DG et al: Thallium-201 myocardial imaging in evaluation of asymptomatic individuals with ischemic ST segment depression on exercise electrocardiogram, *Br Heart J* 42:562-571, 1979.

37. Nolewajk AJ et al: 201 Thallium stress myocardial imaging: an evaluation of fifty-eight asymptomatic males, *Clin Cardiol* 4:134-142, 1981.

38. Uhl GS, Kay TN, Hickman JR: Computer-enhanced thallium-scintigrams in asymptomatic men with abnormal exercise tests, *Am J Cardiol* 48:1037-1046, 1981.

39. Fleg JL et al: Prevalence and prognostic significance of exercise-induced silent myocardial ischemia detected by thallium scintigraphy and electrocardiography in asymptomatic volunteers, *Circulation* 81:428-436, 1990.

40. Langou RA et al: Predictive accuracy of coronary artery calcification and abnormal exercise test for coronary artery disease in asymptomatic man, *Circulation* 62:1196-1202, 1981.

41. Gianrossi R et al: Cardiac fluoroscopy for the diagnosis of coronary artery disease: a meta analytic review, *Am Heart J* 120:1179-1188, 1990.

42. Detrano R, Froelicher V: Diagnosis and treatment: a logical approach to screening for coronary artery disease, *Ann Intern Med* 106:846-852, 1987.

43. Uhl GS et al: Angiographic correlation of coronary artery disease with high density lipoprotein cholesterol in asymptomatic men, *Am J Cardiol* 48:903-911, 1981.

44. Diamond GA, Forrester JS: Analysis of probability as an aid in the clinical diagnosis of coronary artery disease, *New Engl J Med* 300:1350-1359, 1979.

45. Hammermeister KE, De Rouen TA, Dodge HT: Effect of coronary surgery on survival in asymptomatic and minimally symptomatic patients, *Circulation* 62:98-104, 1980.

46. Hickman JR et al: A natural history study of asymptomatic coronary disease, *Am J Cardiol* 45:422-430, 1980.

47. Kent KM et al: Prognosis of asymptomatic or mildly symptomatic patients with coronary artery disease, *Am J Cardiol* 49:1823-1831, 1982.

48. Siscovick DS et al: Sensitivity of exercise electrocardiography for acute cardiac events during moderate and strenuous physical activity, *Arch Intern Med* 151:325-330, 1991.

49. Fagan LF et al: Prognostic value of exercise thallium scintigraphy in patients with good exercise tolerance and a normal or abnormal exercise electrocardiogram and suspected or confirmed coronary artery disease, *Am J Cardiol* 69:607-611, 1992.

50. Gavrielides S et al: Recovery-phase patterns of ST segment depression in the heart rate domain cannot distinguish between anginal patients with coronary artery disease and patients with syndrome X, *Am Heart J* 122(6):1593-1598, 1991.

51. Bruce RA, Fisher LD: Clinical medicine: exercise-enchanced risk factors for coronary heart disease vs. age as criteria for mandatory retirement of healthy pilots, *Aviat Space Environ Med* 27:792-798, 1987.

52. Thompson AJ, Froelicher VF: Kugel's artery as a major collateral channel in severe coronary disease, *Aerospace Med* 45:1276-1280, 1974.

53. Bruce RA, De Rouen TA, Hossack KF: Pilot study examining the motivational effects of maximal exercise testing to modify risk factors and health habits, *Cardiology* 66:111-120, 1980.

CHAPTER 8

Miscellaneous Applications

EVALUATION OF TREATMENTS

The exercise test can be used to evaluate the effects of medical and surgical treatment. The effects of various medications for angina, congestive heart failure, and hypertension, including nitrates, digitalis, and antihypertensive agents, have been evaluated by exercise testing. Exercise testing has also been used to evaluate patients before and after coronary artery bypass surgery (CABS) and percutaneous transluminal coronary angioplasty (PTCA). In serial studies, one problem with using treadmill time or workload rather than measuring maximal oxygen uptake to evaluate cardiovascular function is that individuals learn to perform treadmill walking more efficiently. Consequently, treadmill time or workload can increase during serial studies without any improvement in cardiovascular function. Thus it is important to include the measurement of ventilatory oxygen uptake when the effects of medical or surgical treatment are being evaluated by treadmill testing.

EVALUATION OF ANTIANGINAL AGENTS

Reproducibility

Because studies using standard exercise testing are required by the U.S. Food and Drug Administration (FDA) before approval of antianginal agents, it is important to know the reproducibility of exercise variables in angina patients. To evaluate reproducibility, Sullivan et al[1] at the University of California at San Diego studied 14 angina patients during 3 consecutive days of treadmill testing. A random effects analysis of variance (ANOVA) model was used to measure reliability and to determine any trends in the test results. The intraclass correlation coefficient (ICC), a generalization of the Pearson product-moment correlation coefficient for bivariate data, served as the measure of reliability. The results are summarized in Table 8-1. Prior studies evaluating the changes of work performance in patients with angina pectoris concentrated on improvements in total exercise time. Sklar et al,[2] using moderately severe angina as an endpoint, observed coefficients of variation (standard deviation divided by the mean multiplied by 100) of approximately 5% for

TABLE 8-1.

Standard Deviation (SD) of Change of Two Measurements, ICC, Coefficient of Variation (CV) at Peak Exercise, Onset of Angina, and Gas-Exchange Anaerobic Threshold (ATge)

Variable	Peak Exercise			Onset of Angina			ATge		
	SD	ICC	CV (%)	SD	ICC	CV (%)	SD	ICC	CV (%)
Time (sec)	58	0.70	6 ± 6	65	0.70	11 ± 6	65	0.70	15 ± 9
Vo$_2$ (L/min)	0.150	0.88	6 ± 4	0.152	0.85	6 ± 4	0.113	0.83	7 ± 4
Double product (×10^3)	2.6	0.90	9 ± 5	2.0	0.75	8 ± 5	2.2	0.75	8 ± 6
Heart rate (beats/min)	7	0.94	4 ± 2	6	0.89	4 ± 2	8	0.83	4 ± 4
ST60 X (mV)	0.06	0.80	34 ± 25	0.03	0.79	31 ± 25	0.03	0.78	45 ± 29
ST60 GD (mV)	0.05	0.83	23 ± 21	0.04	0.65	25 ± 16	0.05	0.65	53 ± 34

Vo$_2$, Ventilatory oxygen uptake; ST60, 60 msec after the end of QRS; X, lead X; GD, lead with greatest depression.

total treadmill time. Similar results were obtained by Sullivan et al,[1] who found a coefficient of variation of 6% for peak time. However, when the ICC was determined to test for reproducibility, a rather low value of $r = 0.70$ was obtained. The addition of a given amount of time to each observation of a parameter would increase the mean without affecting the standard deviation and thus would lower the coefficient of variation. During sequential exercise testing, many investigators have noted an increase in total treadmill time in patients with normal results, patients with angina, and patients with congestive heart failure (CHF). In the study by Sullivan et al[1] we observed better reproducibility for oxygen uptake than for time at each analysis point.

Conclusions from the study of Sullivan et al[1] include the following:

1. Measured oxygen uptake should be used instead of total exercise time because it is a more reproducible measure of aerobic exercise capacity.
2. The ventilatory threshold is a reproducible submaximal exercise variable at which to evaluate myocardial ischemia and myocardial oxygen demand.
3. A pretrial exercise test allows the patient to become familiar with the exercise testing staff, the equipment, and the nature of his or her anginal endpoints.
4. The treadmill protocol should be designed for the patient's exercise capacity with 2 metabolic equivalents (METs) or fewer increments per stage.
5. Computerized techniques for electrocardiogram (ECG) analysis provide reproducible measurements of ST-segment displacement.
6. Statistical methods based on the estimate of the measurement error associated with a particular variable can be used by the clinician or investigator to better plan and evaluate an intervention.

Safety of Placebo in Studying Antianginal Agents

Because the safety of withholding standard therapy and enrolling patients with stable angina in placebo-controlled trials was not known, Glasser et al[3] identified all events leading to dropout from trials of 12 antianginal drugs submitted in support of new drug applications to the FDA. Persons who dropped out of the trials were classified as having done so because of adverse cardiovascular events or other causes, without records of their drug assignments. There were 3161 subjects who entered any randomized, double-blind phase of placebo-controlled protocols; 197 (6.2%) withdrew because of cardiovascular events. There was no difference in risk of adverse events between drug and placebo groups. A prospectively defined subgroup analysis showed that groups who received calcium antagonists were at an increased risk of dropout compared with placebo groups, primarily because of a disproportionate number of adverse events in studies of one drug. There were few adverse experiences associated with short-term placebo use. Thus withholding active treatment for angina does not increase the risk of serious cardiac events.

EVALUATION BEFORE AND AFTER PTCA AND CABS

The exercise test has not been able to predict the likelihood of restenosis after PTCA.[4] However, the exercise test has shown an increased exercise capacity after CABS or with medical management after PTCA, as the review of the literature in Table 8-2 shows.

EVALUATION OF PATIENTS FOR SURGERY

Carliner et al[5] performed a prospective study of preoperative exercise testing in 200 patients older that 40 years scheduled for elective major noncardiac surgery under general anesthesia. The exercise test showed ST-segment depression in 32 patients (16%). The exercise test has not been justified as a routine means of evaluating patients before surgery. Nonexercise stressors are frequently used for evaluating patients for vascular surgery because they are limited by claudication.

EVALUATION OF PATIENTS WITH DYSRHYTHMIAS

An exercise test can be used to evaluate patients with dysrhythmias or to induce dysrhythmias in patients with the appropriate symptoms. The dysrhythmias that can be evaluated include premature ventricular contractions (PVCs), sick sinus syndrome, and various degrees of heart block. Ambulatory monitoring or isometric exercise often detects a higher prevalence of dysrhythmias, including more serious dysrhythmias than does dynamic exercise testing. The findings in each of these tests, however, may have different significances.

Young et al[6] argues that maximal exercise testing is useful for detection of dysrhythmias and assessment of antidysrhythmic drug efficacy. Because few reports document the safety of exercise testing in patients with malignant ventricular dysrhythmias, they reviewed the complications of symptom-limited exercise in 263 patients with such dysrhythmias who underwent a total of 1377 maximal treadmill

TABLE 8-2.

Studies that Included Exercise Testing Before and After PTCA or CABG

	Number	Medication	Multi-vessel Disease Before	Exercise Capacity Before	Change (%)	Mean Maximum HR (Beats/Min) Before	After	Maximum Double Product* Before	After	Angina Pectoris During ET Before	After	Abnormal ST-Segment Response (%) Before	After
PTCA													
Rod	14	BB and dig NR	0%	6.2 METs	10%	138	149	27	30	71%	7%	(1.0 mm, 0.2 mm)	
Suzuki	14	Off BB, dig, Nit	0%	14 min	14%	122	145	20	25	57%	21%	36%	7%
Rousing	45	Off BB, dig, Nit	6%	7.6 min	38%					67%	7%	33%	7%
Kent	32	Off BB, Nit	14%	7 ± 2 min	143%					28%	1%	—	—
Scholl	36	Off dig, Nit	17%	7.5 min	37%			21	31	NA	8%	56%	20%
Meier	132	NA	41%	74 watts	86%					97%	23%	72%	21%
Gruenzig	133	NA	42%	47% APN	67%					100%	33%	79%	10%
Vandormael	57	Off medications	84%	6.2 min	35%					56%	11%	75%	32%
Dubach	38	Usual medications	50%	6.8 METs	27%	126	142	21	25	71%	39%	76%	47%
TOTAL / AVERAGE	501		28%		51%	128	145	22	28	68%	19%	61%	21%
CABG													
Guiney	40	Off dig, BB	85%	NA	61%					95%	8%	95%	38%
Gohlke	467	NA	87%	62 watts	47%					54%	5%	79%	28%
Hultgren	190	NA	48%	5.0 min	40%	130	142	19	24	71%	28%	38%	25%
Bartel	123	Dig and BB NR	80%	NA	NA	130	142	21	24	100%	32%	67%	36%
Kloster	38	NA	84%	388 kpm/min	63%	107	119			100%	17%	71%	56%
Lapin	46	NA	64%	NA	16%					85%	20%	73%	26%
Frick	45	BB and Nit NR	100%	569 kpm/min	26%	124	135	21	24	40%	Decrease	(2.8 mm, 1.5 mm)	
Meier	28	NA	41%	68 watts	79%					89%	29%	82%	14%
Dubach	28	Used medications	93%	6.0 METs	37%	122	134	12	14	50%	7%	61%	29%
TOTAL / AVERAGE	1005		80%		41%	123	134	19	22	67%	17%	69%	34%

*Maximum double product = Systolic blood pressure × Heart rate at maximum × 10^3.

HR, Heart rate; ET, exercise test; BB, beta-blocker; dig, digoxin; NR, not restricted; nit, nitrates; NA, not available; APN, age-predicted exercise capacity; km/min, kilogram-meters/minute.

From Dubach P et al: J Cardiovasc Rehabil 10:120-125, 1990.

tests. Of these, 74% had a history of ventricular fibrillation or hemodynamically compromising ventricular tachycardia, and the remainder had experienced ventricular tachycardia after recent myocardial infarction (MI) or in connection with poor left ventricular function. A *complication* was defined as the occurrence of dysrhythmia, such as ventricular fibrillation, ventricular tachycardia, or bradycardia, during exercise testing that mandated immediate medical treatment. Complications were noted in 24 patients (9.1%) during 32 tests (2.3%), whereas 239 patients (90.9%) were free of complications during 1345 tests (97.7%). There were no deaths, MIs, or lasting morbid events. Clinical descriptors associated with complications included the male gender, the presence of coronary artery disease (CAD), and a history of exertional dysrhythmia. Clinical variables previously considered to confer increased risk during exercise, such as poor left ventricular function, high-grade ventricular dysrhythmias before or during exercise, exertional hypotension, and ST-segment depression, did not predict complications. Occurrence of a complication was also unaffected by the use of antidysrhythmic drugs at the time of exercise. Complication frequency in their study group was compared with that in a reference population of 3444 cardiac patients without histories of symptomatic dysrhythmias who underwent 8221 exercise tests. Of these, 4 subjects (0.12%) developed ventricular fibrillation (0.05% of tests) without fatality or lasting morbidity. They concluded that maximal exercise testing could be conducted safely in patients with malignant dysrhythmias and that clinical variables previously considered to confer risk during exercise were not predictive of complications.

Young et al[6] also compared the provocation of PVCs in a standard exercise test with provocation of PVCs in an abbreviated form of testing (Mini) that seemed to approximate more closely the demands of daily activities. In the Mini protocol, the treadmill was kept at 12% elevation, and speed began at 1.7 mph, increasing every 15 seconds from 2.5, 3.4, 4.2, 5.5, and 6.0 to 6.5 mph, where it was then kept until the test was completed. The study involved 52 patients, 42 men and 10 women, average age 49 years, with known or suspected history of ventricular dysrhythmias. Hemodynamic and ST-segment changes were similar during both forms of testing. During the exercise test, 37 patients (71%) exhibited PVCs, whereas 32 (62%) did so during Mini testing. Standard exercise testing and Mini testing provoked the same degree of PVCs in 10 of 13 patients who had repetitive PVCs. In two patients, the yield of these complex forms of PVCs was higher with Mini testing, and in one patient, with standard exercise testing. To assess drug efficacy for the suppression of PVCs, the abbreviated protocol may be useful for patients undergoing serial exercise studies.

EVALUATION OF PATIENTS WITH VALVULAR HEART DISEASE

Exercise testing has been used in the evaluation of patients with valvular heart disease to qualify the amount of disability caused by their disease, to reproduce any exercise-induced symptomatology, and to evaluate their response to medical and surgical intervention. The exercise ECG has been used to identify concurrent

CAD, but there is a high prevalence of false-positive responses (ST-segment depression not due to ischemia) because of the frequent baseline ECG abnormalities and left ventricular hypertrophy. Some physicians have used the exercise test to help decide when surgery is needed. Exercise testing has been used most in patients with aortic stenosis (AS).[7,8]

Patients with Aortic Stenosis

Effort syncope in patients with AS is an important and well-appreciated symptom. During effort syncope, systolic blood pressure is reduced, pulses and apical impulse are absent, and murmurs disappear. Various mechanisms have been hypothesized as the cause for effort syncope in patients with AS, including carotid artery hyperreactivity, inadequate cardiac output leading to cerebral anemia and syncope, and an inability to increase cardiac output during exercise because of left ventricular failure or dysrhythmias.

Most guidelines regarding exercise testing list moderate to severe AS as a contraindication for exercise testing because of concern with syncope and cardiac arrest. Therefore guidelines for monitoring patients with AS during exercise testing and the clinical situations in which exercise testing is performed must be considered. The results of studies of exercise testing performed in patients with AS are reviewed in Table 8-3.

Exercise testing can be clinically useful in the management of patients with AS. Exercise plays an important role in the objective assessment of symptoms, hemodynamic response, and functional capacity. Whether ST-segment depression indicates significant CAD remains unclear. By performing exercise testing before and after surgery, the benefits of surgery and baseline impairment can be quantified. Exercise testing offers the opportunity to evaluate objectively any disparities between history and clinical findings (e.g., in the elderly, asymptomatic subject with physical or Doppler findings of severe AS). Often the echocardiographic studies are inadequate in such patients, particularly when they are smokers. When Doppler echocardiography reveals a significant gradient in the asymptomatic patient with normal exercise capacity, the patient could be followed closely until symptoms develop. In patients with an inadequate systolic blood pressure response to exercise or a fall in systolic blood pressure from the resting value when symptoms occur, surgery appears to be needed.

SUMMARY

The studies evaluating antianginal agents and vasodilators have been greatly hampered by the increase in treadmill time that occurs merely by performing serial tests. For this reason, expired gas analysis is frequently being added to protocols evaluating therapeutic agents. The studies of CABS and PTCA are confounded by differences in medications before and after intervention and by the low rate of abnormal results in preintervention tests in the patients undergoing PTCA who mostly have single-vessel disease. Standard exercise testing does not appear to be

TABLE 8-3.

Studies that Reported Exercise Testing in Patients with AS

Study	No.	Age (yr)	Mode	Mean Value Area (cm²)	Mean Value Gradient (mm Hg)	Maximum HR (Beats/Min)	Exercise Capacity	Angina (%)	>1.0 mm ST-Segment Depression (%)	Abnormal BP Response (%)
Halloran	31	(8-17)‡	Bike	1.22 ± 0.74	50	(160-200)	NA	0	48	NA
Chandramouli	44	(5-19)	Treadmill	NA	(10-11)	NA	NA	0	27	NA
Aronow	19	(35-56)	Treadmill	NA	(53-80)	NA	NA	0	37	NA
Thitmer	23	11	Bike	NA	86 (30-235)	NA	NA	(0-29)	(71-100)	NA
James	65	12	Bike	NA	(30-70)	(183-194)	NA	6	(38-89)	(0-32)
Barton	11	12 (6-20)	Treadmill	NA	38 (14-80)	182	NA	9	54	63
Niemala	14	46 ± 5	Bike	1.0 ± 0.6	NA	150 ± 17	520 kpm/min	0	NA	NA
Kveselis*	12	13 ± 3	Bike	0.60 ± 0.16	59 ± 18	180 ± 17	800 kpm/min	0	100	58
Linderholm†	20	58 ± 14	Bike	NA	57 ± 23	NA	500 kpm/min	35	X = 1.33 mm ± 0.8	NA
Nylander	91	65 (57-78)	Bike	(0.48-1.63)	(18-64)	NA	NA	29	NA	NA

NA, Not available; *HR,* heart rate; *BP,* blood pressure; *kpm/min,* kilogram-meters/minute. X, difference.
Modified from Atwood JE et al: *Chest* 93:1085, 1988.
*Selected subgroup with >1.0 mm ST-segment depression.
†Selected subgroup without CAD.
‡Parenthesis denote range.

very helpful in predicting restenosis. The results from studies determining the risk of exercise-induced PVCs and more serious ventricular dysrhythmias are mixed, but prognosis appears to relate more to the "company they keep" than to the dysrhythmias themselves. Some investigators contend that exercise testing is a better means of evaluating dysrhythmic patients than other testing modalities. Certainly, exercise-induced dysrhythmias are best studied with exercise. From one study, we must conclude that exercise testing has little value in evaluating patients before noncardiac surgery. Further work in this area is needed, but non-exercise stress modalities are playing an important role, particularly in the workup of patients with vascular problems limited by claudication. Other applications of exercise testing include its use for evaluating patients with unstable angina, valvular heart disease, and intermittent claudication.

REFERENCES

1. Sullivan M et al: The reproducibility of hemodynamic, electrocardiographic, and gas exchange data during treadmill exercise in patients with stable angina pectoris, *Chest* 86:375-382, 1984.
2. Sklar J et al: The effects of a cardioselective (metroprolol) and a nonselective (propranolol) beta-adrenergic blocker on the response to dynamic exercise in normal men, *Circulation* 65:894-899, 1982.
3. Glasser SP et al: Exposing patients with chronic, stable, exertional angina to placebo periods in drug trials, *JAMA* 265:1550-1554, 1991.
4. Honan MB et al: Exercise treadmill testing is a poor predictor of anatomic restenosis after angioplasty for acute myocardial infarction, *Circulation* 80:1585-1594, 1989.
5. Carliner NH et al: Routine preoperative exercise testing in patients undergoing major noncardiac surgery, *Am J Cardiol* 56:51-58, 1985.
6. Young DZ et al: Safety of maximal exercise testing in patients at high risk for ventricular arrhythmia, *Circulation* 70:184-191, 1984.
7. Areskog NH: Exercise testing in the evaluation of patients with valvular aortic stenosis, *Clin Physiol* 4:201-208, 1984.
8. Atwood JE et al: Exercise and the heart: exercise testing in patients with aortic stenosis, *Chest* 93:1083-1087, 1988.

CHAPTER 9

Case Examples

Chapter 9 consists of 42 exercise ECG examples, including complete 12-lead averages from selected important times during the exercise test. Although these averages are all that are provided, remember that the proper way to read an exercise test is to observe the raw, unfiltered, unaveraged ECG data. The filtering process can distort the ECG and in fact, it is better when you are aware of the usual motion artifact in the signals. Proper skin preparation, good electrodes, and reliable cables cannot be replaced by signal processing. The raw ECG data should be examined for consistent ST-segment shifts found not in one complex, but in at least 3 complexes in a row. A classic "abnormal" ST-segment response can be seen in almost any exercise test in one ECG complex. Also the ST-segment depression should be consistent with the ECG data that precede and that follow it. The averages are helpful only after confirming consistency with the raw ECG to summarize changes and to highlight particular findings, as in this chapter. Accompanying the ECGs are case summaries under headings that explain the major reason for their inclusion. The management described is not necessarily the "correct" way of approaching the patient, and often more tests are listed as being performed than are necessary. The major purpose of the cases is to illustrate a wide range of examples of exercise ECG responses and to provide some idea of what they are usually associated with clinically.

FIG 9-1.

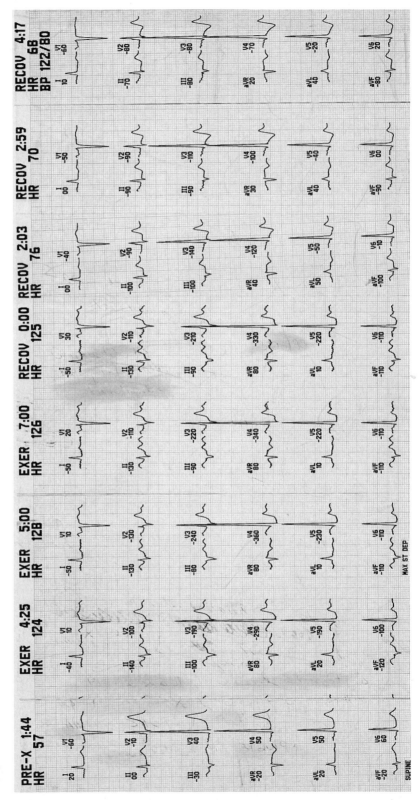

PATIENT B8557 (Fig 9-1): EVALUATION FOR CARDIAC VALVULAR SURGERY

1. History and physical examination/medications/procedures: This patient is a 75-year-old white man with a history of mitral valve prolapse and now with moderate mitral regurgitation who recently noted progressive fatigue and declining exercise capacity.

2. Symptoms/reason for test: Evaluation of change in exercise capacity

3. Resting ECG: Results were normal except for increased voltage and prominent anterior forces. The R wave was greater than the S wave in V_2, which can be caused by RBBB, RVH, WPW, posterior infarct, or as in this patient, a normal variant.

4. Exercise hemodynamics/symptoms: Heart rate increased from 60 to 132 beats/min, and SBP rose from 160 to 180 mm Hg. He reached 7 METs with a Borg scale of 18, and his exercise capacity was above age-predicted normal. No angina occurred during the test.

5. Exercise ECG: During exercise, his QRS major vector shifted laterally, causing R-wave voltage to increase in leads V_4, V_5, and V_6—the same leads that showed the greatest ST-segment depression (3 mm). In recovery, the QRS vector shifted back toward V_2, and the J-junction returned to normal quickly, but the T waves became biphasic and the ST-segment vector was downsloping.

6. Interpretation: This ST pattern usually results from profound ischemia but could be due to LV hypertrophy associated with a supply and demand imbalance; in this case, demand outstripped supply.

7. Recommendations/follow-up: Because of his symptoms and echo findings, he underwent cardiac catheterization. His ventriculogram showed a slightly enlarged ventricular cavity with normal wall thickness, good contractility, and 4+ mitral regurgitation. His LAD coronary artery had two tandem lesions of 15% to 40%, the first diagonal had an 80% lesion, and the first obtuse marginal had subtotal stenosis. During supine exercise, the pulmonary artery pressure rose to 46 mm Hg with a V wave of 60 mm Hg.

8. Comments: The results of thallium scintigraphy were positive for ischemia in the anterolateral wall, corroborating his exercise ECG results. The scintigram was done to confirm the need for CABS, which increases the risk and difficulty of the valvular surgery. Aortic valvular disease can also be evaluated with exercise testing after the gradient has been established with echocardiography. Blood pressure must be carefully monitored during and after exercise.

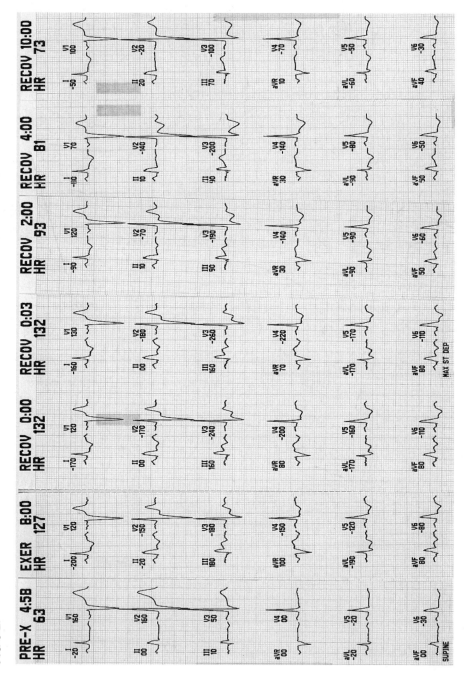

FIG 9-2.

PATIENT F1199 (Fig 9-2): ST-SEGMENT ELEVATION RECIPROCAL TO ST-SEGMENT DEPRESSION

1. History and physical examination/medications/procedures: This patient is a 65-year-old Mexican-American referred for evaluation of dull chest pain, which was precipitated by exercise and anger but occurred occasionally at rest. He reported a heart attack 10 years ago, a family history of premature CAD, and symptoms of peripheral vascular disease. He was on antihypertensive medication and a calcium antagonist.

2. Symptoms/reason for test: Evaluation of atypical angina (50% pretest probability because the MI was undocumented)

3. Resting ECG: The results showed prominent anterior forces (R > S in V_2) and a nonspecific intraventricular conduction delay. There is minor ST-segment depression and lateral T-wave inversion.

4. Exercise hemodynamics/symptoms: Heart rate rose from 63 to 132 beats/min; SBP standing was 140 and dropped to 110 mm Hg at maximum exercise. (Exertional hypotension is associated with increased risk of events during testing and severe CAD.) He had typical angina but stopped because of claudication. Accordingly, he was assigned a Duke Treadmill Angina Index score of 1. (1 point = "angina occurred"; 2 points = "angina was the reason for stopping.") The Duke score relates directly to prognosis and angiographic disease severity.

5. Exercise ECG: Showed ST-segment elevation in leads III and aV_F, as well as ST-segment depression in I and aV_L, ST-segment depression was present in the lateral leads and most notable in V_3, which showed downsloping ST-segment depression that persisted for 10 minutes into recovery.

6. Interpretation: The ST-segment changes persisted until almost 10 minutes into recovery, and the patient exhibited exertional hypotension, both of which are associated with severe CAD.

7. Recommendations/follow-up: Cardiac catheterization revealed triple-vessel disease and normal ventricular function.

8. Comments: The ST-segment elevation is most likely reciprocal to the lateral depression. Some studies have shown that anterior precordial lead ST-segment depression (V_1 to V_3) is associated with LAD disease, but this patient had triple-vessel disease with normal LV function. The VA prognostic score was 3, consistent with a 10% annual cardiovascular mortality. Most of the ST-segment depression occurred in V_3—the lead with the largest R wave.

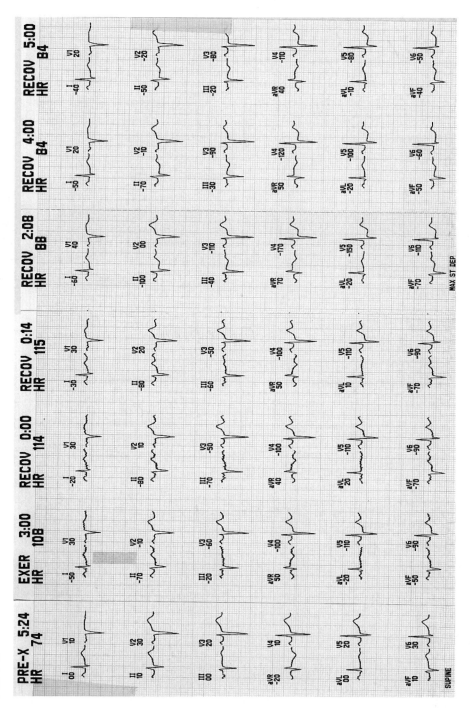

FIG 9-3.

PATIENT G1698 (Fig 9-3): MORE ABNORMAL IN RECOVERY THAN DURING EXERCISE

1. History and physical examination/medications/procedures: This patient is a 47-year-old white man admitted to the hospital with an MI diagnosed by chest pain, a CPK of 550, and transient T-wave changes.

2. Symptoms/reason for test: Angina persisted after this non–Q-wave infarction, and he was started on beta-blockers. The above-exercise ECG test was performed 8 days later, before discharge from the hospital.

3. Resting ECG: Essentially normal results were consistent with a non–Q-wave MI and with normal LV function (i.e., there is a 95% probability that ejection fraction is normal when the resting ECG is normal). Small R waves in V_1 and V_2 were present on a prior ECG.

4. Exercise hemodynamics/symptoms: Heart rate went from 76 to 115 beats/min with exercise, and his SBP went from 100 to 170 mm Hg. This patient had an aerobic capacity about 50% of normal for his age. No angina was reported during testing (Duke TM Angina Score of 0).

5. Exercise ECG: There was more abnormal ST-segment depression in recovery than during exercise. The onset of ST-segment depression began 2 minutes into recovery.

6. Interpretation: Recovery-only changes usually are associated with single- or double-vessel disease. Often when depression is borderline because of upsloping during exercise, it will become clearly abnormal in recovery.

7. Recommendations/follow-up: Patient underwent catheterization, which showed normal ventricular function and total occlusion of the LAD artery. all other arteries were normal.

8. Comments: Our studies have shown that recovery-only ST-segment depression does not represent a false-positive response. A cooldown walk should be avoided, and patients should be placed supine to bring out recovery ST-segment changes.

FIG 9-4.

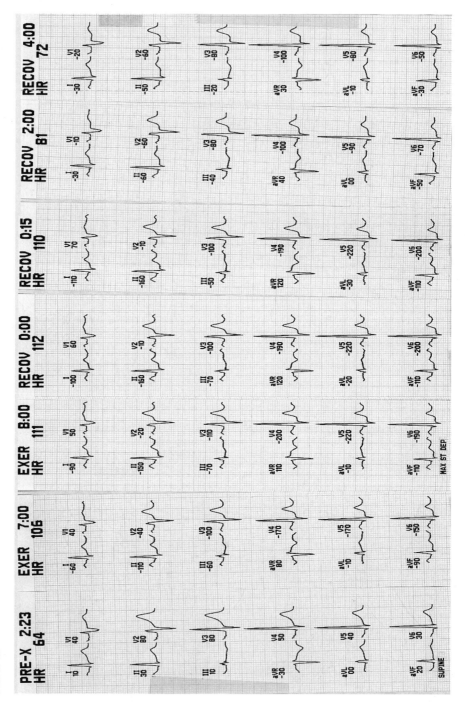

PATIENT T4157 (Fig 9-4): POSITIVE DUE TO LAD ARTERY DISEASE

1. History and physical examination/medications/procedures: This patient is a 38-year-old white man with hypertension and hypercholesterolemia who reported 2 weeks of exertional angina pectoris.

2. Symptoms/reason for test: Recent onset of angina (one of the criteria for unstable angina), which was not a contraindication to testing, since his symptoms were stable as determined by a current medical history assessment

3. Resting ECG: Normal results were consistent with normal ventricular function. Early repolarization is present.

4. Exercise hemodynamics/symptoms: Patient remained on beta-blockers and calcium antagonists for the exercise test. His heart rate increased from 56 to 112 beats/min; his SBP rose from only 120 to 130 and then dropped to 120 mm Hg at maximal exercise. He reached 9 METs with a Borg scale of 11, representing an exercise capacity of 70% of age-predicted normal. Typical angina during exercise and recovery was the reason for stopping the test (Duke Treadmill Angina Index of 2).

5. Exercise ECG: The ST segments in the lateral precordial leads started with early repolarization at baseline, crossed the isoelectric line at 7 minutes of exercise, and dropped 2 mm by the start of recovery. Also there was about 1 mm of horizontal ST-segment depression in the inferior leads, which cleared after 4 minutes of recovery.

6. Interpretation: Abnormal ST-segment depression in multiple leads at a low level of exercise is consistent with profound ischemia.

7. Recommendations/follow-up: Thallium scintigraphy revealed redistribution in the inferior and anterior walls. Cardiac catheterization revealed severe stenosis of the mid-LAD artery, and the ventriculogram was totally normal. Angioplasty successfully reduced the 90% proximal LAD lesion to a 20% lesion.

8. Comments: Often patients still have ST-segment depression in recovery after a successful PTCA. Exercise testing does not appear to be helpful in prediction of restenosis; return of angina is the best indicator.

FIG 9-5.

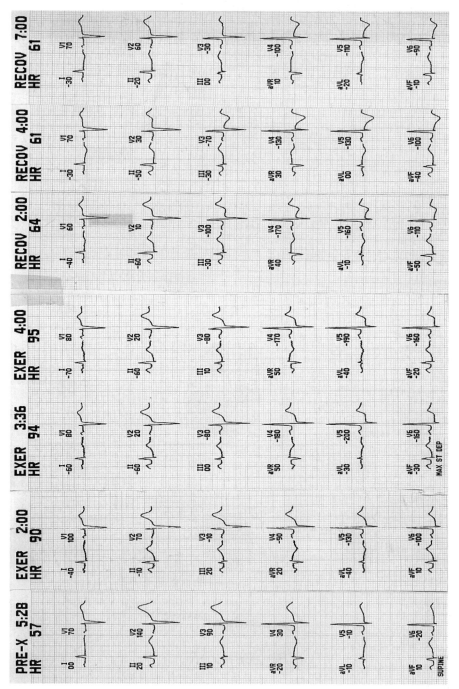

PATIENT M0487 (Fig 9-5) **MARKEDLY ABNORMAL DUE TO SEVERE CAD**

1. History and physical examination/medications/procedures: This patient is a 70-year-old white man referred for evaluation of typical angina. He is currently on a calcium antagonist and has had no previous cardiac events.

2. Symptoms/reason for test: Evaluation for disease severity

3. Resting ECG: Results were normal, except for minor ST-segment depression in the lateral leads.

4. Exercise hemodynamics/symptoms: Typical angina during exercise was the reason for stopping. At a Borg scale of 13, the patient reached 3 METs, which was 50% of expected for his age. Heart rate rose from 57 to 95 beats/min and SBP dropped from 170 to 160 mm Hg.

5. Exercise ECG: There was nearly 2 mm of ST-segment depression in V_4, V_5, and V_6. At 4 minutes of recovery, he still had at least 1 mm of ST-segment depression with inverted T waves. This depression cleared by 12 minutes of recovery.

6. Interpretation: There was markedly positive ST-segment depression extending into recovery.

7. Recommendations/follow-up: He was found to have triple-vessel coronary disease consistent with his marked ST-segment depression at a low heart rate and with evolutionary ST-T wave changes in recovery. He was referred for CABS.

8. Comments: The presence of typical angina in this case made the pretest probability of CAD very high and the possibility of a false-positive test very low, irrespective of the exercise response. However, evolutionary ST-T wave changes in recovery can be helpful in ruling out a false-positive response. His VA prognostic score of 3 is associated with an annual cardiovascular mortality of 10%, making him a candidate for surgery.

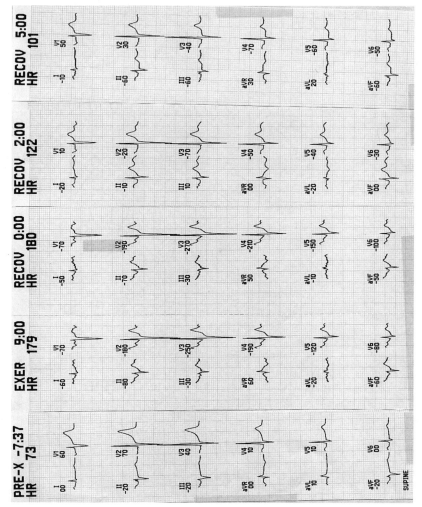

FIG 9-6.

PATIENT BD7614 (Fig 9-6): RECOVERY-ABNORMAL ST-SEGMENT RESPONSE WITH ANGINA

1. History and physical examination/medications/procedures: This is a 42-year-old white male inpatient with a 20-pack-year smoking history who currently abstains. He has a family history of coronary disease before age 65. He had no previous MIs, catheterizations, or procedures.

2. Symptoms/reason for test: Evaluation for possible coronary disease after stabilization of chest pain syndrome

3. Resting ECG: Results were normal; thus there is a high probability that he has normal ventricular function.

4. Exercise hemodynamics/symptoms: Heart rate rose from 73 to 180 beats/min, and SBP increased from 130 to 188 mm Hg for a double product of 33.5. At a Borg perceived-exertion score of 19, the patient achieved 8 METs, which is 68% of his age-predicted exercise capacity. Angina occurred during testing.

5. Exercise ECG: Minor, upsloping ST-segment depression during exercise becomes downsloping in recovery.

6. Interpretation: Borderline, downsloping ST-segment depression occurred only during recovery but with typical angina.

7. Recommendations/follow-up: Cardiac catheterization revealed an isolated 85% lesion of his first marginal and normal ventricular function. He was treated medically.

8. Comments: Previous investigators proposed that abnormal ST-segment depression confined to the recovery period represents a false-positive response or possibly coronary spasm. However, recent studies report that its predictive value is just as high as other patterns. Although the exact mechanism is uncertain, such "recovery-only" ST-segment depression is usually associated with mild CAD. Though this patient had nonsignificant junctional ST-segment depression (>0.1 mm), his ST segments were downsloping in recovery. Slope may be more powerful for prediction of CAD than amplitude.

FIG 9-7.

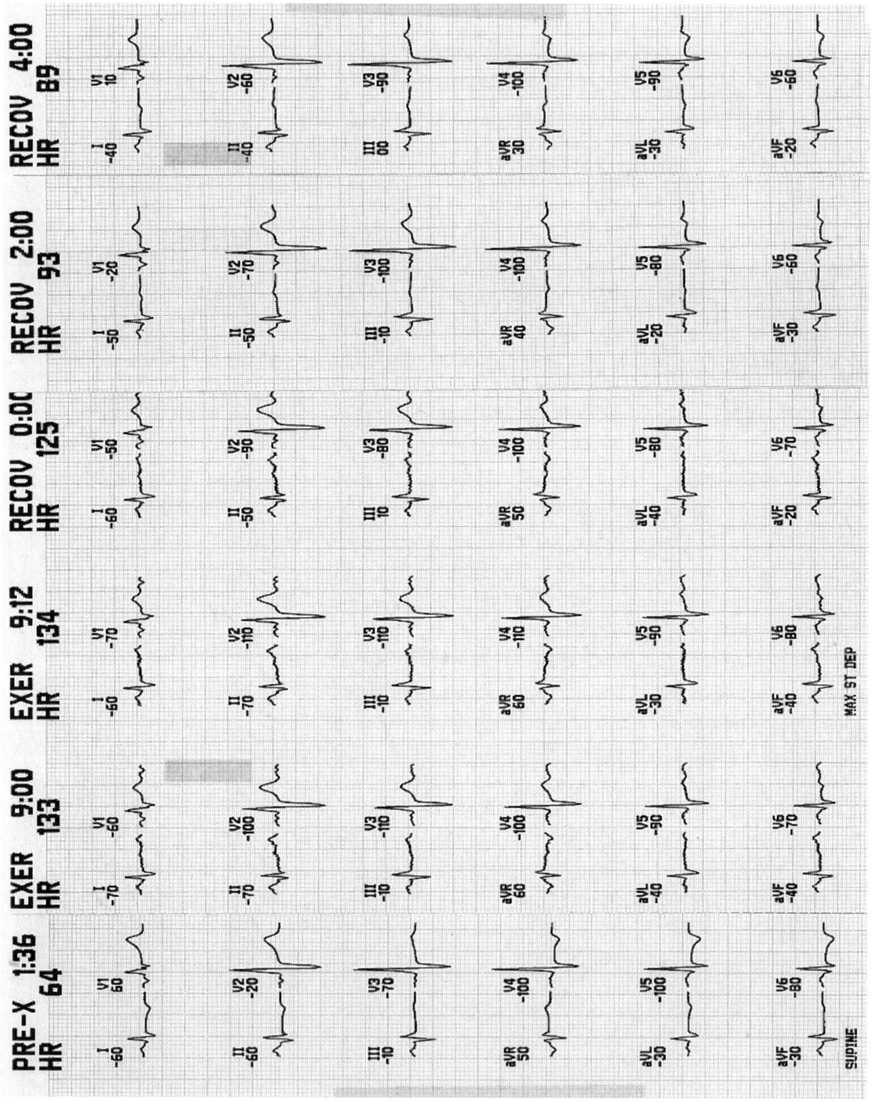

PATIENT KD8625 (Fig 9-7): T-WAVE NORMALIZATION AFTER CORONARY ARTERY BYPASS SURGERY

1. History and physical examination/medications/procedures: This patient is a 57-year-old white male outpatient referred for evaluation of atypical angina. He has insulin-dependent diabetes and a 20-pack-year history of cigarette smoking but currently abstains. He had a bypass 2 years before evaluation and now has developed chest pain again.

2. Symptoms/reason for test: Evaluation of atypical angina that returned after successful bypass

3. Resting ECG: Inferior Q waves with an R greater than S in V_1 as a result of posterior extension. Lateral ST-segment depression and T-wave inversion are also present.

4. Exercise hemodynamics/symptoms: Heart rate rose from 64 to 134 beats/min, and SBP increased from 124 to 230 mm Hg. At a Borg-perceived exertion scale of 19, he achieved 10 METs, which is a little above expected for his age. No angina or other chest pain occurred during testing.

5. Exercise ECG: During exercise the T waves in most leads rose, causing previously inverted T waves to appear normal, as in lead V_5. The ST segments returned to baseline by 4 minutes of recovery.

6. Interpretation: T-wave inversion normalized.

7. Recommendations/follow-up: The patient was reassured because of his lack of chest pain and the absence of further ST-segment depression. He returned to work and felt no limitations or continued chest pain.

8. Comments: If the patient's T-wave normalization had been accompanied by chest pain, this would have been called *pseudonormalization* and been consistent with ischemia. However, based on his excellent exercise capacity, good double product, and absence of chest pain, the response is just caused by normalization. Although some guidelines suggest that patients with a baseline ST-T–wave abnormality of this sort should undergo thallium scintigraphy, the expense of that study was averted by the negative results of a standard exercise test.

FIG 9-8.

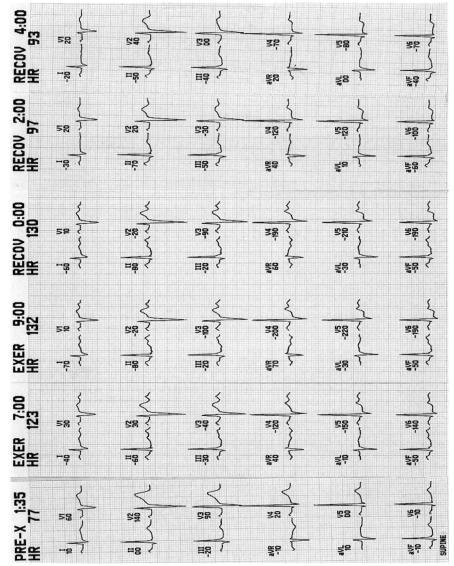

PATIENT CG7666 (Fig 9-8): MORE THAN 2 MM ST-SEGMENT DEPRESSION TREATED WITH MEDICAL MANAGEMENT BECAUSE OF GOOD HEMODYNAMIC RESPONSE

1. History and physical examination/medications/procedures: This patient is a 46-year-old male outpatient with typical angina, chronic obstructive lung disease, a 30-pack-year history of cigarette smoking, and current tobacco use. He reports a family history of premature CAD and elevated cholesterol. He had an MI 6 years before testing.

2. Symptoms/reason for test: Evaluation of typical angina for severity of CAD

3. Resting ECG: Results were entirely normal.

4. Exercise hemodynamics/symptoms: His heart rate and SBP increased from 77 to 132 beats/min and from 125 to 135 mm Hg, respectively. At a Borg scale of 20, he achieved 8 METs, which is 70% of expected for his age. The test was terminated due to ST-segment changes. He had typical angina during exercise and recovery.

5. Exercise ECG: Approximately 2 mm of horizontal or downsloping ST-segment depression was present in leads V_5 and V_6 at maximal exercise; abnormal ST-segment depression cleared by 4 minutes of recovery.

6. Interpretation: Downsloping ST-segment depression of 2 mm in the lateral precordial leads accompanied by angina pectoris is usually associated with severe CAD.

7. Recommendations/follow-up: Patient underwent coronary catheterization and was found to have double-vessel CAD and normal ventricular function. It was decided to manage him medically.

8. Comments: His angina was treated with a calcium antagonist instead of a beta-blocker because of his lung disease. On this regimen, he rarely developed angina and was able to increase his exercise capacity to 12 METs with a vigorous walking program.

FIG 9-9.

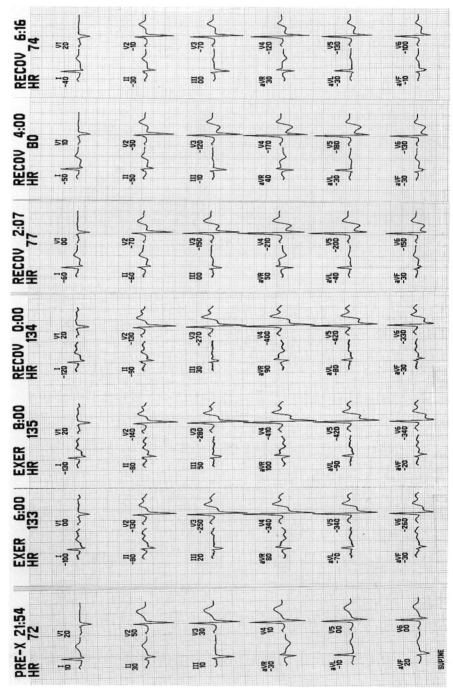

PATIENT CR1788 (Fig 9-9): **MARKEDLY POSITIVE AFTER EPISODE OF UNSTABLE ANGINA**

1. History and physical examination/medications/procedures: This patient is a 44-year-old male inpatient who was admitted for evaluation of unstable angina. His unstable angina stabilized with beta-blockers and antihypertensives, but the cause and severity of his then typical angina remained uncertain. He has a family history of premature CAD and elevated cholesterol levels. He has never smoked.

2. Symptoms/reason for test: Evaluation of the cause of his chest pain after stabilization of unstable angina and demonstration of the severity of his CAD if it is the cause

3. Resting ECG: Results were normal; there were no diagnostic Q waves.

4. Exercise hemodynamics/symptoms: His SBP dropped 40 mm Hg at peak exercise from a submaximal high of 220 mm Hg; his heart rate and SBP increased from 72 to 135 beats/min and from 154 to 180 mm Hg, respectively. At a Borg scale of 17, he reached 8 METs, which was 70% of expected for his age. The test was terminated due to ST-segment changes and typical angina.

5. Exercise ECG: He developed 4 mm of horizontal ST-segment depression in the precordial leads that became downsloping at maximal exercise and continued into recovery. Abnormal ST changes persisted for longer than 6 minutes into recovery.

6. Interpretation: This was a markedly positive exercise test with downsloping ST-segment depression of over 3 mm in multiple leads accompanied by angina pectoris and an SBP drop.

7. Recommendations/follow-up: Patient underwent cardiac catheterization and was found to have severe triple-vessel CAD but good ventricular function. He then underwent bypass surgery.

8. Comments: Downsloping ST-segment depression of a marked degree in multiple leads is highly predictive of triple-vessel or left main CAD. Furthermore, exertional hypotension is a marker for severe CAD and poor prognosis.

FIG 9-10.

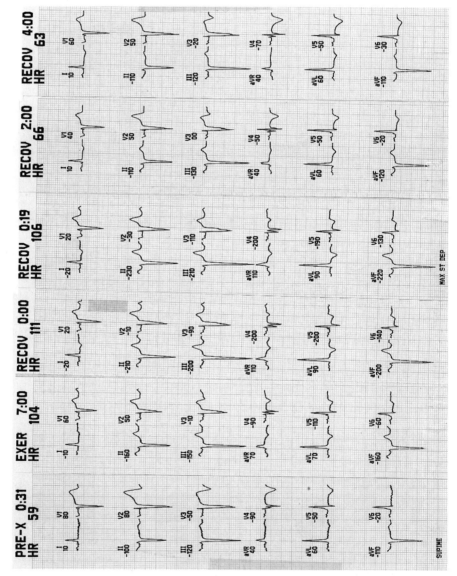

PATIENT JW7324 (Fig 9-10): NEGATIVE FOR SEVERE CAD WITH RESTING ST-SEGMENT DEPRESSION

1. History and physical examination/medications/procedures: This patient is a 68-year-old male outpatient referred for atypical angina. He is on beta-blockers and a nitrate. He is a nonsmoker and has a questionable history of an MI 10 years before this evaluation.

2. Symptoms/reason for test: Evaluation of atypical angina

3. Resting ECG: ECG showed left axis deviation, IVCD, T-wave inversion in the lateral precordial leads, and probable LVH (R wave in $aV_L > 11$ mm). The small, anterior R waves suggest myocardial damage. (NOTE: After a Q-wave infarct, 15% of infarct patients grow back R waves). Also, there is minor ST-segment depression in the lateral precordial leads at rest.

4. Exercise hemodynamics/symptoms: This patient's heart rate increased from 59 to 111 beats/min, and his SBP rose from 130 to 170 mm Hg. At a Borg-perceived exertion scale of 16, he reached 5 METs, which is 66% of predicted for his age. Typical angina occurred during exercise and persisted into recovery.

5. Exercise ECG: During exercise, 2 mm of additional ST-segment depression developed in the lateral precordial leads, but it cleared rapidly by 2 minutes of recovery.

6. Interpretation: In the presence of an abnormal baseline ECG, the exercise ECG still indicates severe disease if there is more than 2 mm of additional depression that persists into recovery. This patient's ST-segment changes neither persisted long in recovery nor reached 2 additional millimeters. Therefore no further studies were performed.

7. Recommendations/follow-up: Medical management continued. He did well without any symptoms or problems.

8. Comments: The diagnostic criterion for severe CAD in postinfarct patients with abnormal baseline ST segments is 2 mm of additional depression that persists into recovery. This patient's test results did not meet this criterion.

FIG 9-11.

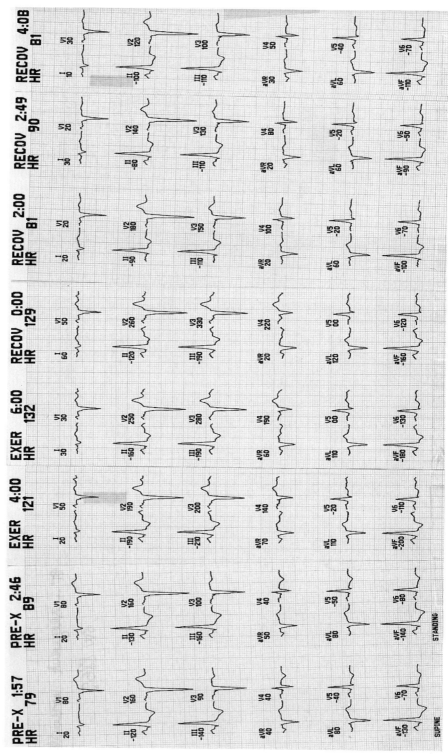

PATIENT SW8869 (Fig 9-11): ST-SEGMENT ELEVATION OVER Q WAVES

1. History and physical examination/medications/procedures: This patient is a 56-year-old male outpatient referred for evaluation of typical angina. He had an MI in March 1991. This exercise test was performed 6 weeks after his MI to evaluate his exercise capacity. His medications include nitrates, calcium blockers, and antihypertensives. He has never smoked, but his cholesterol level is elevated.

2. Symptoms/reason for test: A 1-month post-MI evaluation of continued chest pain and exercise capacity for return to full activities

3. Resting ECG: There are anterior Q waves with T-wave inversion in the anterior and inferior leads. A periinfarctional intraventricular conduction defect is also present.

4. Exercise hemodynamics/symptoms: Heart rate increased from 79 to 132 beats/min, and SBP rose from 139 to 162 mm Hg. The patient reported a Borg scale of 13 at a submaximal effort of 4 METs. Typical angina occurred during the test.

5. Exercise ECG: There were no additional ST-segment changes, except for a slight increase in the ST-segment elevation over his anterior Q waves, particularly at maximal exercise and recovery.

6. Interpretation: Increase in the ST-segment elevation over anterior Q waves was associated with chest pain in this patient.

7. Recommendations/follow-up: He underwent further testing with thallium scintigraphy and cardiac catheterization. He was found to have an anterior wall aneurysm with complete occlusion of his LAD artery. There was 70% stenosis of his circumflex (LCX) artery and right coronary artery (RCA), and his ejection fraction was 38%. He was recommended for CABS.

8. Comments: Additional elevation over anterior Q waves is "normal" after an MI and reflects the amount of underlying wall motion abnormality due to ventricular damage. Such Q-wave ST-segment elevation is thought to conceal lateral depression and cause false-negative results. This patient had typical angina pectoris and was found to have significant additional CAD and a lowered ejection fraction. His ECG also reflected considerable myocardial damage, including an intraventricular conduction defect, which has been implicated in nonischemic ST-segment depression with exercise (i.e., with false-positive results).

FIG 9-12.

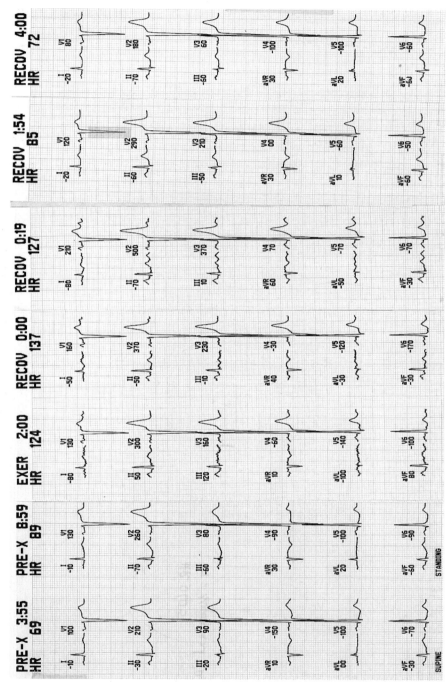

PATIENT HR0105PA (Fig 9-12): LVH WITH STRAIN AND WITHOUT EXERCISE-INDUCED ST CHANGES

1. History and physical examination/medications/procedures: This patient is a 60-year-old white male outpatient with no prior cardiovascular symptoms or procedures. He is taking no cardiac medications and has a history of a 60-pack-year habit of cigarette smoking but currently abstains.

2. Symptoms/reason for test: Recent typical angina

3. Resting ECG: The results were abnormal, showing LVH with strain (downsloping ST-segment depression in the lateral leads).

4. Exercise hemodynamics/symptoms: Heart rate increased from 69 to 137 beats/min, and SBP rose from 160 to 200 mm Hg. He reported a Borg scale of 19 on reaching 4 METs, which is 50% of his age-predicted exercise capacity. No angina occurred during testing.

5. Exercise ECG: Although junctional depression occurred during exercise, the ST-segment slope improved (i.e., it went from downsloping to horizontal). In recovery, the ST segments returned very quickly to their baseline levels. There were no T-wave changes or other ST-segment changes.

6. Interpretation: The ST-segment slope improved while the junctional depression worsened. This response was not diagnostic for severe CAD.

7. Recommendations/follow-up: Though a false-negative test was not suspected, cardiac catheterization was performed when his symptoms recurred. No coronary lesions were found.

8. Comments: Typically, ST-segment depression during exercise is accompanied by a worsening of the ST slope (i.e., a change from upsloping to downsloping) and not the reverse, as in this case. Also, despite his abnormal resting ST-segment depression, this patient's negative exercise test response is still very reliable for ruling out severe CAD. That is, specificity is reduced by the presence of resting ST-segment depression, whereas sensitivity remains good.

FIG 9-13.

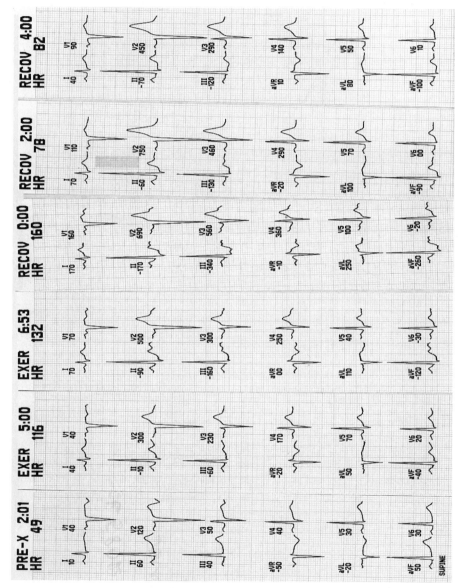

PATIENT GL5802 (Fig 9-13): ISOLATED INFERIOR LEAD (II, III, aV$_F$) DEPRESSION

1. History and physical examination/medications/procedures: This patient is a 44-year-old white male inpatient who underwent screening for a high-level exercise program. He has a 10-pack-year history of cigarette smoking and is still smoking. He has a family history of premature coronary disease, and his cholesterol level has been elevated in the past. He has had no previous cardiac events or procedures.

2. Symptoms/reason for test: Screening for high-level exercise program

3. Resting ECG: Results were normal.

4. Exercise hemodynamics/symptoms: His heart rate increased from 49 to 160 beats/min, and his SBP rose from 130 to 190 mm Hg. At a Borg-perceived exertion scale of 16, he reached 16 METs, which is 140% of expected for his age (i.e., supranormal). He developed noncardiac chest pain during testing.

5. Exercise ECG: More than 2 mm of horizontal ST-segment depression occurred in the inferior leads (II, III, and aV$_F$) during and after exercise. There was no depression in the lateral leads, but there was elevation in the anterior leads. All changes cleared after 2 minutes of recovery. This was an instance of normal, anterior ST-segment elevation associated with ST-segment depression being isolated to the inferior limb leads. There was no evidence that atrial repolarization caused this ST-segment depression.

6. Interpretation: This is most likely a false-positive study.

7. Recommendations/follow-up: Thallium scintigraphy was normal.

8. Comments: Isolated, inferior-lead, exercise-induced ST-segment depression when there is a normal baseline ECG usually represents a false-positive response. Atrial repolarization is often the cause but not in this case.

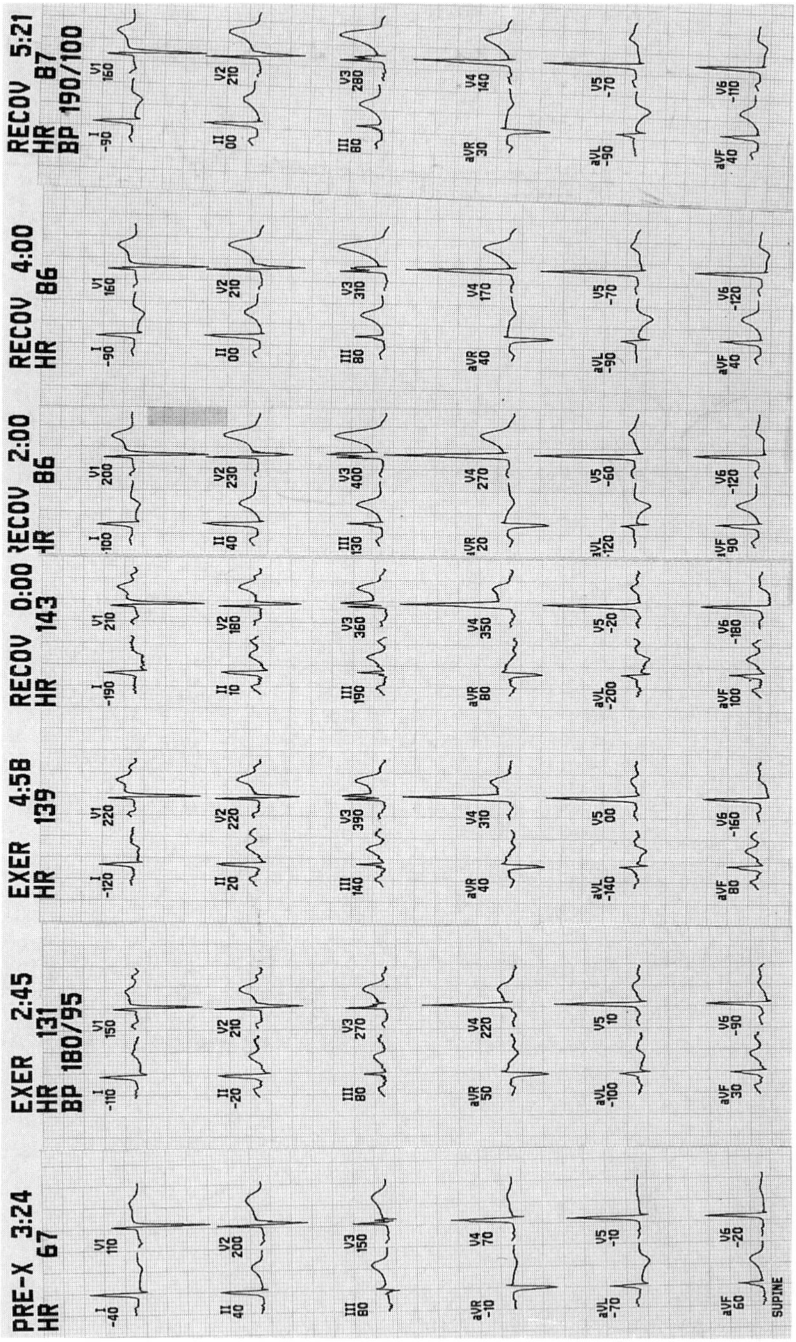

FIG 9-14.

PATIENT CM8308 (Fig 9-14): EXERCISE-INDUCED ST-SEGMENT ELEVATION ACCOMPANIED BY ST-SEGMENT DEPRESSION WITHOUT DIAGNOSTIC Q WAVES

1. History and physical examination/medications/procedures: This patient is a 73-year-old white male outpatient referred for evaluation of typical angina. He is taking an antihypertensive. He is not a cigarette smoker. He had an MI 2 years before this evaluation and only recently developed angina.

2. Symptoms/reason for test: Typical angina pectoris

3. Resting ECG: Results were largely normal, with low-amplitude T waves and mild ST-segment depression in limb leads I and aV_L.

4. Exercise hemodynamics/symptoms: His heart rate increased from 82 to 143 beats/min, and his SBP dropped from 170 to 155 mm Hg. At a Borg scale of 18, he reached 8 METs, which is above average for his age. No angina occurred during testing, but he did exhibit exertional hypotension.

5. Exercise ECG: During exercise, there is striking ST-segment elevation in V_3 and V_4, accompanied by increased R-wave amplitude. There is also downsloping ST-segment depression in lateral leads V_5 and V_6. No PVCs occurred.

6. Interpretation: Non–Q wave ST-segment elevation representing acute transmural ischemia. This finding localizes the subtending coronary artery (in this case the LAD artery) and is known to be very dysrhythmogenic. Manifestations of this transmural ischemia respond very well to a calcium antagonist because it is caused by coronary artery spasm in either a "normal" segment or near a fixed lesion. The "normal" segment does not have a lesion seen by angiography but has a defect that sensitizes it to thrombus resulting in a coronary "cough."

7. Recommendations/follow-up: Patient underwent catheterization and was found to have an 85% proximal LAD lesion. There were no other lesions. He underwent PTCA and was treated with a calcium antagonist.

8. Comments: The associated ST-segment depression in leads V_5 and V_6 made the presence of other lesions more likely, but catheterization revealed only the LAD stenosis.

FIG 9-15.

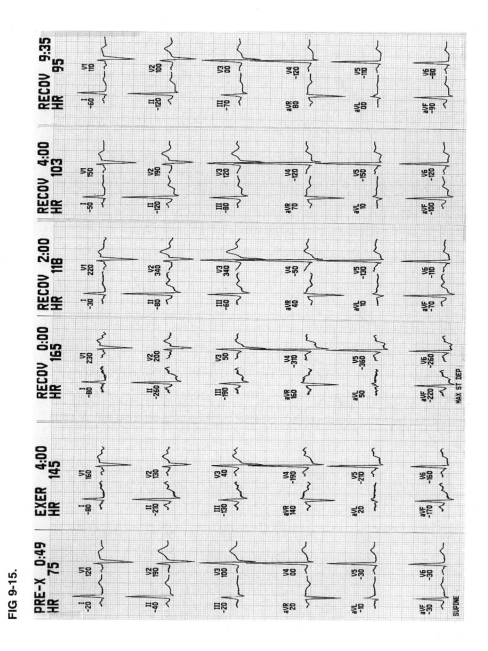

PATIENT BE7892 (Fig 9-15): **FALSE-POSITIVE TEST**

1. History and physical examination/medications/procedures: This patient is a 60-year-old white male outpatient referred for evaluation of noncardiac chest pain of uncertain origin. He was receiving a calcium antagonist for hypertension. He does not smoke, but his cholesterol level is elevated. He has had no previous cardiac events or procedures.

2. Symptoms/reason for test: Evaluation of patient with chest pain and a low probability of CAD

3. Resting ECG: The results were entirely normal.

4. Exercise hemodynamics/symptoms: Heart rate increased from 75 to 165 beats/min, and SBP rose from 130 to 210 mm Hg. At a Borg scale of 16, the patient reached 11 METs, which is 124% of expected for his age. Angina did not occur, and the test was terminated due to ST-segment changes.

5. Exercise ECG: Approximately 2 to 3 mm of horizontal and even downsloping ST-segment depression developed during exercise and persisted into recovery.

6. Interpretation: Markedly abnormal exercise test exhibited more than 2 mm of horizontal or downsloping ST-segment depression in exercise and recovery.

7. Recommendations/follow-up: The patient underwent thallium scintigraphy, and it was entirely normal. (NOTE: Thallium scintigraphy is often the first line of secondary evaluation in such individuals, although exercise echocardiography could be used.)

8. Comments: It is remarkable that such a dramatically abnormal test can, in fact, be a false-positive response. However, he did have a very good exercise capacity and was asymptomatic. In my experience, in most instances, false-positive results do not have a disease process but can be considered normal variants.

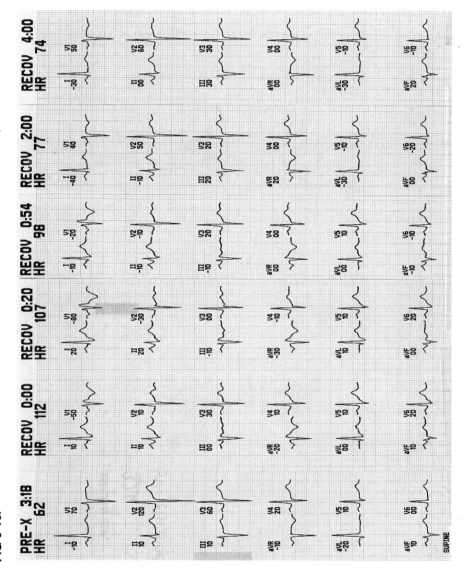

FIG 9-16.

PATIENT MR4924 (Fig 9-16):   EXERCISE-INDUCED RIGHT BUNDLE BRANCH BLOCK (RBBB)

1. History and physical examination/medications/procedures: This patient is a 57-year-old man not taking any cardiac medications who was referred for evaluation of atypical angina. He is a 5-pack-year current cigarette smoker and has elevated cholesterol levels. He has had no prior cardiac events or procedures.

2. Symptoms/reason for test: Atypical angina (50% pretest probability of CAD)

3. Resting ECG: Results were normal.

4. Exercise hemodynamics/symptoms: The heart rate increased from 62 to 112 beats/min, and his SBP rose from 160 to 250 mm Hg. At a Borg scale of 17, the patient reached 7 METs, which was 75% of expected for his age. He did not develop chest pain during the test.

5. Exercise ECG: There were no ST-segment changes during exercise, but at the start of the recovery period, he developed an RBBB pattern without ST-segment depression. It cleared by 2 minutes of recovery.

6. Interpretation: This is not a rate-dependent block, since it occurred in recovery when the heart rate was decreasing.

7. Recommendations/follow-up: This RBBB pattern was not provoked by ischemia, as evidenced by the absence of ST-segment depression or angina.

8. Comments: Rate-dependent LBBBs or RBBBs usually occur during exercise and not at slower heart rates in recovery, as in this case. Perhaps a postexercise rise in pulmonary artery pressure can account for this phenomenon.

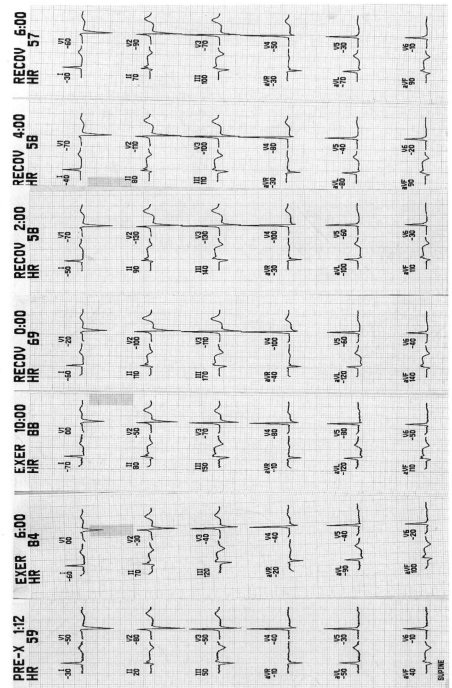

FIG 9-17.

PATIENT C4915 (Fig 9-17): AFTER THROMBOLYSIS FOR MI WITH ST-SEGMENT ELEVATION OVER INFERIOR Q WAVES

1. History and physical examination/medications/procedures: This patient is a 60-year-old man who was admitted to the hospital with an MI. His CPK rose to 1000, and he was given thrombolysis and started on beta-blockers.

2. Symptoms/reason for test: Predischarge assessment after uncomplicated MI treated with thrombolysis. He was asymptomatic and taking beta-blockers at the time of his submaximal test, 6 days after his infarct.

3. Resting ECG: Inferior Q waves with T-wave inversion and ST-segment elevation consistent with an aneurysm and ST-segment depression in the anterior precordial leads were present.

4. Exercise hemodynamics/symptoms: Heart rate increased from 59 to 88 beats/min, and SBP rose from 90 to 110 mm Hg. At a Borg score of 13, he reached 6 METs, which was 70% of normal for his age. He had no angina during the test.

5. Exercise ECG: During exercise, there was further ST-segment elevation in the inferior leads as well as 1 mm of additional ST-segment depression in the anterior precordial leads.

6. Interpretation: ST-segment elevation over pathological Q waves is a normal finding after MI and is produced by wall motion abnormality secondary to damaged myocardium.

7. Recommendations/follow-up: He did well and was successfully rehabilitated after his uncomplicated MI. He is back to work full-time and without symptoms. However, complaints of fatigue prompted discontinuation of the beta-blockers and subsequent alleviation of this side effect.

8. Comments: His risk of another cardiac event was so low that beta-blockers were judged to offer too little added benefit in view of the unpleasant side effects. Predischarge tests are usually performed using a submaximal target such as a Borg score of 15.

FIG 9-18.

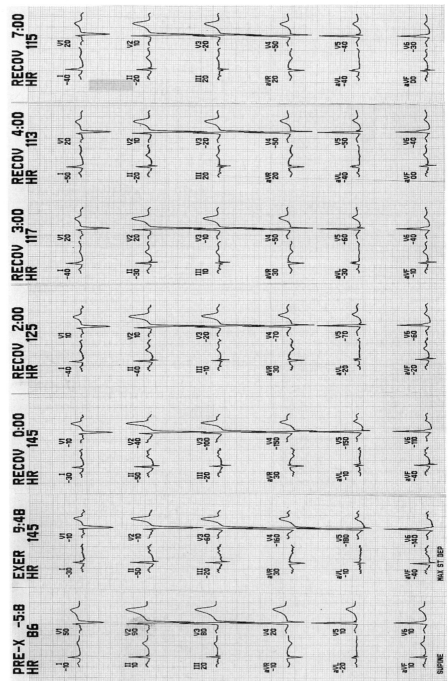

PATIENT SU2927 (Fig 9-18): ST "COVING"

1. History and physical examination/medications/procedures: This patient is a 52-year-old white man taking nitrates. He is a 40-pack-year current cigarette smoker and has an elevated cholesterol level. He had bypass surgery 3 years before this evaluation and now is having chest pain of uncertain origin.

2. Symptoms/reason for test: Follow-up after coronary bypass with recurrence of chest pain

3. Resting ECG: Results were normal.

4. Exercise hemodynamics/symptoms: Heart rate increased from 86 to 146 beats/min, and SBP rose from 120 to 184 mm Hg. At a Borg scale of 19, the patient reached 5 METs, which was 50% of expected for his age. Typical angina occurred during exercise and recovery.

5. Exercise ECG: Normal ST-segment levels occurred at baseline and early exercise; ST "coving" depression developed at the onset of recovery, particularly in lead V_5. Interestingly, the magnitude of this ST-segment depression is not apparent because atrial repolarization has distorted the PR interval, thus obscuring the isoelectric line.

6. Interpretation: The results were abnormal by ST-level criteria, but the ST coving pattern confounds calculation of the ST slope.

7. Recommendations/follow-up: Thallium scintigram exhibited a septal defect that reperfused.

8. Comments: Coving occurs rarely and is of uncertain significance; it has received little attention in the literature. The ST coving seen in this patient appears to be associated with ischemia (abnormal thallium test results and angina). However, early reports of this pattern may have been misleading, since the ST coving resulted from the poor frequency response of the older recorders. Also, it is unusual to see atrial repolarization affect the lateral leads, as in this test.

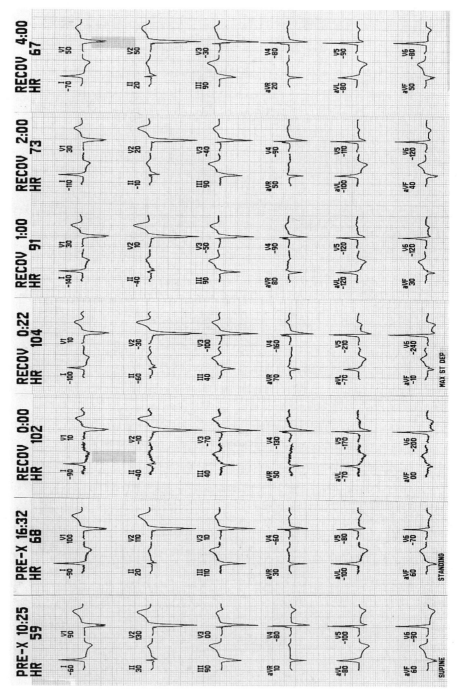

FIG 9-19.

PATIENT C8256 (Fig 9-19): PREOPERATIVE EVALUATION WITH ABNORMAL RESTING ECG

1. History and physical examination/medications/procedures: This patient is a 72-year-old white man with a prior MI and CABS. He was referred for clearance for elective knee arthroplasty. His most recent MI was in 4-20-92, and his bypass was 10 years before this evaluation. Currently, he has typical angina and is being treated with calcium antagonists, nitrates, and antihypertensives.

2. Symptoms/reason for test: Evaluation of ischemia before elective surgery.

3. Resting ECG: His resting ECG is consistent with inferior and anterior Q-wave MIs and also shows T-wave inversion and ST-segment depression in the lateral and high lateral leads (V_4 through V_6, I, and aV_L). His anteroseptal, Q-wave, ST-segment elevation is consistent with LV aneurysm.

4. Exercise hemodynamics/symptoms: His heart rate increased from 59 to 104 beats/min, and his SBP rose from 120 to 164 mm Hg. His exercise capacity was 2 METs, or a third of what was expected for his age. He did not have angina pectoris, but the test was terminated due to claudication.

5. Exercise ECG: At maximal exercise there was 1 mm of additional ST-segment depression in lead V_6, which normalized by the first minute of recovery.

6. Interpretation: There was no evidence of serious ischemia at a low workload and low double product. Double product equals SBP times heart rate and is proportional to myocardial oxygen demand.

7. Recommendations/follow-up: Because he did not have 2 mm of additional ST-segment depression persisting into recovery, the judgment was that he did not have significant myocardium in jeopardy. He was cleared for surgery, which proceeded without complications.

8. Comments: A nonexercise stress test may have been more effective in producing ECG signs of ischemia in this patient. However, persantine-thallium testing should not routinely replace exercise testing except in preoperative patients who fulfill the screening criteria (i.e, patients with chest pain or CHF symptoms or signs but who cannot exercise). Most perioperative events occur in the 72 hours after surgery and are difficult to predict.

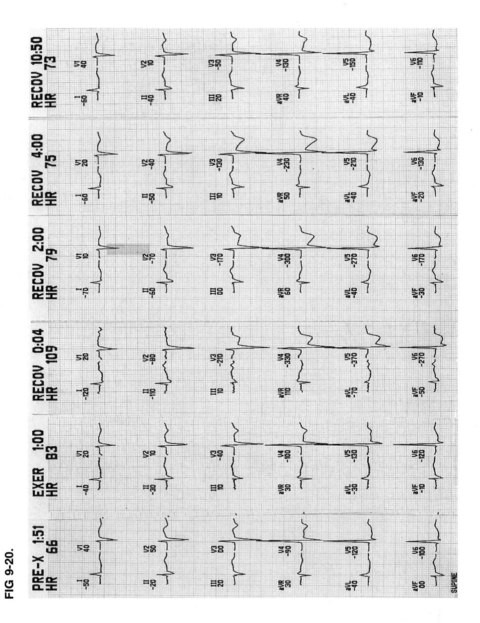

FIG 9-20.

PATIENT SA7094 (Fig 9-20): EXERTIONAL HYPOTENSION DUE TO ISCHEMIA; RESTING ST-SEGMENT DEPRESSION POSSIBLY DUE TO DIGOXIN

1. History and physical examination/medications/procedures: This patient is a 70-year-old white man who underwent bypass surgery 16 years before this evaluation. He is currently taking digoxin for intermittent atrial fibrillation as well as a beta-blocker.

2. Symptoms/reason for test: Onset of atypical angina 16 years after bypass surgery had successfully relieved his typical angina

3. Resting ECG: There was left-axis deviation, anterior T-wave inversion, and 1 mm lateral ST-segment depression.

4. Exercise hemodynamics/symptoms: Heart rate increased from 66 to 109 beats/min, and SBP dropped from 155 to 145 mm Hg. The patient reported a Borg score of 13 on reaching 4 METs, which was 60% of his age-predicted exercise capacity. No angina occurred during the test.

5. Exercise ECG: As much as 2 mm of additional downsloping ST-segment depression occurred in the lateral precordial leads; it persisted more than 10 minutes into recovery.

6. Interpretation: This abnormal exercise response is consistent with ischemia, particularly because his ST-segment depression was downsloping, persisted more than 5 minutes into recovery, and was accompanied by exertional hypotension.

7. Recommendations/follow-up: Thallium scintigraphy later revealed a septal reperfusion defect. Subsequent catheterization showed occlusion of his left anterior descending graft, prompting referral for a bypass procedure, this time with an internal mammary artery. Revascularization reversed his exertional hypotension.

8. Comments: Some guidelines have recommended that such patients with resting ST-segment depression or those on digoxin should proceed directly to a non-ECG exercise study. However, we have found that if the changes are more than an additional 2 mm persisting into recovery, the predictive accuracy for severe CAD is still very good. That is, there appears to be no decrease in sensitivity for the prediction of coronary disease. However, concerns have been raised regarding a decline in specificity, resulting in more false-positive results. Therefore had this test been negative, the scintigram could have been avoided. It appears that routine exercise ECG testing can still be an effective and economical first line of evaluation for such patients.

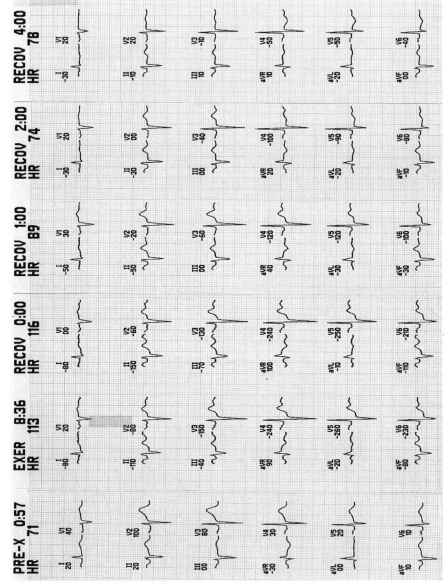

FIG 9-21.

PATIENT G7503 (Fig 9-21): RCA DISEASE ONLY

1. History and physical examination/medications/procedures: The patient is a 70-year-old white man referred for evaluation of typical angina.

2. Symptoms/reason for test: Evaluation of disease severity and consideration for further treatment of typical angina.

3. Resting ECG: There was left axis deviation, which is the most common normal variant.

4. Exercise hemodynamics/symptoms: Heart rate increased from 74 to 116 beats/min, and SBP rose from 140 to 200 mm Hg. He reached 4 METs, which was 60% of predicted for his age. Typical angina occurred during exercise and recovery, although ST-segment depression was the reason for stopping.

5. Exercise ECG: At maximal exercise there was approximately 2 mm of mildly upsloping ST-segment depression in the lateral precordial leads (V_4 through V_6). By 4 minutes of recovery, these leads showed about 0.5 mm of junctional depression downsloping into inverted T waves.

6. Interpretation: Marked junctional ST-segment depression during exercise diminishes rapidly in recovery but becomes downsloping with concomitant T-wave inversion.

7. Recommendations/follow-up: Cardiac catheterization was recommended because his symptoms were unstable. There was 100% occlusion of his RCA with collateral filling. He was treated medically.

8. Comments: These test results suggested more serious disease. Nonetheless, a block in a large RCA can produce such signs of ischemia. Although this patient's junctional depression normalized rapidly in recovery, the development of downsloping ST segments and T-wave inversion is consistent with ischemia. Rapid normalization usually indicates less severe disease. Isolated RCA disease is usually the most difficult lesion to detect because of collateralization.

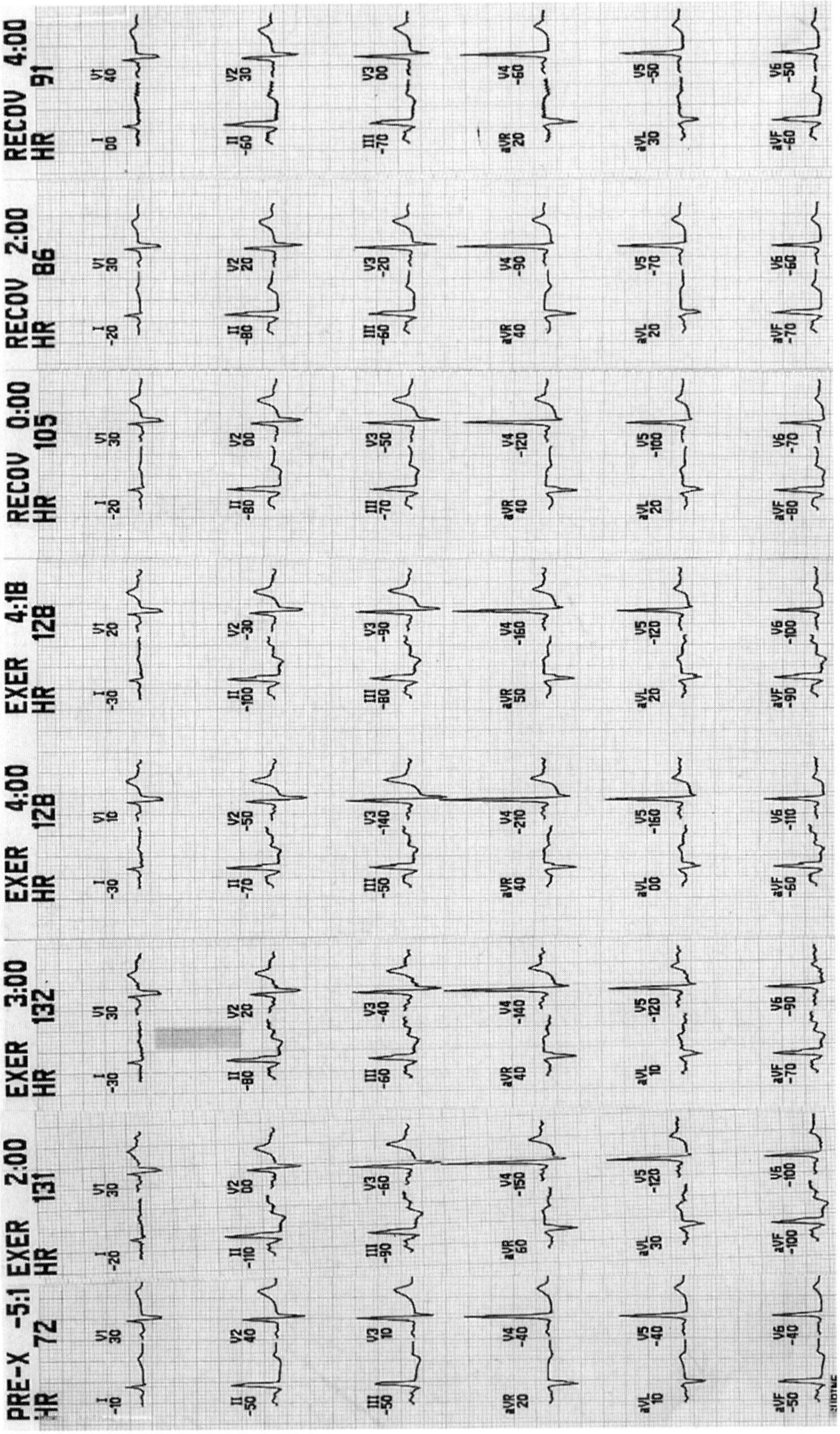
PRE-X -5:1
HR 72
EXER 2:00
HR 131
EXER 3:00
HR 132
EXER 4:00
HR 128
EXER 4:18
HR 128
RECOV 0:00
HR 105
RECOV 2:00
HR 86
RECOV 4:00
HR 91

FIG 9-22.

PATIENT M7563 (Fig 9-22): PROGNOSTIC TESTING

1. History and physical examination/medications/procedures: This patient is a 70-year-old white man, tested for evaluation of occasional typical chest pain since his MI in 1984. He has a history of CHF and is on nitrates and a calcium antagonist.

2. Symptoms/reason for test: Evaluation of the severity of CAD

3. Resting ECG: There is minor ST-segment depression in the inferior and lateral leads, but otherwise the results are normal.

4. Exercise hemodynamics/symptoms: Heart rate increased from 72 to 131 beats/min, and SBP from 120 to 140 mm Hg. At a Borg scale of 20, he reached 3 METs, which was 40% of expected for his age. Typical angina occurred during exercise and recovery.

5. Exercise ECG: During exercise, he had nearly 1 mm of additional horizontal ST-segment depression in the lateral leads and 0.5 mm in the inferior leads. This cleared by 2 minutes of recovery and returned to baseline.

6. Interpretation: Despite a mildly abnormal ST-segment response, his VA prognostic score was 5, which is associated with a projected annual mortality of 10%.

7. Recommendations/follow-up: This patient was offered cardiac catheterization to evaluate his suitability for CABS because his exercise capacity was limited and his projected mortality high.

8. Comments: Despite only minor ST-segment depression, a patient may still be assigned a poor prognostic score when his test is accompanied by other abnormal exercise responses and there is a history of CHF.

FIG 9-23.

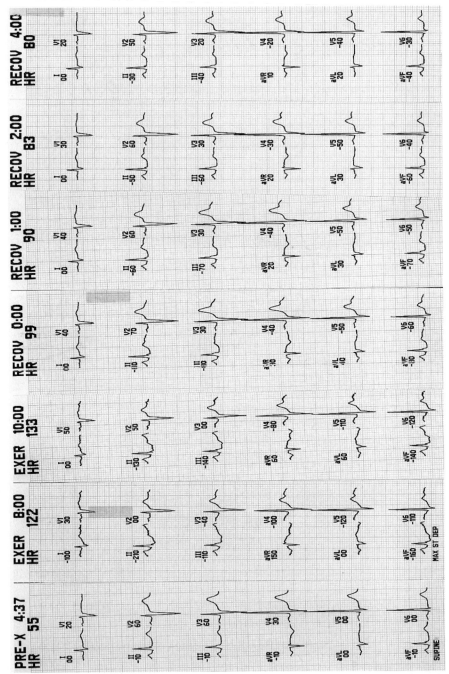

PATIENT C7789 (Fig 9-23): AFTER PTCA TESTING WITH EXERCISE-INDUCED ST-SEGMENT DEPRESSION IN THE INFERIOR LEAD ONLY

1. History and physical examination/medications/procedures/diagnosis: This patient is a 53-year-old white man who reported for evaluation 1 month after a PTCA. He was on nitrates and calcium antagonists.

2. Symptoms/reason for test: Recurrence of chest pain after successful relief of angina by PTCA

3. Resting ECG: Results were normal.

4. Exercise hemodynamics/symptoms: His heart rate increased from 55 to 133 beats/min, and SBP rose from 155 to 190 mm Hg. At a Borg score of 18, he reached 10 METs, which was normal for his age. No angina occurred during testing.

5. Exercise ECG: Approximately 1 mm of horizontal ST-segment depression developed in the inferior limb leads (II, III, and aV_F) during exercise and cleared rapidly by 1 minute of recovery. The lateral precordial leads also developed 1 mm of junctional ST-segment depression but remained upsloping throughout the test.

6. Interpretation: Isolated abnormal depression in the inferior leads.

7. Recommendations/follow-up: He had no further chest pain and was able to work full-time without medications. A thallium scintigram was negative.

8. Comments: Anxious patients reporting chest pain can be reassured by a negative exercise test. However, restenosis after PTCA cannot be predicted by exercise ECG parameters, although it can be recognized by recurrence of chest pain during the test. ST-segment changes isolated to the inferior leads are likely to be false positives, particularly if these changes occur only during exercise. This test showed only inferior lead ST-segment depression associated with a normal resting ECG and therefore was likely to be a false positive. Alternatively, isolated inferior changes are often indicative of ischemia when accompanied by a lateral or anterior infarction pattern (Q waves) in the resting ECG.

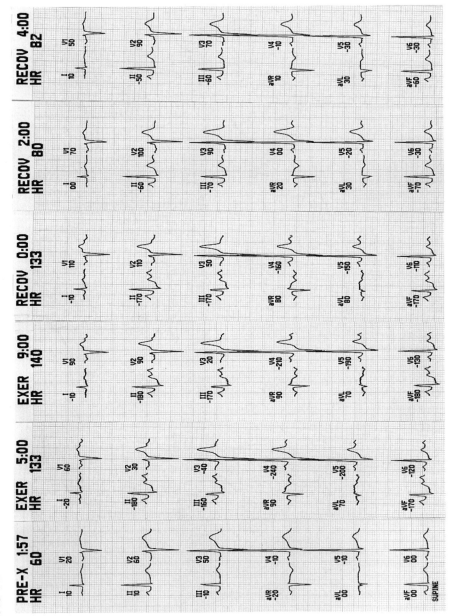

FIG 9-24.

PATIENT PF4340 (Fig 9-24): UPSLOPING ST-SEGMENT DEPRESSION

1. History and physical examination/medications/procedures: This patient is a 61-year-old white male outpatient referred for evaluation of atypical angina. He underwent a cardiac catheterization 3 years before this evaluation, has no other risk factors, and is not smoking. He is currently taking a calcium antagonist.

2. Symptoms/reason for test: Evaluation of atypical angina

3. Resting ECG: Results were normal.

4. Exercise hemodynamics/symptoms: Heart rate increased from 60 to 140 beats/min, and SBP rose from 120 to 210 mm Hg. At a Borg scale of 20, he reached 11 METs, which was 125% of expected for his age (25% above average).

5. Exercise ECG: Upsloping ST-segment depression during exercise returned to normal by 2 minutes of recovery. The mild ST-segment elevation in a V_L during exercise appears to be reciprocal to the inferior ST-segment depression in leads II, III, and aV_F. No angina occurred during the test.

6. Interpretation: According to some criteria that disregard ST slope (e.g., ST_{60} or ST integral), this test would be considered abnormal. The inclusion of upsloping ST-segment depression as a criterion for an abnormal result decreases test specificity but increases sensitivity. This patient's response is normal or, at worse, borderline.

7. Recommendations/follow-up: He did well; no further evaluation was necessary. In retrospect, he was a nervous individual whose pain pattern (sharp and stabbing) indicated a low probability for serious CAD.

8. Comments: His cardiac catheterization in 1989 was normal; progression to significant CAD is unlikely without serious risk factors.

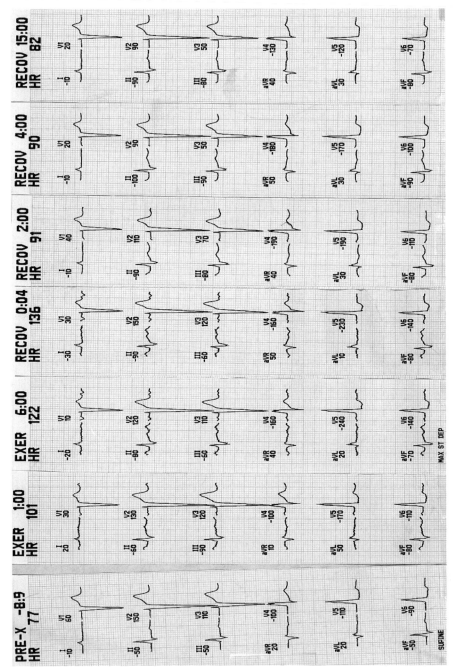

FIG 9-25.

PATIENT BR8594 (Fig 9-25): RESTING ST-SEGMENT DEPRESSION AND DIGOXIN ADMINISTRATION AFTER MI

1. History and physical examination/medications/procedures: This patient is a 62-year-old white male outpatient referred for evaluation of atypical angina. He had an MI 3 years before and is taking digoxin, nitrates, and an antihypertensive. His cholesterol is elevated, and he is a 60-pack-year cigarette smoker.

2. Symptoms/reason for test: Evaluation of patient with prior MI and recent history of atypical angina for signs of ischemia and disease severity

3. Resting ECG: One mm of horizontal ST-segment depression in the lateral leads but no diagnostic Q waves. However, the narrow R waves in leads V_1, V_2, and V_3 suggested an old anteroseptal, Q-wave infarct which had "grown back" small R waves.

4. Exercise hemodynamics/symptoms: His heart rate increased from 77 to 136 beats/min, and his SBP rose from 125 to 160 mm Hg. At a Borg scale of 19, he reached 6 METs, which was 70% of his age-predicted exercise capacity. No angina occurred during testing.

5. Exercise ECG: Patient demonstrated an additional 1.5 mm of ST-segment depression in V_5, which was downsloping and persisted for a short time into recovery.

6. Interpretation: His treadmill score of 1 is associated with an annual cardiovascular mortality of approximately 6%. Persistent and downsloping ST-segment depression is consistent with multivessel disease even in the presence of baseline ST-segment depression and digoxin administration.

7. Recommendations/follow-up: Cardiac catheterization revealed triple-vessel disease.

8. Comments: Resting ST-segment depression does not invalidate the use of the standard exercise ECG. It is still the most cost-effective first step in the evaluation of such patients.

FIG 9-26.

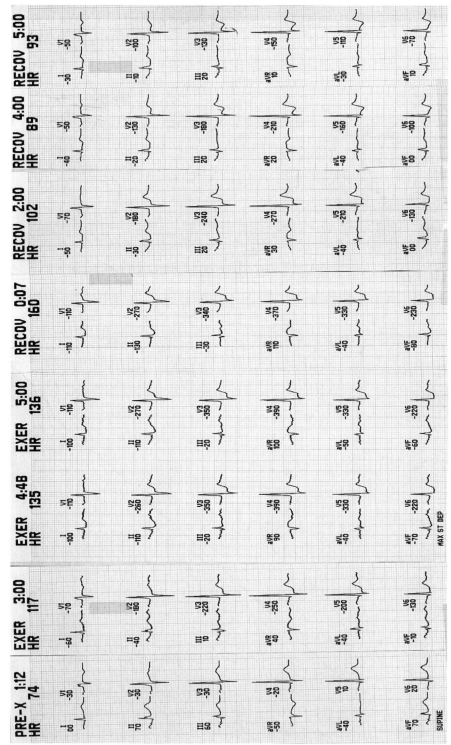

PATIENT SG6458 (Fig 9-26): MARKEDLY POSITIVE ST-SEGMENT RESPONSE AFTER MI HAS BEEN RULED OUT

1. History and physical examination/medications/procedures: This patient is a 68-year-old white male inpatient referred for evaluation after being ruled out for an MI. He is taking nitrates and is a heavy smoker. He has a family history of CAD, although he himself has had no events

2. Symptoms/reason for test: Evaluation of atypical angina

3. Resting ECG: Normal; minor ST-segment elevation is present in the inferior limb leads (II, III, and aV_F).

4. Exercise hemodynamics/symptoms: Heart rate increased from 82 to 136 beats/min, and SBP increased from 130 to 160 mm Hg. At a Borg score of 15, he reached 4 METs, which was 50% of expected for his age. Typical angina occurred during exercise and recovery.

5. Exercise ECG: As much as 2 to 3 mm of horizontal ST-segment depression developed during exercise in precordial leads V_2 to V_6. These ST segments became downsloping in recovery, with this condition persisting beyond 5 minutes after exercise.

6. Interpretation: This profound ST-segment depression was consistent with multivessel disease.

7. Recommendations/follow-up: His VA prognostic score was associated with an elevated annual cardiovascular mortality rate of 6%. For this reason, he was urged to undergo cardiac catheterization and was found to have triple-vessel disease with good LV function.

8. Comments: This patient's noninvasive VA prognostic score led to CABS, since his Parsonett-estimated surgical mortality was very low. He did well with surgery and has increased his exercise capacity.

FIG 9-27.

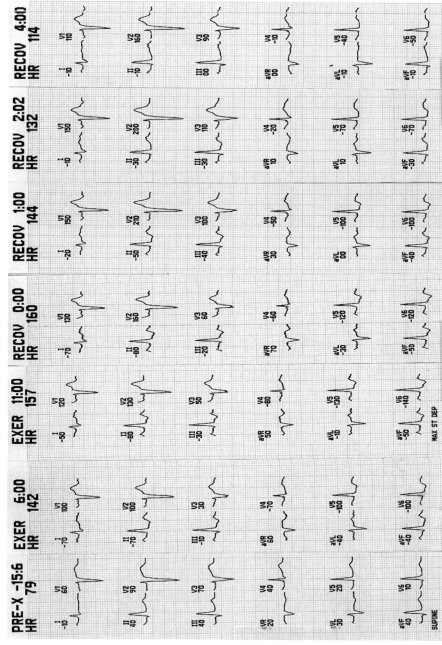

PATIENT HR7784 (Fig 9-27): AFTER CABS; DOWNSLOPING ST-SEGMENT DEPRESSION AT A HIGH HEART RATE

1. History and physical examination/medications/procedures: This patient is a 66-year-old outpatient referred for evaluation of recent onset of angina after an asymptomatic recovery from a bypass operation 2 years before this test. He is currently on a calcium antagonist and has never smoked.

2. Symptoms/reason for test: Return of chest pain after a bypass

3. Resting ECG: There were small inferior Q waves, but otherwise the test was normal.

4. Exercise hemodynamics/symptoms: His heart rate increased from 90 to 158 beats/min, and his SBP rose from 165 to 190 mm Hg, resulting in a double product of 30,000. At a near maximal effort (Borg scale of 19), he reached 10 METs, which was 125% of what is expected for his age. No angina occurred during testing.

5. Exercise ECG: Patient developed downsloping ST-segment depression in leads V_5 and V_6 during exercise, which persisted for about 1 minute into recovery and then quickly normalized.

6. Interpretation: Abnormal downsloping ST-segment depression occurring at a high double product and workload is consistent with mild ischemia.

7. Recommendations/follow-up: This patient's angina was controlled with medications.

8. Comments: Although ST-segment depression after bypass has limited prognostic value, exercise capacity remains important prognostically. Regardless of whether abnormal exercise-induced ST-segment depression occurred, every bypass patient tested in our laboratory who has exceeded 10 METs has survived beyond 3 years. Risk stratification of these patients is complicated by a variety of factors that could affect prognosis (e.g., time since bypass, underlying disease, and risk factor changes.) Downsloping ST-segment depression usually is ominous but does not usually occur at high heart rates.

FIG 9-28.

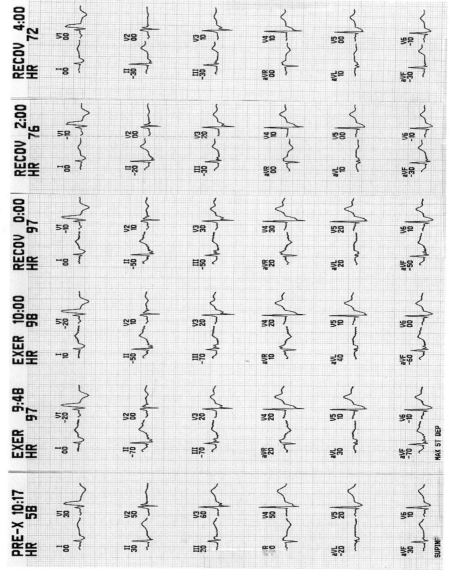

PATIENT WH4391 (Fig 9-28): CHRONIC OBSTRUCTIVE PULMONARY DISEASE (COPD), RIGHT BUNDLE BRANCH BLOCK (RBBB), AND CHEST PAIN

1. History and physical examination/medications/procedures: This patient is a 73-year-old white man referred for evaluation of chest pain. He has COPD and a 90-pack-year habit of cigarette smoking but currently abstains. He has an elevated cholesterol level and is taking a calcium antagonist and an antihypertensive. He has no history of prior MIs, bypass surgery, or heart catheterizations.

2. Symptoms/reason for test: Atypical angina thought to be secondary to pulmonary hypertension

3. Resting ECG: Results reveal RBBB.

4. Exercise hemodynamics/symptoms: His heart rate increased from 64 to 98 beats/min, and SBP from 118 to 155 mm Hg. At maximal exertion (Borg scale of 20), the patient only achieved 3 METs, which was less than half of expected for his age. Typical angina occurred during exercise and recovery and was the reason for stopping the test, which produced a Duke Treadmill Angina Score of 2.

5. Exercise ECG: There was no abnormal ST-segment depression in V_5 or in the anterior precordial leads.

6. Interpretation: Patient had exercise-induced chest pain, which was most likely a consequence of his pulmonary disease in which dilation of the pulmonary artery was caused by pulmonary hypertension.

7. Recommendations/follow-up: A thallium scintigram was negative.

8. Comments: During exertion, patients with pulmonary disease frequently experience chest pains that simulate angina. This is thought to be due to pulmonary artery dilation in response to pulmonary hypertension. Thallium scintigraphy is often helpful for ruling out ischemia because the baseline ECG in pulmonary patients is often distorted. With RBBB, ST-segment depression frequently occurs in the anterior leads as a normal finding, and lateral ST-segment depression is associated with ischemia.

FIG 9-29.

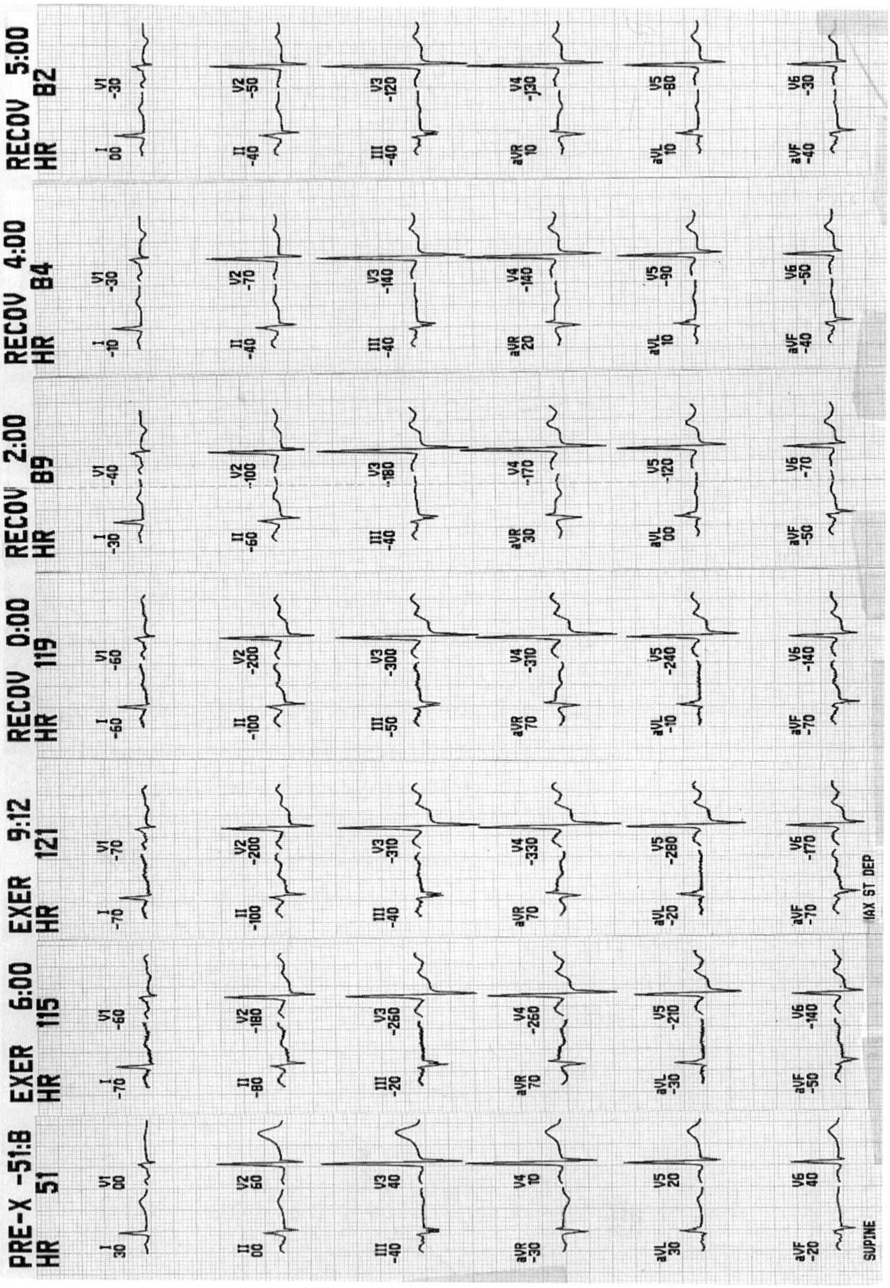

PATIENT PL8707 (Fig 9-29): SILENT ISCHEMIA DURING THE TREADMILL TEST AND PROMINENT ANTERIOR FORCES

1. History and physical examination/medications/procedures: This patient is a 78-year-old white man referred for evaluation of typical angina. He was taking a beta-blocker.

2. Symptoms/reason for test: Evaluation of typical angina

3. Resting ECG: Prominent anterior forces with an R greater than S in V_2 (differential, including RVH, RBBB, WPW type A, posterior MI, normal variant). This appears to be a normal variant, though it could be caused by RVH or a posterior infarct.

4. Exercise hemodynamics/symptoms: His heart rate increased from 51 to 110 beats/min, and SBP rose from 150 to 200 mm Hg; his double product was only 22. This patient reached 7 METs, which was normal for his age. Angina did not occur during testing, and the test was terminated due to ST-segment depression.

5. Exercise ECG: During exercise, he had significant junctional depression across the anterior precordium, including V_2. These ST segments changed from mildly upsloping to horizontal by maximum exercise and persisted as downsloping ST-segment depression through 5 minutes of recovery.

6. Interpretation: ST-segment depression of more than 2 mm and downsloping in multiple leads is consistent with severe CAD.

7. Recommendations/follow-up: Patient was found to have triple-vessel CAD but good ventricular function. His predicted annual mortality rate was only 2%, and he was satisfied with his exercise capacity. Medical management was recommended, and he has done well.

8. Comments: ST-segment depression usually occurs in the lead with the greatest R wave (i.e., along the left ventricle's major vector of activation and repolarization). For example, when there are prominent anterior forces, the major ST-segment depression occurs anteriorly (V_2 and V_3). Many patients being evaluated for angina will not have their pain during the exercise test. True silent ischemia is rare. Beta-blockers can take away anginal pain and sometimes exacerbate exercise-induced ST-segment depression.

FIG 9-30.

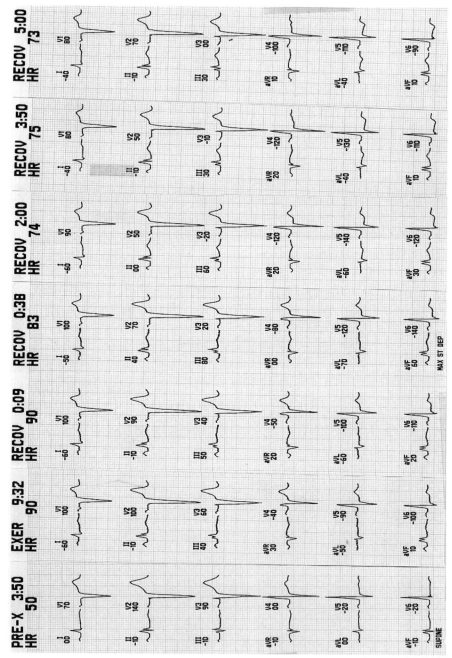

PATIENT RB20068 (Fig 9-30): RESTING ST-SEGMENT DEPRESSION, DIGOXIN, AFTER MI WITH ANTERIOR Q-WAVES, AND RECOVERY-ONLY DEPRESSION

1. History and physical examination/medications/procedures: This patient is a 50-year-old male outpatient referred for evaluation of ischemia. He is taking digoxin, beta-blockers, and an antihypertensive. He is a 35-pack-year, current cigarette smoker. He has a family history of coronary heart disease, and his cholesterol level is elevated. He had a cardiac catheterization and PTCA 4 years before this evaluation and an MI several months before.

2. Symptoms/reason for test: Evaluation after a recent MI

3. Resting ECG: ST-segment elevation over anterior Q waves was accompanied by minor ST-segment depression in the lateral precordial leads.

4. Exercise hemodynamics/symptoms: Heart rate increased from 59 to 90 beats/min, and his SBP rose from 150 to 170 mm Hg, resulting in a double product of only 15,000. With a maximal effort (Borg scale of 20), he reached 6 METs, which was about 60% of expected for his age. No angina occurred during testing.

5. Exercise ECG: At maximal exercise, lead V_6 exhibited 1 mm of horizontal ST-segment depression, which became markedly abnormal by 2 minutes of recovery with 1.5 mm of downsloping ST-segment depression. Leads V_4 and V_6 developed similar, recovery-only ST-segment depression. There was no further elevation over the anterior Q waves.

6. Interpretation: Recovery-only ST-segment changes are still significant predictors of CAD.

7. Recommendations/follow-up: Because of his low exercise capacity and a predicted annual mortality rate of 10%, it was recommended that he undergo a cardiac catheterization, which revealed severe triple-vessel disease and an ejection fraction of about 40%.

8. Comments: Although his abnormal ST-segment depression was isolated to the recovery period, this response was still associated with severe disease. Furthermore, his history of prior MI increased his risk of death. This test also showed an anterior Q-wave infarct with no further elevation over the Q waves. ST-segment elevation over Q waves is a common and normal finding associated with a wall motion abnormality.

FIG 9-31.

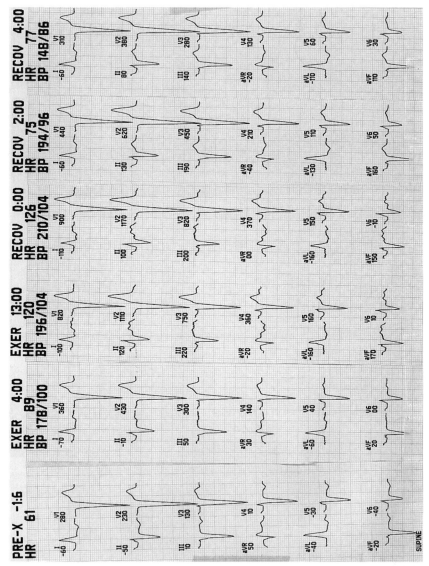

PATIENT AP0100 (Fig 9-31): ST-SEGMENT ELEVATION OVER ANTERIOR Q WAVES

1. History and physical examination/medications/procedures: This patient is a 57-year-old white male outpatient referred for testing for typical angina pectoris. He had an MI several years before, which was followed by bypass surgery. Medications include beta-blockers and a calcium antagonist. He has a family history of CAD and an elevated cholesterol level. He is not a smoker.

2. Symptoms/reason for test: Typical angina

3. Resting ECG: Results showed intraventricular conduction defect; anterior Q waves; very small R waves in V_3, III, and aV_F; and lateral ST-segment depression.

4. Exercise hemodynamics/symptoms: Heart rate went from 73 to 126 beats/min, and at a Borg scale of 17, 8 METs was reached, which is 85% of what is expected for age. No angina occurred during testing.

5. Exercise ECG: ST-segment elevation over the anterior leads, V_3 particularly, with no additional depression in the lateral leads.

6. Interpretation: This finding is consistent with a wall motion abnormality rather than ischemia. The small R waves were associated with the myocardial damage, which was confirmed by the Q waves adjacent in V_1 and V_2.

7. Recommendations/follow-up: Usual management after MI and CABS was not recommended.

8. Comments: If angina had occurred, further workup would have been indicated. The ST-segment elevation may lessen as time progresses. It had been thought that this elevation could pull up lateral ST-segment depression and cause false negatives, but this is probably not the case.

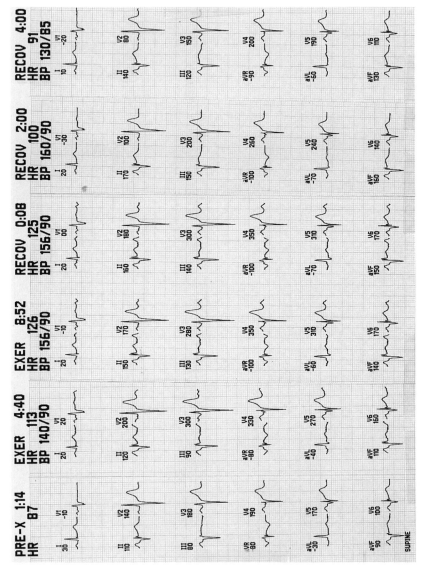

FIG 9-32.

PATIENT HB0134 (Fig 9-32): **ST-SEGMENT ELEVATION OVER INFERIOR AND LATERAL Q WAVES**

1. History and physical examination/medications/procedures: This patient is a 58-year-old male in-patient who was referred for predischarge exercise testing 8 days after an MI. His medications include nitrates and a calcium antagonist. He has a 35-pack-year history of cigarette smoking and is currently smoking. He has been having atypical angina after his infarct.

2. Symptoms/reason for test: Predischarge submaximal exercise test

3. Resting ECG: Inferior and lateral Q waves are diagnostic of an inferior and lateral recent MI. Inferior ST-segment elevation is consistent with an inferior aneurysm.

4. Exercise hemodynamics/symptoms: Heart rate went from 83 to 125 beats/min, and SBP from 110 to 160; the test was stopped at 5 METs, and no chest pain occurred.

5. Exercise ECG: There is ST-segment elevation over the inferior and lateral Q waves.

6. Interpretation: This elevation is due to wall motion abnormality rather than ischemia. When retested 2 months after his infarct, there was less elevation, and the patient has done well.

7. Recommendations/follow-up: Usual follow-up and medical therapy were recommended.

8. Comments: ST-segment elevation frequently occurs after a Q-wave infarct. It may hide ischemia by pulling up depression and adjacent leads. When typical angina occurs during testing, periinfarct ischemia is suggested, regardless of whether there is ST-segment depression.

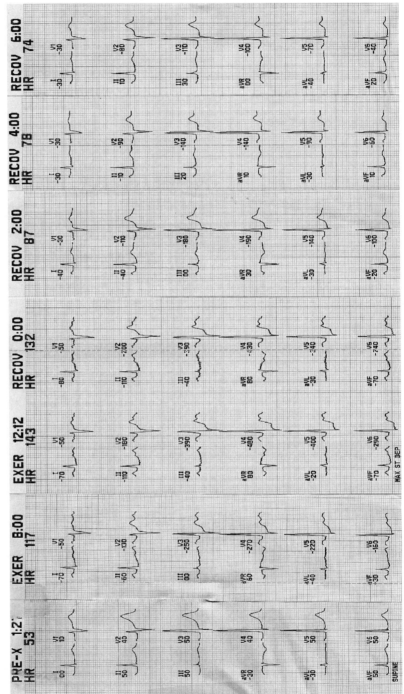

FIG 9-33.

PATIENT GA5197 (Fig 9-33): **MARKEDLY POSITIVE ST-SEGMENT RESPONSE WITH GOOD PROGNOSIS**

1. History and physical examination/medications/procedures: This patient is a 70-year-old white male nonsmoker with an elevated cholesterol level. He takes no cardiac medications, and he underwent a PTCA in July 1990. He has been asymptomatic until the recent onset of atypical chest pain.

2. Symptoms/reason for test: Evaluation of chest pain occurring 3 years after PTCA

3. Resting ECG: Results were entirely normal

4. Exercise hemodynamics/symptoms: Heart rate rose from 53 to 143 beats/min, and SBP increased from 130 to 170 mm Hg. At a Borg scale score of 17, the patient reached 13 METs, which was twice his age-predicted exercise capacity. He was asymptomatic during the test, which was stopped because of ST-segment changes.

5. Exercise ECG: By a heart rate of 120 beats/min, the patient had 2 mm of junctional ST-segment depression in leads V_3 through V_6. By a heart rate of 140, he had developed up to 5 mm of horizontal ST-segment depression in V_4 through V_6. Even lead V_3, which showed upsloping depression at maximal exercise, became downsloping by 4 minutes of recovery and persisted with 1 mm of ST-segment depression until the sixth minute of recovery.

6. Interpretation: This was a markedly abnormal exercise test ECG despite an excellent exercise capacity and probable normal ventricular function.

7. Recommendations/follow-up: This patient has an exercise capacity that is exceptional for his age and a cardiovascular annual mortality rate of less than 2% based on the VA prognostic score. Although the test suggested severe ischemia, his prognosis is excellent.

8. Comments: A beta-blocker and an exercise program would be appropriate management.

FIG 9-34.

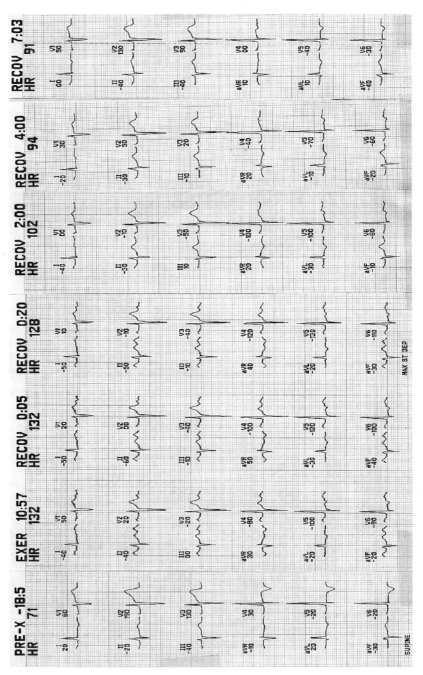

PATIENT WD4558 (Fig 9-34): PSEUDONORMALIZATION VERSUS NORMALIZATION

1. History and physical examination/medications/procedures: This patient is a 51-year-old white man with no prior cardiac events or procedures. He has a 15-pack-year history of smoking, is currently a nonsmoker, and takes no medications. This was a follow-up test.

2. Symptoms/reason for test: Routine follow-up

3. Resting ECG: Abnormal ECG showed T-wave inversion in the lateral precordial leads and "normal" ST elevation in leads V_2 and V_3. He did not meet the voltage criteria for LVH.

4. Exercise hemodynamics/symptoms: Heart rate rose from 71 to 132 beats/min, and his SBP increased from 148 to 195 mm Hg. At a Borg scale score of 20, the patient reached 10 METs, which was his age-predicted exercise capacity. No angina occurred during testing.

5. Exercise ECG: By a heart rate of 132 beats/min, the T waves had normalized in lead V_4 and had become less downsloping in leads V_5 and V_6. There was no significant ST-segment depression with exercise.

6. Interpretation: Normalization of T waves can be a manifestation of ischemia. However, with the absence of angina and a negative thallium scan it is unlikely that this patient has ischemia. He likely had a non–Q-wave infarct and now has no additional ischemia. ST-segment elevation in the precordial leads that depresses to the baseline during exercise is quite normal.

7. Recommendations/follow-up: Patient will be followed. A thallium scintigram was negative.

8. Comments: If there were signs or symptoms of ischemia, this pattern would be called *pseudonormalization* but instead is called *normalization*. In cases of pseudonormalization, patients may have their most normal appearing ST and T waves during periods of ischemia.

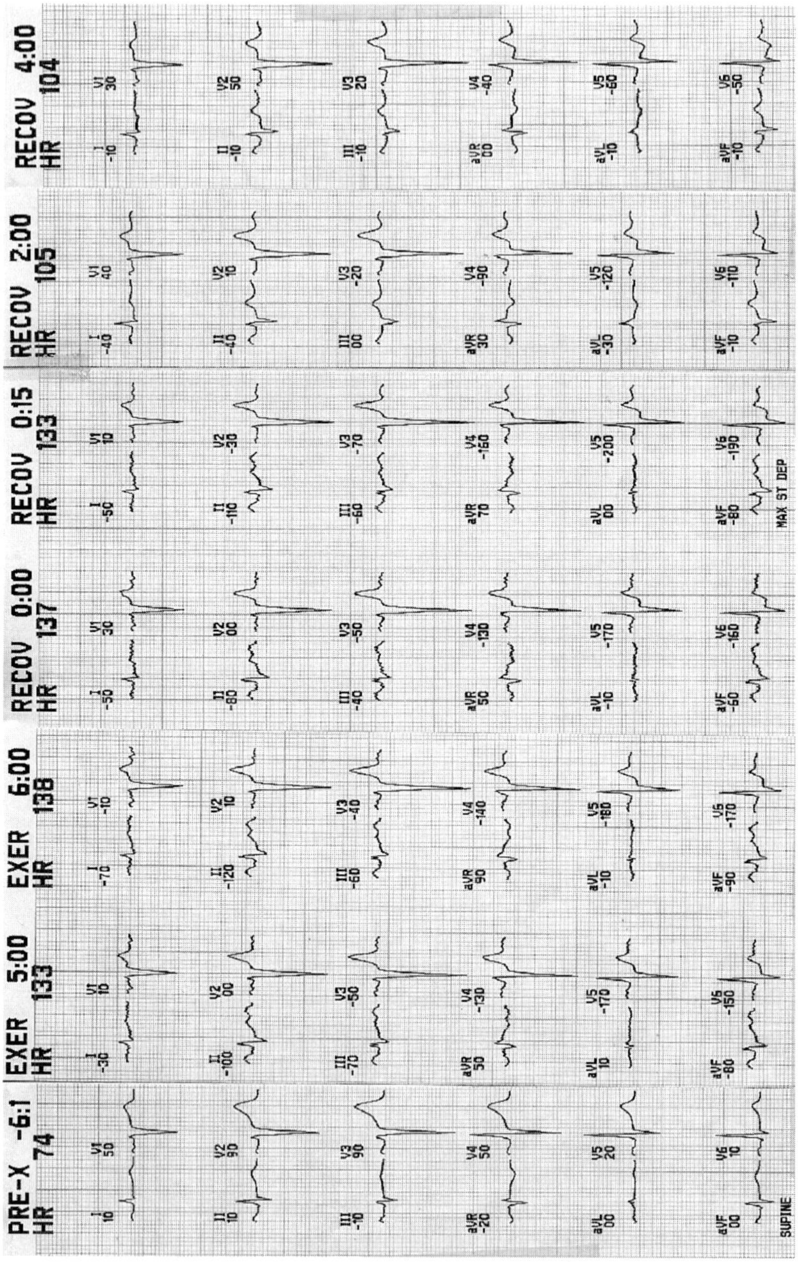

FIG 9-35.

PATIENT SK9773 (Fig 9-35): MARKEDLY ABNORMAL ST-SEGMENT RESPONSE WITHOUT ANGINA (SILENT ISCHEMIA)

1. History and physical examination/medications/procedures: This is a 64-year-old male outpatient with no previous cardiac events or procedures who has an elevated cholesterol level and over 90-pack-years of cigarette smoking, although he is not currently smoking. His medications include a calcium antagonist given for chest pain.

2. Symptoms/reason for test: Evaluation of noncardiac or uncertain chest pain

3. Resting ECG: Results showed poor R progression from leads V_1 to V_3, but otherwise the results were normal.

4. Exercise hemodynamics/symptoms: Heart rate increased from 74 to 138 beats/min, and his SBP rose from 146 to 185 mm Hg. At a Borg scale score of 20, the patient reached 3 METs, which was about 40% of normal for his age. No angina occurred during testing.

5. Exercise ECG: By a heart rate of 134 beats/min there is 1 mm of nearly horizontal ST-segment depression in leads V_4 and V_5. At maximal exercise there is almost 2 mm of horizontal ST-segment depression in only these leads. In immediate recovery, this becomes downsloping and stays downsloping beyond 4 minutes of recovery.

6. Interpretation: This was a markedly abnormal exercise test with downsloping ST-segment depression localized to leads V_4 and V_5 and persisting into recovery. This patient has a limited exercise capacity and signs of severe ischemia.

7. Recommendations/follow-up: The primary concern in this individual is his poor exercise tolerance, so because his projected survival rate is good, the first approach is to try a beta-blocker and an exercise program.

8. Comments: Contrary to early exaggerated concerns regarding silent ischemia, it has become apparent that patients with this abnormality usually have milder CAD than their counterparts with angina.

FIG 9-36.

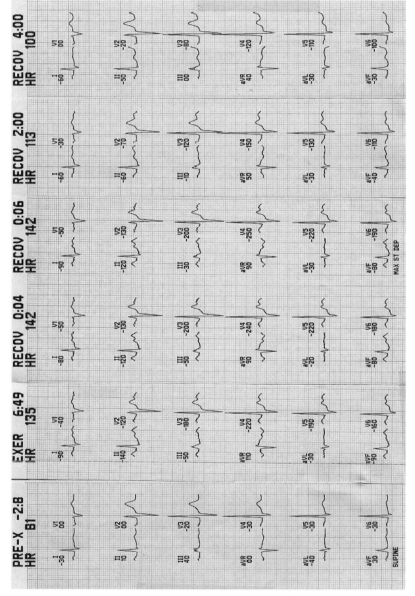

PATIENT CF8793 (Fig 9-36): **ST-SEGMENT DEPRESSION ABNORMAL ONLY IN RECOVERY**

1. History and physical examination/medications/procedures: This patient is a 64-year-old inpatient currently taking antihypertensive medications. He has an elevated cholesterol level, has never smoked, and has had no previous cardiovascular events or procedures. He was referred after being admitted to rule out an MI. Enzyme tests and ECGs were negative.

2. Symptoms/reason for test: Evaluation for one episode of uncertain chest pain before discharge

3. Resting ECG: The results were entirely normal.

4. Exercise hemodynamics/symptoms: His heart rate rose from 81 to 142 beats/min, and his SBP increased from 150 to 220 mm Hg. He reported a Borg scale score of 18 on reaching 6 METs, which is about 75% of what is expected for his age. He developed angina during the test.

5. Exercise ECG: Upsloping ST-segment depression developed in the lateral and inferior leads. Atrial repolarization appeared to contribute to the ST-segment depression in the inferior leads. All ST depression remained upsloping until 4 minutes of recovery, when the lateral precordial leads showed slightly greater than 1 mm of horizontal to downsloping ST-segment depression.

6. Interpretation: This patient is one of the 10% who have abnormal results and who develop their abnormal ST-segment depression only in recovery. This is usually associated with milder CAD but does not ensure a false-positive result.

7. Recommendations/follow-up: Patient visited again in 1 month with chest pain and underwent cardiac catheterization. He was found to have single-vessel CAD involving a large RCA. He did well on medical management.

8. Comments: ST-segment depression in recovery only was once thought to be a false-positive test. To the contrary, most studies have found it to be as predictive of CAD as other patterns. In general, however, depression occurring only at maximal exercise is associated with the mildest disease and lowest probability for predicting disease, whereas depression in exercise and recovery is considered a more serious pattern. Recovery-only ST depression is intermediate in terms of severity of disease and predictive value.

FIG 9-37.

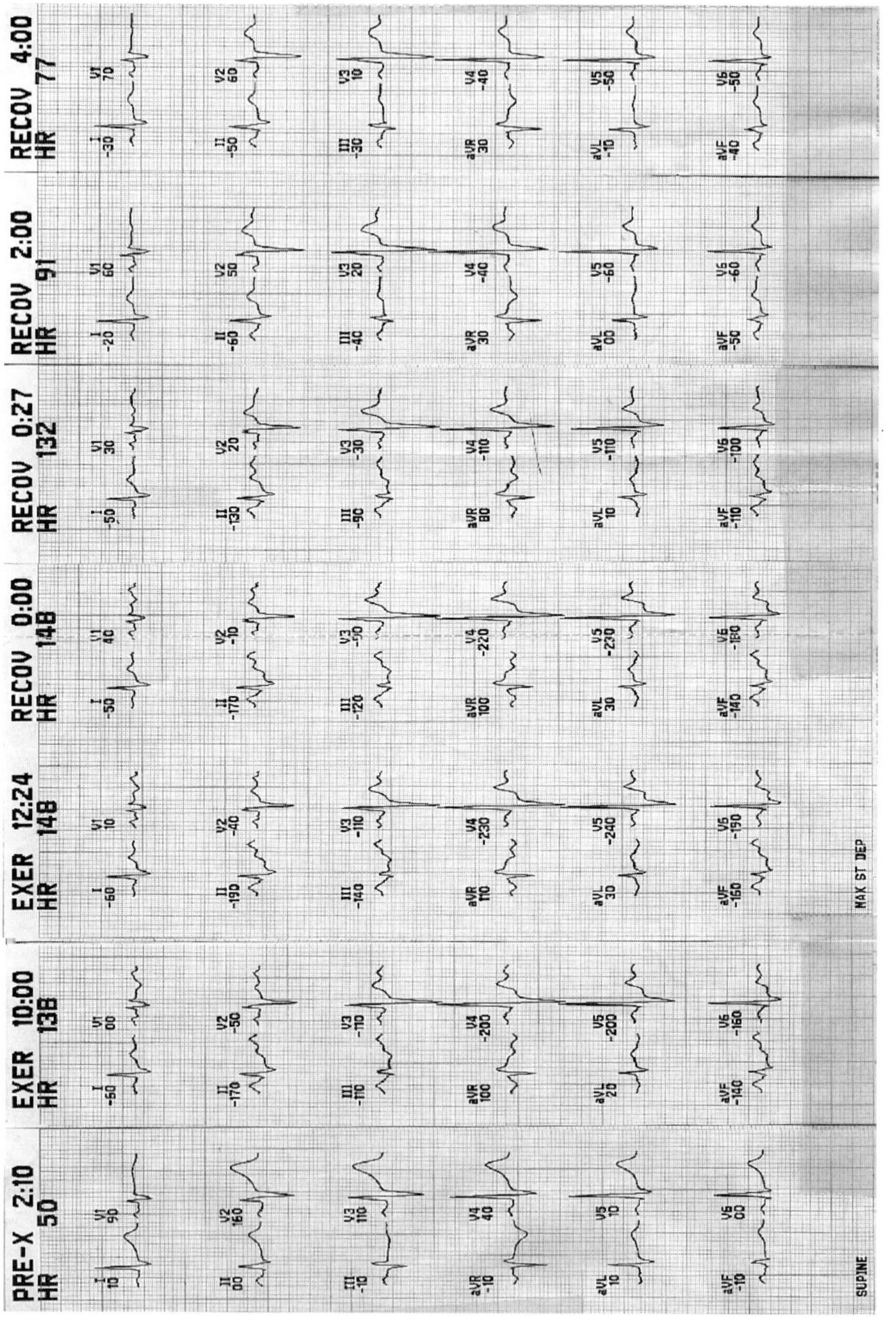

PATIENT DJ4415 (Fig 9-37): EVALUATION AFTER PTCA

1. History and physical examination/medications/procedures: Patient is a 46-year-old male outpatient referred for evaluation of chest pain after a successful PTCA. He had a cardiac catheterization in December 1992 and a PTCA shortly thereafter. He has a 40-pack-year history of cigarettes smoking but quit a month ago and has an elevated cholesterol level. His medications include a beta-blocker and a calcium antagonist.

2. Symptoms/reason for test: Recurrence of angina after PTCA

3. Resting ECG: Results were entirely normal.

4. Exercise hemodynamics/symptoms: His heart rate rose from 50 to 148 beats/min, and his SBP increased from 112 to 165 mm Hg. At a Borg scale score of 20, the patient reached 12 METs, which was slightly above what was expected for his age. No angina occurred during testing.

5. Exercise ECG: He evolved ST-segment depression in the lateral precordial leads that became almost 2.5 mm and downsloping at maximal exercise. He also developed about 1.5 mm of horizontal ST-segment depression in the inferior leads. This abnormal ST depression resolved rapidly in immediate recovery.

6. Interpretation: This pattern represents an abnormal exercise response with rapid normalization in recovery. An abnormal response isolated to maximal exercise is usually associated with milder forms of CAD.

7. Recommendations/follow-up: The patient was catheterized because of the return of symptoms after his prior PTCA. Results showed significant restenosis of his proximal LAD artery and prompted a repeat PTCA. A subsequent exercise test was normal.

8. Comments: ST-segment depression during exercise only is usually associated with milder forms of CAD and a good prognosis. Exercise testing is unable to predict who will reocclude after PTCA but can be helpful if symptoms recur, particularly atypical angina.

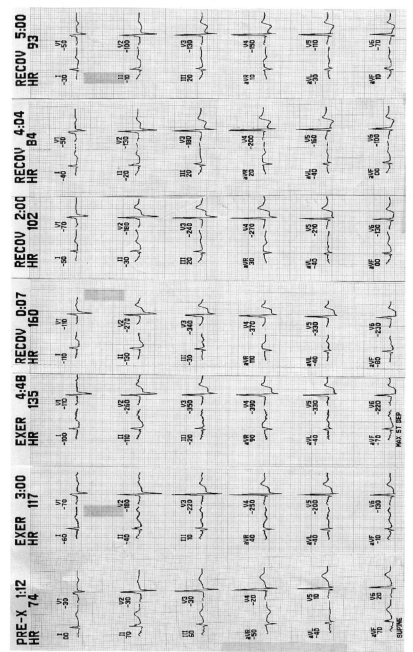

FIG 9-38.

PATIENT SG6458 (Fig 9-38): EVALUATION AFTER BEING RULED OUT FOR AN MI

1. History and physical examination/medications/procedures: This patient is a 68-year-old inpatient who was admitted to rule out a possible MI. ECGs and isoenzyme tests did rule out MI; this treadmill test was performed before discharge.

2. Symptoms/reason for test: Recent rule-out of MI

3. Resting ECG: Results showed prominent anterior forces but were otherwise normal.

4. Exercise hemodynamics/symptoms: Heart rate increased from 74 to 160 beats/min, and his blood pressure rose from 130 to 160 mm Hg, giving a double product of 22,000. At maximal exercise, the patient reported a Borg scale score of 15 and reached 9 METs, which was 20% greater than expected for his age. Typical angina occurred during exercise and recovery.

5. Exercise ECG: By 5 minutes of exercise, there was as much as 4 mm of horizontal ST-segment depression in multiple precordial leads and limb lead I. The ST-segments became downsloping in recovery, with abnormal ST-segment depression persisting beyond 5 minutes of recovery.

6. Interpretation: Marked ST-segment depression qualified by a normal hemodynamic response resulted in a VA prognostic score associated with a cardiovascular mortality rate of less than 2% a year.

7. Recommendations/follow-up: Patient chose medical management and has done well during follow-up.

8. Comments: Marked ST-segment depression is predictive of angiographic disease and the presence of ischemia, whereas exercise capacity and hemodynamic responses are more closely associated with prognosis and severity of ischemia.

FIG 9-39.

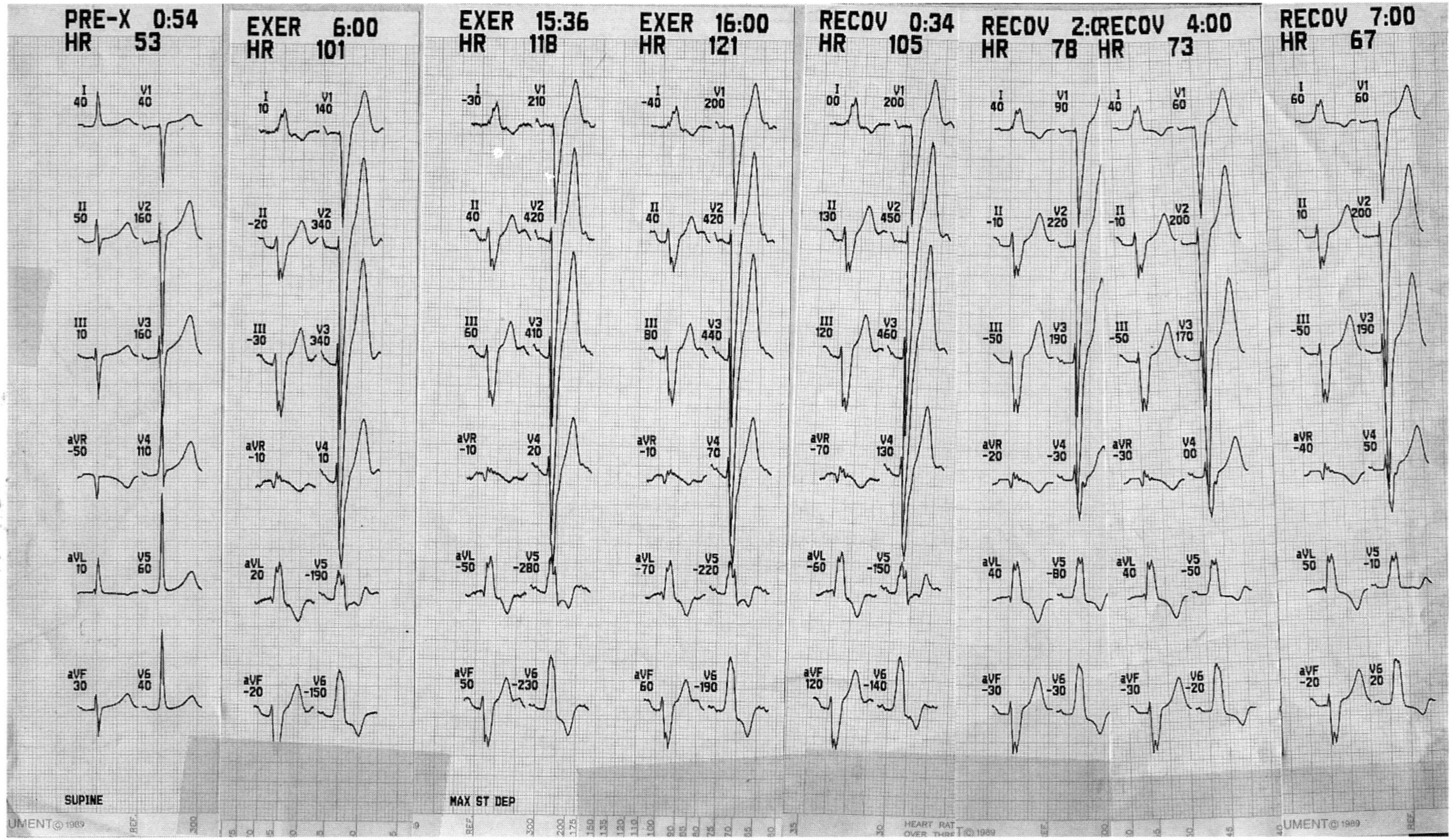

PATIENT PJ2303 (Fig 9-39): **RATE-DEPENDENT LEFT BUNDLE BRANCH BLOCK (LBBB)**

1. History and physical examination/medications/procedures: This patient is a 73-year-old male outpatient on beta-blockers with 10-pack-years of cigarette smoking but who currently does not smoke. He has a family history of premature CAD and an elevated cholesterol level. He has no prior cardiac events or procedures.

2. Symptoms/reason for test: Evaluation of noncardiac or uncertain chest pain

3. Resting ECG: Results showed a mild intraventricular conduction defect and prominent voltage but otherwise were normal.

4. Exercise hemodynamics/symptoms: Results heart rate rose from 53 to 121 beats/min, and SBP increased from 170 to 188. At a Borg scale score of 15, he reached 10 METs, which was 150% of normal (50% above age-predicted average). He had no chest pain during the test.

5. Exercise ECG: Patient developed LBBB pattern at a heart rate of 100 beats/min during exercise. The marked ST-segment depression is not indicative of ischemia.

6. Interpretation: Rate-dependent LBBB is said to be more predictive of CAD when it occurs at a heart rate under 125 beats/min. This patients' LBBB appeared at a heart rate of 101 beats/min.

7. Recommendations/follow-up: Patient had a thallium scintigram, which showed a mild septal defect but no evidence of reperfusion.

8. Comments: LBBB is usually associated with a poor outcome in the older population. In contrast, U.S. Air Force pilots were usually returned to flying despite this abnormality because cardiac catheterization typically revealed normal coronaries. Because this patient was relatively asymptomatic and had an excellent exercise capacity, we felt that his thallium scintigram confirmed a good prognosis. Recently, another patient with LBBB arrested during an exercise test. Although this is highly unusual, it is a reminder that in some individuals, profound LV dysfunction may accompany an LBBB pattern.

FIG 9-40.

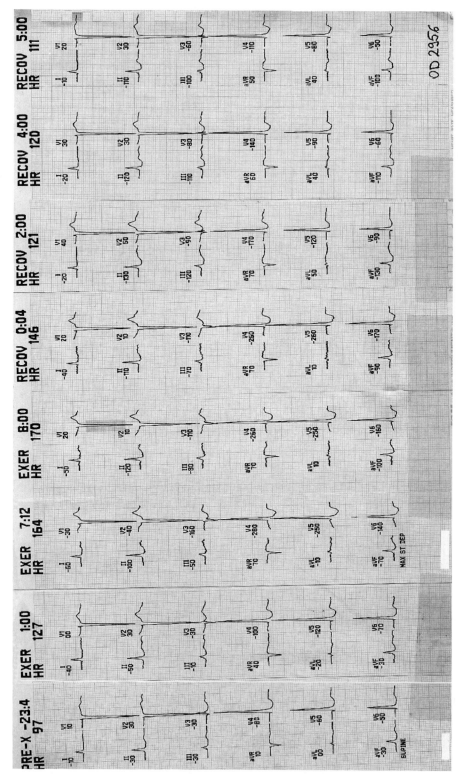

PATIENT OD2956 (Fig 9-40): EVALUATION OF AORTIC STENOSIS

1. History and physical examination/medications/procedures: This patient is a 64-year-old male in-patient referred for evaluation of valvular heart disease. He is a nonsmoker and is taking digoxin and an antihypertensive. He has had a mild systolic murmur, which has been closely followed. His echocardiogram did not show serious aortic stenosis.

2. Symptoms/reason for test: Evaluation of exercise capacity in patient with mild aortic stenosis and atypical angina

3. Resting ECG: ECG showed LVH with strain and atrial fibrillation.

4. Exercise hemodynamics/symptoms: Heart rate rose from 97 to 170 beats/min, and his SBP increased from 98 to 130 mm Hg. The patient reported a Borg scale score of 19 on reaching 4 METs, which was 50% of expected for his age. He reported no chest pain during testing.

5. Exercise ECG: Abnormal ST-segment depression occurred in multiple leads.

6. Interpretation: During exercise, the patient developed additional ST-segment depression, which cleared by 2 minutes of recovery. The SPB response and exercise capacity were consistent with a mild aortic gradient.

7. Recommendations/follow-up: This study confirmed the mild status of his aortic stenosis. A thallium scintigram was normal.

8. Comments: Significant aortic stenosis is a contraindication for exercise testing. It is essential to screen for it with a physical examination and evaluate any systolic murmur that appears significant before exercise testing. If the gradient is severe, exercise testing is contraindicated.

FIG 9-41.

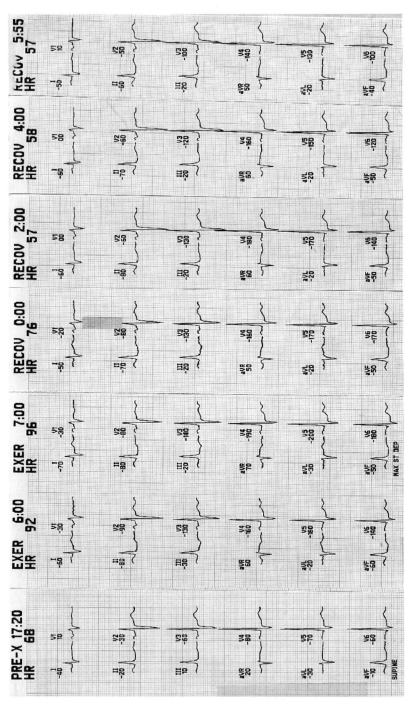

PATIENT SA4317 (Fig 9-41): THALLIUM SCAN TO LOCALIZE AND DETERMINE THE DEGREE OF A CORONARY LESION

1. History and physical examination/medications/procedures: This patient is a 64-year-old outpatient being treated for angina with nitrates and calcium antagonist. He is a nonsmoker but has a family history of coronary disease and an elevated cholesterol level. He has no prior cardiac events.

2. Symptoms/reason for test: Evaluation of typical angina for disease severity

3. Resting ECG: Results were entirely normal.

4. Exercise hemodynamics/symptoms: The patient's heart rate rose from 68 to 96 beats/min, and his SBP increased from 155 to 180 mm Hg. He reached 8 METs with a Borg scale score of 18.

5. Exercise ECG: Typical angina occurred during the test. At a heart rate of 96 beats/min, he had 1.5 mm of horizontal ST-segment depression in the lateral leads. Abnormal ST-segment depression persisted for 6 minutes into recovery.

6. Interpretation: ST-segment depression occurred at a low double product consistent with severe CAD.

7. Recommendations/follow-up: Patient underwent cardiac catheterization and was found to have double-vessel CAD, including a 70% proximal PDA lesion. There were 50% to 60% stenosis of two diagonals and the proximal RCA. Thallium scintigraphy was performed to determine the significance of these lesions. Stress images revealed a perfusion defect involving the inferior wall that redistributed on the delayed images. This confirmed that his only significant lesion was the stenosis of his proximal PDA.

8. Comments: ST-segment depression does not localize, whereas thallium scintigraphy localizes the ischemic vessel and is often helpful in determining whether obstructions are significant. This patient had only one significant lesion, which was in the proximal PDA. He had normal cardiac function.

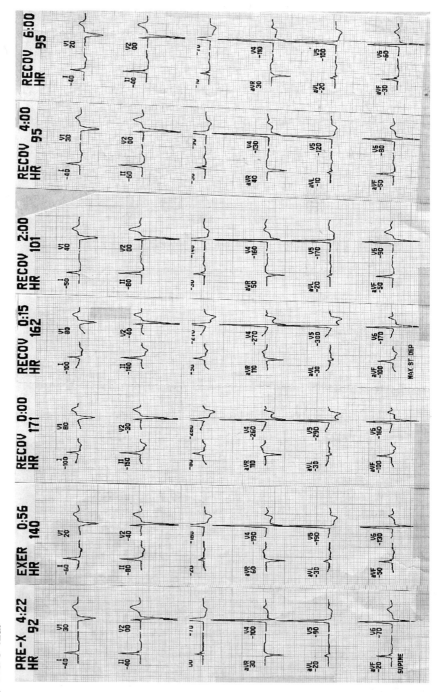

FIG 9-42a.

FIG 9-42b.

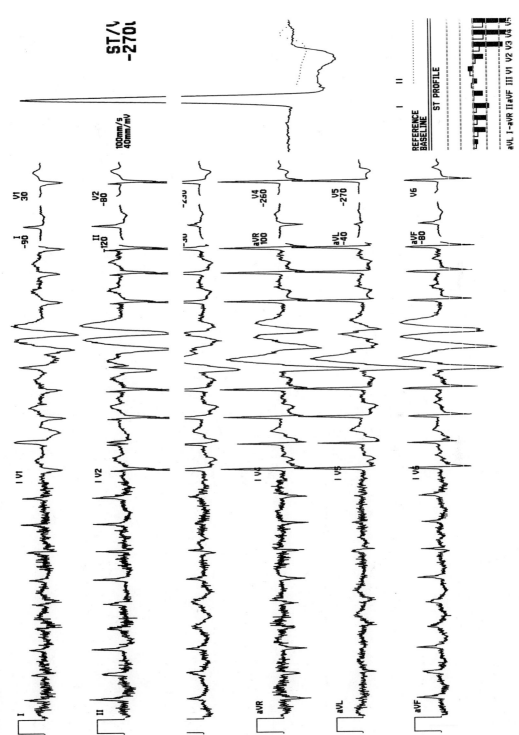

FIG 9-42c.

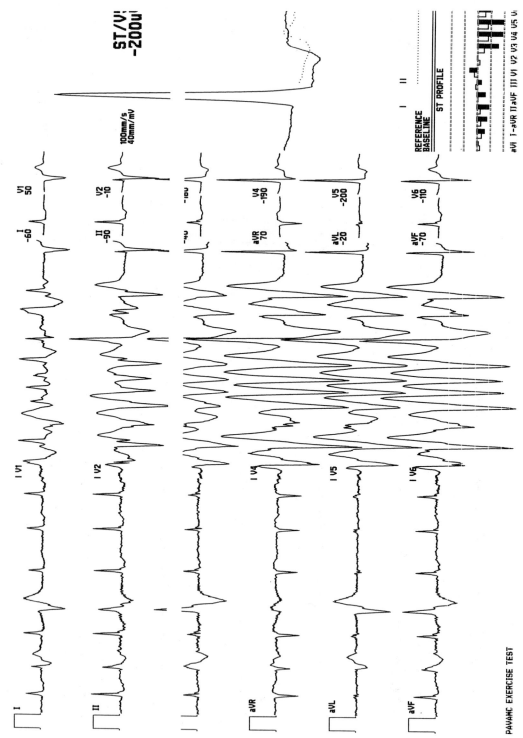

PAVAHC EXERCISE TEST

FIG 9-42d.

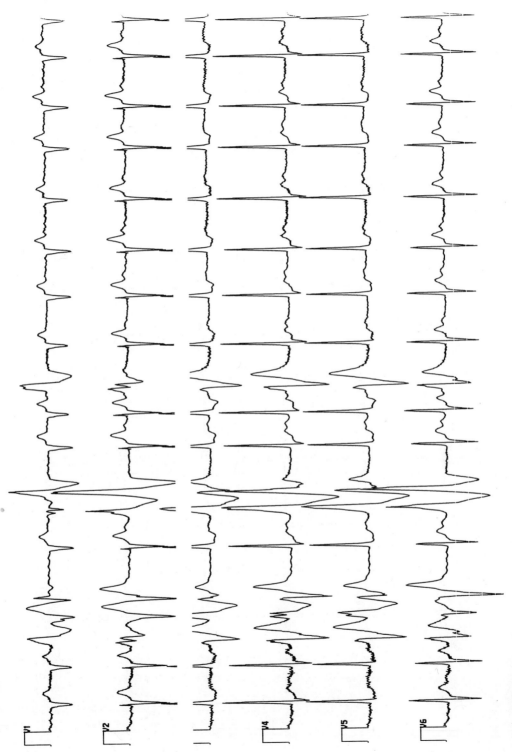

V1 V2 V4 V5 V6

PAVAHC EXERCISE TEST

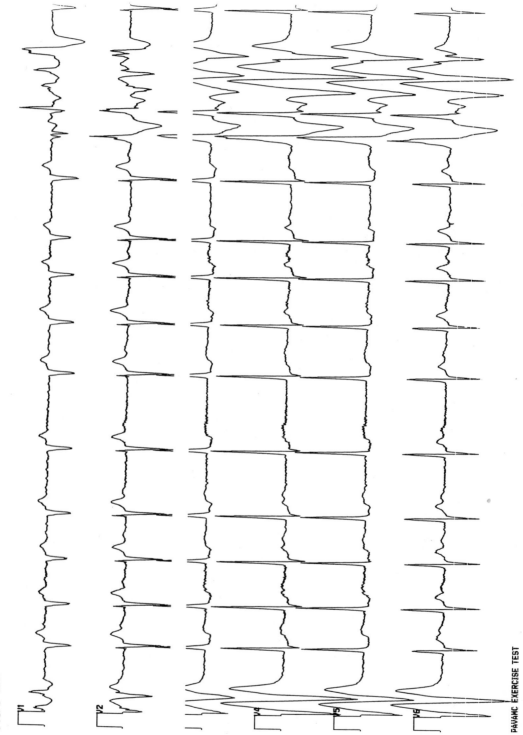

FIG 9-42e.

PAVAMC EXERCISE TEST

PATIENT RM7790 (Fig 9-42): EXERCISE-INDUCED VENTRICULAR TACHYCARDIA

1. History and physical examination/medications/procedures: This patient is a 70-year-old male in-patient with 20-pack-years of smoking but who currently abstains. He underwent bypass surgery in 1980 and a cardiac catheterization in 1989. He is taking a calcium antagonist. He reported the recent return of exertional chest pain and two dizzy spells.

2. Symptoms/reason for test: Evaluation of recurrent typical angina

3. Resting ECG: Results showed LVH with strain and atrial fibrillation.

4. Exercise hemodynamics/symptoms: Patient reached a Borg scale score of 19 and 4 METs, which was 60% of expected. His heart rate at rest was 92 beats/min and rose to 171 beats/min, and his SBP increased from 140 to 190 mm Hg.

5. Exercise ECG: During exercise, the ST segments in the lateral precordial leads and limb leads II and aV_F depressed as much as 2 mm and became partially downsloping. This abnormal ST-segment depression cleared by 2 minutes of recovery. The patient did not have angina pectoris, and the test was terminated because of claudication.

6. Interpretation: During exercise, he had multiple PVCs and then developed ventricular tachycardia. There was no hemodynamic compromise during the episode. He also had marked ST-segment depression, which could result from digoxin or LVH.

7. Recommendations/follow-up: His catheterization was normal, showing good flow through his grafts.

8. Comments: Nonsustained, exercise-induced ventricular tachycardia occurring during exercise testing has not been independently associated with future cardiac events. However, most guidelines consider three or more consecutive PVCs as grounds for terminating testing. This has been my policy only in high-risk patients.

Epilogue

Now for some updates to our friends both old and new. Jon Myers, Eddie Atwood, and I are back together again and practicing at Stanford. Jon is working on a gas-analysis manual, and Eddie has become an even a more masterful teacher. Alisa Hideg and Doug Walsh are in medical school at Loma Linda and University of California at Irvine, respectively. Kiernan Morrow and Jeff Thomas will be entering medical school at Pennsylvania State and UCSF, respectively. Tianna Uhman and Dat Do are doing the day-to-day laboratory work here now and, I hope, will get into medical school next year. Susan Quaglietti, a cardiac nurse practioner, has become CEO for coordination of patient care, our research studies, and conferences (and social events). Paul Ribisl, Bill Herbert, and Paul Dubach are still collaborators and friends though far away.

The QUEXTA project is poised to begin but lacks the final personnel funding. The optical disc data loggers sit at 10 VAMCs waiting for the study to begin. Ken Lehmann waits patiently for our project to begin while on sabbatical in Rotterdam. A flurry of publications closed out our Long Beach experience: writings regarding the 3000 Veteran follow-ups, the nomogram, the Ramp treadmill (or Tramp), and computer ECG scores. Things have been slow because of a lack of funding, but we did function as an ECG core laboratory for the Gensia project and are trying to get a magnetic resonance imaging exercise training study funded. Well, that's all for now; I hope you enjoy the book and that it is a help to you.

Victor F. Froelicher

Index

A

B